Antimicrobial and Antiviral Materials

Antimicrobial and Antiviral Materials

Polymers, Metals, Ceramics, and Applications

Edited by
Peerawatt Nunthavarawong, Sanjay
Mavinkere Rangappa, Suchart Siengchin and
Mathew Thoppil-Mathew

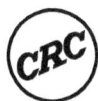

CRC Press
Taylor & Francis Group
Boca Raton London New York

CRC Press is an imprint of the
Taylor & Francis Group, an **informa** business

First edition published 2022
by CRC Press
6000 Broken Sound Parkway NW, Suite 300, Boca Raton, FL 33487–2742

and by CRC Press
2 Park Square, Milton Park, Abingdon, Oxon, OX14 4RN

© 2022 Taylor & Francis Group, LLC

CRC Press is an imprint of Taylor & Francis Group, LLC

Library of Congress Cataloging-in-Publication Data
Names: Nunthavarawong, Peerawatt, editor.
Title: Antimicrobial and antiviral materials : polymers, metals, ceramics, and applications / edited
    by Peerawatt Nunthavarawong, Sanjay Mavinkere Rangappa, Suchart Siengchin, and Mathew
    Thoppil-Mathew.
Description: First edition. | Boca Raton, FL : CRC Press, 2022. | Includes bibliographical
    references and index.
Identifiers: LCCN 2021042419 (print) | LCCN 2021042420 (ebook) | ISBN 9780367697440 (hbk) |
    ISBN 9780367697495 (pbk) | ISBN 9781003143093 (ebk)
Subjects: LCSH: Anti-infective agents.
Classification: LCC RM267 .A546 2022 (print) | LCC RM267 (ebook) | DDC 615.7/92—dc23
LC record available at https://lccn.loc.gov/2021042419
LC ebook record available at https://lccn.loc.gov/2021042420

ISBN: 978-0-367-69744-0 (hbk)
ISBN: 978-0-367-69749-5 (pbk)
ISBN: 978-1-003-14309-3 (ebk)

DOI: 10.1201/9781003143093

Typeset in Times LT Std
by Apex CoVantage, LLC

Contents

Preface

Despite having continued research into the development of new materials for microbial/viral inactivation, scientific progress has been challenging to gain pace with the rapid high resistance of bacteria/viruses. This has led to a surge in the number of papers, patents, and reviews. Therefore, state-of-the-art emerging antimicrobial/antiviral technologies, several vital aspects aim to inactivate microbial/viral infections. Consequently, we believe it is essential to have a book on "Antimicrobial/Antiviral Materials: Polymers, Metals, Ceramics, and Applications." Eminent scholars have contributed various chapters for this book. We hope that the present book will be very informative for scientists, academic staff, faculty members, researchers, and students working in antimicrobial and antiviral materials.

The book consists of 11 chapters that shed light on antimicrobial and antiviral materials. Chapter 1 focuses on various materials such as polymers, metals, and ceramics, which are used for antimicrobial/antiviral applications. Chapter 2 discusses the antibacterial, antiviral, and antioxidant properties of metal nanoparticles. Chapter 3 discusses about the reducing agents used to prepare silver nanoparticles from plant extracts and explains about the antimicrobial and antilarvicidal properties. Chapter 4 describes the infection by microbes and viruses from the viewpoint of biofilms and materials. Chapter 5 focuses on the preparation, properties, and applications of the bioreduction method of nanocomposite polymer films and fabrics. Chapter 6 gives an overview of research activities about antibacterial ceramics in the past, in the current situation, and to be carried out in the future. Chapter 7 exposes advanced synchrotron radiation techniques on investigating the antimicrobial material structures and relevant properties. Chapter 8 aims to gather information related to the current technologies of nanomaterials and the applications of emerging antimicrobial/antiviral technologies in biomedical fields. Chapter 9 describes recent advances in antimicrobial/antiviral nanoparticle titanium dioxide coatings for medical applications. Chapter 10 depicts the forefront research of conducting polymer micropump, aiming at antimicrobial and antiviral transdermal drug delivery applications. Chapter 11 emphasizes on recent advances in antimicrobial/antiviral activities of bulk copper, copper particles, copper thin films, and thermal-sprayed copper coatings, mainly focusing on the reasons as to why antimicrobial and antiviral copper cold spray coatings are beneficial for the disinfection of coronavirus disease.

The editors are thankful to the authors for their contributions and the CRC Press editorial team for their support and guidance.

Dr. Peerawatt Nunthavarawong (Thailand)
Dr. Sanjay Mavinkere Rangappa (Thailand)
Prof. Dr.-Ing. habil. Suchart Siengchin (Thailand)
Prof. Dr. Mathew Thoppil-Mathew (USA)

Acknowledgments

The work was financially supported by Thailand Science Research and Innovation Fund and King Mongkut's University of Technology North Bangkok (KMUTNB), Thailand, with Contract No. KMUTNB-63-KNOW-039 and KMUTNB-FF-65–19.

Author/Editor Biographies

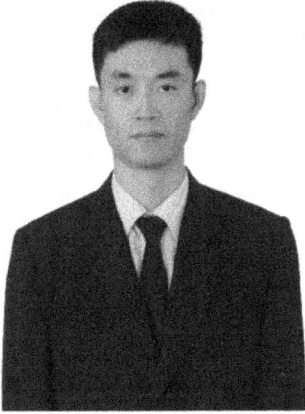

Dr. Peerawatt Nunthavarawong, Assistant Professor in Mechanical Engineering (Tribology), Tribo-Systems for Industrial Tools and Machinery Research Laboratory, Department of Teacher Training in Mechanical Engineering, King Mongkut's University of Technology North Bangkok, Bangkok, Thailand.

Dr. Nunthavarawong is currently Assistant Professor in Mechanical Engineering (Tribology) at the Department of Teacher Training in Mechanical Engineering, King Mongkut's University of Technology North Bangkok (KMUTNB), Bangkok, Thailand, and is currently Research Lecturer for a Ph.D. program at The Sirindhorn International Thai–German Graduate School of Engineering, KMUTNB. He has earned a doctorate in Mechanical Engineering, Applied Mechanics, and a specialty in Friction & Wear of Materials from Kasetsart University, Bangkok, Thailand, in 2012. A few years thereafter, in 2015, he began to work on his post-doctorate program at the University of the Witwatersrand (Wits), Johannesburg, South Africa. During the second year of his fellowship, he studied a short course and received his certificate of competence in Tribology: Friction, Wear, and Lubrication, achieving as the NQF level 9 (equivalent to a master's degree) from Wits in November 2016. He has been appointed as a working committee member of the Thai Tribology Association and the Secretary-General of the Association of Tribologists and Lubrication Engineers of Thailand since 2014 and 2018, respectively. Currently, he is a member of the Society of Tribologists and Lubrication Engineers in the USA, and is a member of the Cold Spray Club–MINES ParisTech in France. Dr. Peerawatt's research and contributions with more than 30 publications mainly involved friction and wear of materials, contact, and damage mechanics, cold gas dynamic spraying, thermal spraying, applied nuclear physics for material processing, and computational methods for engineered materials. He has also delivered several keynotes and invited lectures in various international conferences and workshops. Furthermore, he served as a reviewer for the *Jurnal Tribologi* by the Malaysian Tribology Society and the *Journal of Bio- and Tribo-Corrosion* by Springer. He is also the co-inventor of the ion-implanted hard-metal-cemented carbide cold-sprayed coatings. This invention was primarily granted by the World Intellectual Property Organization (2018), and was extensively patented in Canada (2018), Australia (2019), the USA (2020), and Japan (2020).

(https://scholar.google.co.th/citations?user=65F4XGUAAAAJ&hl=en)

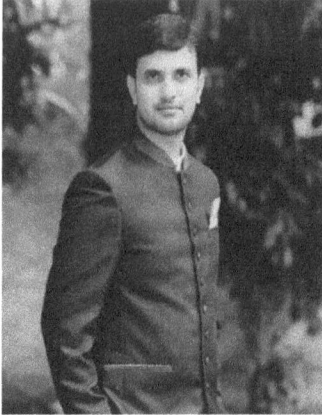

Dr. Sanjay Mavinkere Rangappa, Senior Research Scientist, Natural Composites Research Group Lab, Academic Enhancement Department, King Mongkut's University of Technology North Bangkok, Bangkok, Thailand.

Dr. Rangappa is currently working as Senior Research Scientist and also as "Advisor within the office of the President for University Promotion and Development toward International goals" at King Mongkut's University of Technology North Bangkok, Bangkok, Thailand. He received the B.E. (Mechanical Engineering) in the year 2010, M.Tech. (Computational Analysis in Mechanical Sciences) in the year 2013, Ph.D. (Faculty of Mechanical Engineering Science) from Visvesvaraya Technological University, Belagavi, India, in the year 2018, and Post-Doctorate from King Mongkut's University of Technology North Bangkok, Thailand, in the year 2019. He is a Life Member of Indian Society for Technical Education (ISTE) and an Associate Member of Institute of Engineers (India). He is also acting as a Board Member of various international journals in the fields of materials science and composites. He is a reviewer for more than 85 international journals (for Nature, Elsevier, Springer, Sage, Taylor & Francis, Wiley, American Society for Testing and Materials, American Society of Agricultural and Biological Engineers, IOP, Hindawi, NC State University, USA, ASM International, Emerald Group, Bentham Science Publishers, and Universiti Putra, Malaysia), and also a reviewer for book proposals and international conferences. In addition, he has published more than 140 articles in high-quality international peer-reviewed journals indexed by SCI/Scopus, 5 editorial corners, 40 book chapters, 1 book as an author, and 15 books as an editor (published by lead publishers such as Elsevier, Springer, Taylor & Francis, and Wiley), and also presented research papers at national/international conferences. In 2021, his 17 articles have got top-cited article status in various top journals (*Journal of Cleaner Production*, *Carbohydrate Polymers*, *International Journal of Biological Macromolecules*, *Journal of Natural Fibers*, and *Journal of Industrial Textiles*). He is a Lead Editor of special issues "Artificial intelligence and machine learning in composites and metamaterials," Frontiers in Materials (ISSN 2296–8016) indexed in Web of Science and also "Trends and Developments in Natural Fiber Composites," Applied Science and Engineering Progress (ASEP) indexed in Scopus. He has delivered many keynotes and invited talks in various international conferences and workshops. His current research areas include natural fiber composites, polymer composites, and advanced material technology. He is a recipient of the DAAD Academic exchange-PPP Program between Thailand and Germany to Institute of Composite Materials, University of Kaiserslautern, Germany. He has received a "Top Peer Reviewer 2019" Award, Global Peer Review awards, Powered by Publons, Web of Science Group. The KMUTNB selected him for the "Outstanding Young Researcher" Award 2020. He is recognized by Stanford University's list of the world's top 2% of the most cited scientists in Single Year Citation Impact 2019.

(https://scholar.google.com/citations?user=al91CasAAAAJ&hl=en)

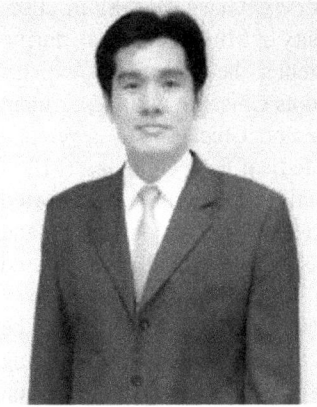

Prof. Dr.-Ing. habil. Suchart Siengchin, President of King Mongkut's University of Technology North Bangkok, Department of Materials and Production Engineering (MPE), The Sirindhorn International Thai–German Graduate School of Engineering (TGGS), King Mongkut's University of Technology North Bangkok, Bangkok, Thailand.

Prof. Siengchin has received his Dipl.-Ing. in Mechanical Engineering. He has received his Dipl.-Ing. in Mechanical Engineering from University of Applied Sciences Giessen/Friedberg, Hessen, Germany, in 1999, M.Sc. in Polymer Technology from the University of Applied Sciences Aalen, Baden-Wuerttemberg, Germany, in 2002, M.Sc. in Material Science from the University of Erlangen-Nürnberg, Bayern, Germany, in 2004, Doctor of Philosophy in Engineering (Dr.-Ing.) from the Institute for Composite Materials, University of Kaiserslautern, Rheinland-Pfalz, Germany, in 2008, and Postdoctoral Research from Kaiserslautern University and School of Materials Engineering, Purdue University, USA. In 2016, he received the habilitation at Chemnitz University in Sachen, Germany. He worked as Lecturer for Production and Material Engineering Department at The Sirindhorn International Thai–German Graduate School of Engineering (TGGS), KMUTNB. He has been full Professor at KMUTNB and became the President of KMUTNB. He won the Outstanding Researcher Award in 2010, 2012, and 2013 at KMUTNB. His research interests include polymer processing and composite material. He is the Editor-in-Chief of *KMUTNB International Journal of Applied Science and Technology* and the author of more than 250 peer-reviewed journal articles, 8 editorial corners, 50 book chapters, 1 book as an author, and 20 books as an editor. He has participated in presentations in more than 39 international and national conferences with respect to materials science and engineering topics. He has been recognized and ranked among the world's top 2% scientists listed by prestigious Stanford University.

(https://scholar.google.com/citations?user=BNZEC7cAAAAJ&hl=en)

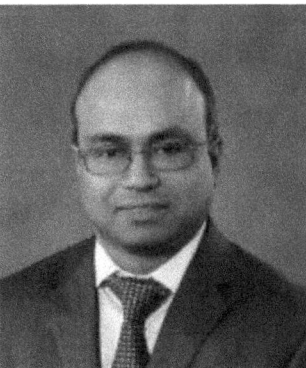

Prof. Dr. Mathew Thoppil-Mathew, Director of Faculty Research, Cedric W. Blazer Endowed Professor of Biomedical Sciences, Department of Biomedical Sciences, University of Illinois College of Medicine Rockford, University of Illinois at Chicago, Rockford, IL, USA.

Prof. Mathew is currently the Cedric W. Blazer Endowed Professor and is leading the Regenerative Medicine and Disability Research Lab within the Department of Biomedical Sciences at the University of Illinois College of Medicine at Rockford. He received his Ph.D. in Mechanical

Engineering (Tribocorrosion) from Strathclyde University, Glasgow, UK, in 2005, and he was Postdoctoral Research Fellow from University of Minho, Portugal, during 2005–2008. Dr. Mathew also holds a faculty appointment at the College of Dentistry and Department of Bioengineering, University of Illinois Chicago, and Department of Orthopedic Surgery, Rush University Medical Center, Chicago. He developed graduate-level courses for the Master of Science in Medical Biotechnology (MBT) Program in Rockford and Bioengineering Ph.D. students. His research is supported by National Institutes of Health (NIH), National Science Foundation (NSF), and research foundations. His research is mainly in areas of biomedical implants and tribocorrosion science. He has published more than 200 papers in refereed journals, books, and conference proceedings. He is now Co-Editor-in-Chief of the *Journal of Bio- and Tribo-Corrosion* by Springer and was instrumental in initiating an international research institute called "Institute of Biomaterials, Tribocorrosion and Nanomedicine" (IBTN), which is a joint venture between University of Illinois Chicago and Sao Paulo State University, Brazil.

(https://scholar.google.com/citations?user=ZHG6Q44AAAAJ&hl=en)

1 Introduction to Antimicrobial and Antiviral Materials

Nunthavarawong P, Sanjay M R,
Siengchin S, and Thoppil-Mathew M

CONTENTS

1.1 INTRODUCTION

The fight against emerging microbial/viral infections remains a worldwide challenge. According to the World Health Organization (WHO), infectious disease control regarding microbial/viral inactivation continues to be a matter for serious concern. Infections caused by microorganisms are a significant source of concern in a variety of industries, including medical devices, drugs, hospital surfaces/furniture, dental restoration and surgery equipment, health care products and hygienic applications, water purification systems, textiles, food packaging, and storage, major or domestic appliances, aeronautics, and so forth [1].

Microbial/viral contaminants are viable on any contacting surfaces that become harmful to health and safety. Antimicrobial/antiviral technologies can be well defined as stuff that enables to harm or disable the progression and replication of bacteria/viruses. Recently, polymeric-, metallic-, and ceramic-based composite materials that are resistant to microorganisms have received much attention.

Among all kinds of materials, polymeric materials, including natural polymers, are suitable for preparing antimicrobial materials such as films and coatings [2]. Antiviral polymers are made by combining an organic backbone with electrically charged moieties like polyanions (such as carboxylate-containing polymers) or poly-cations (such as quaternary ammonium containing polymers) to produce ion-containing polymers with antiviral characteristics [3].

Interestingly, natural materials like copper and wood are the most effective at both killing germs and stopping bacteria from reproducing. Copper and its alloys, such as brass and bronze, have the intrinsic capacity to kill a wide range of dangerous bacteria relatively quickly and effectively [4–5]. Many herbal antimicrobial agents are available in nature, such as clove, portulaca, Tribulus, eryngium, cinnamon,

DOI: 10.1201/9781003143093-1

turmeric, ginger, thyme, pennyroyal, mint, fennel, chamomile, burdock, eucalyptus, primrose, lemon balm, mallow, and garlic [6].

Of the unique features of metals, metal-based antimicrobial macromolecules are emerging as a viable alternative to traditional platforms because they combine many modes of action into a single platform [7]. Because of the primary microbicidal properties associated with these materials, viz. silver, silver oxide, titanium, zinc oxide, nickel, copper, copper oxide, gold, aluminum oxide, magnesium oxide, antimicrobial metallic materials, and their uses have grown tremendously [4].

Antiviral and viricidal coatings are developed using various ways, including altering the surface of a substrate with antiviral polymers, including metal ions/oxides, and using functional nanoparticles [8]. Antibacterial and antiviral materials of diverse kinds, such as small-molecule organics, synthetic, and biodegradable polymers, silver, TiO_2, and copper-derived compounds, play an important role in treating infectious diseases caused by bacteria and viruses, both expected and unforeseen [9].

Positively charged polymers with hydrophobic chains promise antibacterial reagents with a broad antimicrobial spectrum and long persistence [10]. Poly(para-phenylene ethynylene) (PPE), poly(para-phenylene vinylene) (PPV), and poly(diacetylene) (PDA) are conjugated polymeric materials with unique size and structure-dependent chemical and photophysical properties, as well as strong photoinducible antibacterial activity [11]. In a recent study, sodium pentaborate pentahydrate and triclosan are applied to cotton fabrics in order to gain antimicrobial and antiviral properties [12].

Metals or metal nanoparticles can be used to make antibacterial polymeric materials, which have many potentials. Antibacterial polymer-based materials are especially true in situations involving food contact and packaging [13]. Antibacterial, antifungal, antiviral, and antimatrix metalloproteinase properties have all been discovered in quaternary ammonium compounds [14]. Significant discoveries in the field of nanobiomedicine have occurred in areas and numbers that indicate that metal oxide nanoparticles have immense application potential and market value [15]. Graphene and graphene-related materials (GRMs) have a wide range of exciting physicochemical, electrical, optical, antiviral, antibacterial, and other properties [16].

Recent breakthroughs in plasma-assisted surface functionalization of polymer surfaces show that plasma-assisted surface functionalization techniques for synthesizing antiviral polymers with targeted antiviral applications spanning from *in vitro* prevention to *in vivo* therapy are promising [17]. The antimicrobial study found that antimicrobial efficiency was influenced by zinc oxide content, with antimicrobial materials having the most action against gram-negative bacteria [18]. *N,N*-dodecyl, methyl-polyurethane (Quat-12-PU), a polyurethane-based antimicrobial polymer, with high antiviral and antibacterial activity when coated onto surfaces and antibacterial activity when electrospun into nanofibers [19].

For industrial and biomedical applications, antibacterial gum-based biocomposites were employed. Microbial gums, plant exudate gums, and seed gums are all types of antimicrobial gums. In the biomedical field, naturally occurring gum polysaccharides have various uses [20]. The as-synthesized star polymers show promise in antibacterial and antiviral applications [21]. Photoinduced antimicrobial vitamin K compounds-containing nanofibrous membranes (VNFMs) could offer fresh insights into the production of non-toxic, reusable photoinduced antimicrobial materials that could be used in personal protective equipment to increase biological protection [22].

REFERENCES

1. Muñoz-Bonilla, A., & Fernández-García, M. (2012). Polymeric materials with antimicrobial activity. *Progress in Polymer Science*, *37*(2), 281–339. DOI:10.1016/j.progpolymsci.2011.08.005.
2. Mallakpour, S., Azadi, E., & Hussain, C. M. (2021). Recent breakthroughs of antibacterial and antiviral protective polymeric materials during COVID-19 pandemic and post-pandemic: Coating, packaging, and textile applications. *Current Opinion in Colloid & Interface Science*, 101480. DOI:10.1016/j.cocis.2021.101480.
3. Jarach, N., Dodiuk, H., & Kenig, S. (2020). Polymers in the medical antiviral frontline. *Polymers*, *12*(8), 1727. DOI:10.3390/polym12081727.
4. Makvandi, P., Wang, C. Y., Zare, E. N., Borzacchiello, A., Niu, L. N., & Tay, F. R. (2020). Metal-based nanomaterials in biomedical applications: Antimicrobial activity and cytotoxicity aspects. *Advanced Functional Materials*, *30*(22), 1910021. DOI:10.1002/adfm.201910021.
5. Zare, E. N., Jamaledin, R., Naserzadeh, P., Afjeh-Dana, E., Ashtari, B., Hosseinzadeh, M., . . . Makvandi, P. (2019a). Metal-based nanostructures/PLGA nanocomposites: Antimicrobial activity, cytotoxicity, and their biomedical applications. *ACS Applied Materials & Interfaces*, *12*(3), 3279–3300. DOI:10.1021/acsami.9b19435.
6. Parham, S., Kharazi, A. Z., Bakhsheshi-Rad, H. R., Nur, H., Ismail, A. F., Sharif, S., . . . Berto, F. (2020). Antioxidant, antimicrobial and antiviral properties of herbal materials. *Antioxidants*, *9*(12), 1309. DOI:10.3390/antiox9121309.
7. Abd-El-Aziz, A. S., Agatemor, C., & Etkin, N. (2017). Antimicrobial resistance challenged with metal-based antimicrobial macromolecules. *Biomaterials*, *118*, 27–50. DOI:10.1016/j.biomaterials.2016.12.002.
8. Pemmada, R., Zhu, X., Dash, M., Zhou, Y., Ramakrishna, S., Peng, X., & Nanda, H. S. (2020). Science-based strategies of antiviral coatings with viricidal properties for the COVID-19 like pandemics. *Materials*, *13*(18), 4041. DOI:10.3390/ma13184041.
9. Balasubramaniam, B., Prateek, R. S., Saraf, M., Kar, P., Singh, S. P., . . . Gupta, R. K. (2020). Antibacterial and antiviral functional materials: Chemistry and biological activity toward tackling COVID-19-like pandemics. *ACS Pharmacology & Translational Science*, *4*(1), 8–54. DOI:10.1021/acsptsci.0c00174.
10. Pan, Y., Xia, Q., & Xiao, H. (2019). Cationic polymers with tailored structures for rendering polysaccharide-based materials antimicrobial: An overview. *Polymers*, *11*(8), 1283. DOI:10.3390/polym11081283.
11. Wang, Y., Canady, T. D., Zhou, Z., Tang, Y., Price, D. N., Bear, D. G., . . . Whitten, D. G. (2011). Cationic phenylene ethynylene polymers and oligomers exhibit efficient antiviral activity. *ACS Applied Materials & Interfaces*, *3*(7), 2209–2214. DOI:10.1021/am200575y.
12. Iyigundogdu, Z. U., Demir, O., Asutay, A. B., & Sahin, F. (2017). Developing novel antimicrobial and antiviral textile products. *Applied Biochemistry and Biotechnology*, *181*(3), 1155–1166. DOI:10.1007/s12010-016-2275-5.
13. Randazzo, W., Fabra, M. J., Falcó, I., López-Rubio, A., & Sánchez, G. (2018). Polymers and biopolymers with antiviral activity: Potential applications for improving food safety. *Comprehensive Reviews in Food Science and Food Safety*, *17*(3), 754–768. DOI:10.1111/1541-4337.12349.
14. Jiao, Y., Niu, L. N., Ma, S., Li, J., Tay, F. R., & Chen, J. H. (2017). Quaternary ammonium-based biomedical materials: State-of-the-art, toxicological aspects and antimicrobial resistance. *Progress in Polymer Science*, *71*, 53–90. DOI:10.1016/j.progpolymsci.2017.03.001.
15. Nikolova, M. P., & Chavali, M. S. (2020). Metal oxide nanoparticles as biomedical materials. *Biomimetics*, *5*(2), 27. DOI:10.3390/biomimetics5020027.
16. Srivastava, A. K., Dwivedi, N., Dhand, C., Khan, R., Sathish, N., Gupta, M. K., . . . Kumar, S. (2020). Potential of graphene-based materials to combat COVID-19: Properties,

perspectives and prospects. *Materials Today Chemistry*, 100385. DOI:10.1016/j. mtchem.2020.100385.

17. Ma, C., Nikiforov, A., De Geyter, N., Dai, X., Morent, R., & Ostrikov, K. K. (2021). Future antiviral polymers by plasma processing. *Progress in Polymer Science*, 101410. DOI:10.1016/j.progpolymsci.2021.101410.

18. López de Dicastillo, C., Patiño Vidal, C., Falcó, I., Sánchez, G., Márquez, P., & Escrig, J. (2020). Antimicrobial bilayer nanocomposites based on the incorporation of as-synthetized hollow zinc oxide nanotubes. *Nanomaterials*, *10*(3), 503. DOI:10.3390/nano10030503.

19. Park, D., Larson, A. M., Klibanov, A. M., & Wang, Y. (2013). Antiviral and antibacterial polyurethanes of various modalities. *Applied Biochemistry and Biotechnology*, *169*(4), 1134–1146. DOI:10.1007/s12010-012-9999-7.

20. Zare, E. N., Makvandi, P., Borzacchiello, A., Tay, F. R., Ashtari, B., & Padil, V. V. (2019b). Antimicrobial gum bio-based nanocomposites and their industrial and biomedical applications. *Chemical Communications*, *55*(99), 14871–14885. DOI:10.1039/C9CC08207G.

21. Pan, Y., Xue, Y., Snow, J., & Xiao, H. (2015). Tailor-made antimicrobial/antiviral star polymer via ATRP of cyclodextrin and guanidine-based macromonomer. *Macromolecular Chemistry and Physics*, *216*(5), 511–518. DOI:10.1002/macp.201400525.

22. Zhang, Z., El-Moghazy, A. Y., Wisuthiphaet, N., Nitin, N., Castillo, D., Murphy, B. G., & Sun, G. (2020). Daylight-induced antibacterial and antiviral nanofibrous membranes containing vitamin K derivatives for personal protective equipment. *ACS Applied Materials & Interfaces*, *12*(44), 49416–49430. DOI:10.1021/acsami.0c14883.

2 Recent Advances in Materials Science and Engineering Contributing to the Infection Diseases

Sabarish Radoor, Aswathy Jayakumar, Jasila Karayil, Jyothi Mannekote Shivanna, Jyotishkumar Parameswaranpillai and Suchart Siengchin

CONTENTS

2.1 INTRODUCTION

Pathogens such as bacteria, viruses, and fungi are mainly responsible for causing infectious diseases. Infectious diseases can transmit either directly or indirectly and, in most cases, are contagious. For instance, flu, chickenpox, AIDS, etc. are contagious and termed the global killer. Recently, COVID-19, a highly infectious disease caused by the corona virus, has shaken the entire world. In a short period, nearly 40 lakhs of people have lost their life due to COVID. The antiviral drug has been employed to treat infectious diseases; however, many bacterial and viral strains become resistant to the drug and increase mortality. Also, some pathogens (for example corona) show genetic variation over time, and finding an appropriate drug for such a disease is a tedious job. Hence, it is high time to find novel materials that have the efficiency to

DOI: 10.1201/9781003143093-2

curb infectious diseases. Nanomaterials possess excellent antibacterial properties. The antibacterial property of the nanomaterials could be tuned by varying their size and structure. Metal nanoparticles have been successfully employed to destroy disease-causing bacteria such as *Escherichia coli*, *Pseudomonas aeruginosa*, *Klebsiella pneumoniae*, and *Staphylococcus aureus* [1–3].

In this chapter, we discuss the antibacterial, antiviral, and antioxidant properties of various metal nanoparticles. The wound healing application of the nanocomposites is also discussed. Finally, we have shed some light on the antibacterial activity of graphene nanoparticles, which is one of the well-studied materials.

2.2   TITANIUM DIOXIDE NANOPARTICLES

Among metal nanoparticles, titanium nanoparticles have a particular interest due to their unique features such as photocatalytic activity, antibacterial activity, mechanical, thermal, electrical stability, non-toxicity, and high surface area [4–8]. Titanium nanoparticles are one of the most produced nanoparticles after silicon dioxide and zinc oxide nanoparticles. Titanium nanoparticles play an essential role in wound healing applications [9–10]. Sivaranjani and Philominathan [11] developed titanium nanoparticles through green synthesis from *Moringa oleifera* leaves and employed them for wound healing. The *in vitro* studies were conducted on albino rats. The incision wound on the mice was healed (percentage of wound healing: 93%) within 12 days. The authors thus claimed that titanium nanoparticles could be employed for the treatment of wounds and skin infections. Similarly, Santhoshkumar et al. [12] synthesized titanium nanoparticles from *Psidium guajava* extract and evaluated their antioxidant and antibacterial activity. The nanoparticles showed a maximum zone of inhibition around gram-positive (*S. aureus*) and gram-negative (*E. coli*) bacteria. The hydrogen peroxide released from titanium nanoparticles is responsible for its antibacterial activity. 1,1-diphenyl-2-picrylhydrazyl (DPPH) radical scavenging assay revealed that synthesized nanoparticle possesses good free-radical scavenging efficiency (21.4 µg ml^{-1}).

Seydi et al. [13] reported titanium nanoparticles (TiNP) synthesis using *Allium eriophyllum* aqueous extract. The developed nanoparticles exhibit excellent antifungal and antibacterial properties. The TiNP is superior to the control antibiotic, and a significant inhibition effect was noticed for all tested bacteria and fungi. The cytotoxic studies are usually conducted to understand the effect of nanoparticles on healthy cells. In the present work, the cytotoxicity of TiNP was tested using a model cell, human umbilical vein endothelial cells (HUVECs). The cytotoxic analysis revealed that HUVEC cell is viable up to 1000 µg ml^{-1} of TiNP and therefore is safe to use for therapeutic applications. The authors have compared the cutaneous wound healing efficiency of TiNPs ointment with *A. eriophyllum* and TiO$_2$ ointment. Owing to its high antioxidant property, TiNPs reduce the inflammation cells such as neutrophils, macrophages, and lymphocytes and thereby speed the wound healing process. Therefore, the authors claimed that modified titanium nanoparticles are a promising candidate for wound healing applications.

Azadirachta indica leaf extract was employed to synthesize titanium dioxide nanoparticles [14]. The morphological analysis showed that synthesized nanoparticles are spherical, with sizes ranging from 15 to 50 nm. The antibacterial activity test confirmed the strong antibacterial activity of nanoparticles against *E. coli*, *S. aureus*, *Bacillus subtilis*, *Salmonella typhi*, and *K. pneumoniae*. The maximum activity was against *E. coli* with an inhibition diameter of 27.67 mm. The minimum inhibitory (MIC) and minimum bactericidal concentration (MBC) followed the disc diffusion method. The lowest MIC value was obtained for *S. aureus* and *E. coli* (10.42). Akhtar et al. [15] developed titanium dioxide nanocolloid by sonochemical method. The Microplate Alamar Blue Assay (MABA) and disc diffusion method were employed to identify the antibacterial property of the nanocolloid against *E. coli* and *S. aureus*, which is gram-negative and gram-positive bacteria, respectively. MABA test indicates that nanocolloid is more effective in destroying the population of gram-negative bacteria (*P. aeruginosa* (67.3%)) than gram-positive bacteria (*B. subtilis* [percentage inhibition; 63%]). However, the disc diffusion method shows that a maximum inhibition zone was observed for *B. subtilis* (34.21 mm). The antiviral activity of the nanoparticle was also tested, and the result indicates that titanium nanocolloid is quite effective in destroying the activity of the newcastle virus (NDV). The titanium nanocolloid destroyed the glycoprotein spikes on the virus envelope, responsible for initiating infection in healthy cells. The biosynthesis of titanium nanoparticles is receiving significant attention as this method is cheap and eco-friendly. In one of the studies, fungus (*Aspergillus flavus*) was employed to develop titanium dioxide nanoparticles [16]. Here *A. flavus* act as capping/reducing agent and convert the titanium oxide to titanium oxide nanoparticle. The nanoparticles exhibit superior antibacterial activity, and the zones of inhibition and MIC for different gram-positive and gram-negative bacteria are as follows: *S. aureus* (25 mm, MIC 40 g ml^{-1}), *E. coli* (35 MIC 40 g ml^{-1}), *P. aeruginosa* (27 mm, MIC 80 g ml^{-1}), *K. pneumoniae* (18 mm, MIC 70 g ml^{-1}), and *B. subtilis* (22 mm, MIC 45 g ml^{-1}). The authors thus suggested titanium dioxide nanoparticles as a potential candidate to curb the population of pathogenic bacteria (Figure 2.1) [16].

Hassan et al. [17] employed the electrospinning technique to synthesis titania nanorods and tested its antibacterial activity. The nanorods exhibit good crystallinity along with high thermal and photocatalytic properties. Concentration-dependent antibacterial activity was noted. The 45 μg ml^{-1} TiO$_2$ nanorods solution displayed the highest inhibition when compared with other concentrations. The mechanism of action of titanium nanoparticles on bacteria was proposed as follows. Initially, the nanorods get attached to the outer layer of the bacterial cell. The reactive hydroxyl radical generated from titanium nanorods induces cell rupture and destroys the bacterial DNA. The proposed mechanism is well supported by morphological analysis. The aggregated DNA is clearly visible in the SEM micrograph.

2.3 NANOCLAY NANOPARTICLES

Nanoclay is a naturally occurring aluminosilicate with at least one dimension in the order of 1–100 nm. It has a three-dimensional network structure and possesses high

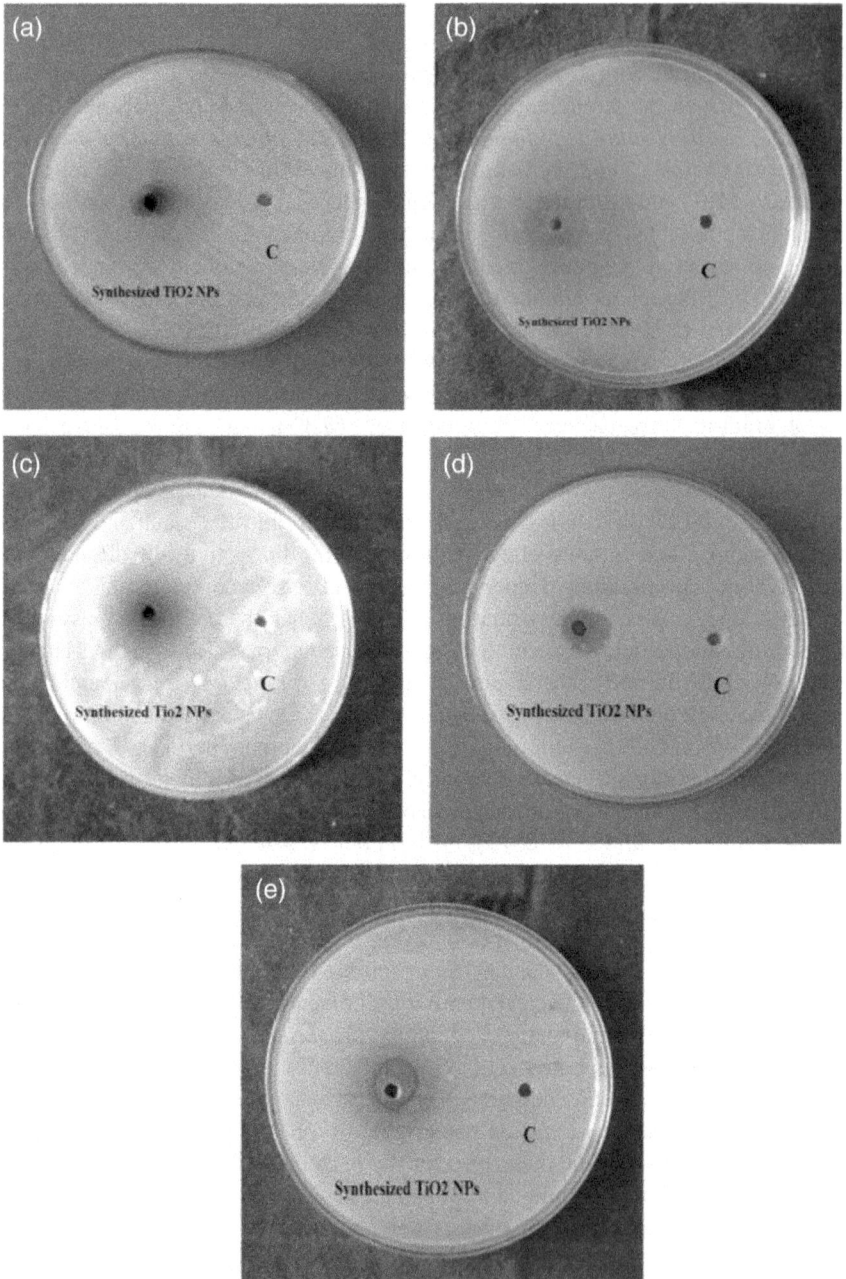

FIGURE 2.1 Antibacterial activity of TiO$_2$ NPs against (a) *S. aureus*, (b) *E. coli*, (c) *P. aeruginosa*, (d) *K. pneumoniae*, and (e) *B. subtilis*.

Source: Reproduced with permission from Elsevier, License Number: 5101300981442

TABLE 2.1

Inhibition Zone of KC/5%clay/x%ZEO against Different Bacteria

Film	Inhibition zone (mm²)				
	S. aureus	B. cereus	E. coli	S. typhimurium	P. aeruginosa
KC/5%clay	0.00	0.00	0.00	0.00	0.00
KC/5%clay/1%ZEO	50.76±2.76	10.11±0.99	35.43±2.66	35.62±1.86	0.00
KC/5%clay/2%ZEO	153.55±22.38	119.21±6.19	110.76±10.25	95.09±1.19	30.19±0.41
KC/5%clay/3%ZEO	538.27±27.59	480.58±15.54	359.12±12.11	243.35±10.34	168.40±15.19

Source: Reproduced with permission from Elsevier, License Number: 5101380510393

surface area, thermal stability, and chemical resistance. Being non-toxic, economical, and readily available, nanoclay has been widely explored to fabricate several polymer composites [18–19]. Previous reports show that nanoclay particles could be adequately dispersed in the polymer matrix, thereby improving mechanical, thermal, and water barrier properties [20–21]. Nanoclays and their composites have been studied for biomedical applications such as bone cement, tissue engineering, drug delivery, wound healing, enzyme immobilization, and so on [22–23].

Shojaee-Aliabadi et al. [24], in one of their previous works, observed that *Zataria multiflora Boiss* essential oil (ZEO) is compatible with kappa-carrageenan (KC) polymer matrix. This prompted the authors to study the synergistic effect of (ZEO) and montmorillonite (MMT) nanoclay on the properties of KC polymer composite. The study shows that MMT and ZEO-loaded composite possesses good mechanical, barrier, and antibacterial properties. The nanocomposite exhibits superior antibacterial activity against five different bacteria (Table 2.1). The authors thus suggested that KC/ZEO/MMT composite could be used as an antibacterial agent in biomedical applications. Entezam et al. [25] incorporated chitosan-modified nanoclay into polyvinyl alcohol hydrogels and investigated its wound dressing application. The modified nanocomposite possesses good mechanical, physical, and antibacterial properties. Due to the inherent antibacterial property of chitosan, the chitosan-modified hydrogel contains excellent antibacterial activity and ultimately destroys the bacterial population. Heydary et al. [26] developed Iranian gum tragacanth (IGT)/ polyvinyl alcohol (PVA)/nanoclay composite through the electrospinning technique. The nanoclay incorporated bio composite exhibits good chemical and mechanical stability. Moreover, 3-wt.% nanoclay-incorporated composite exhibits better wound healing ability than plain biocomposite. Therefore, the authors claimed that the IGT/ PVA/nanoclay bio-composite could be a promising candidate for wound healing studies. A similar result was observed for polyvinyl alcohol/chitosan/montmorillonite nanocomposite. The nanocomposite possesses desirable features (good antibacterial activity, biocompatibility and swelling behavior) for wound healing application [27].

2.4 COPPER NANOPARTICLES

A copper nanoparticle is considered one of the promising candidates for biological applications. Owing to its small size and high surface-to-volume ratio, copper nanoparticles could interact more effectively with microbes and possess good anti-microbial activity [28–29]. Moreover, they contain good mechanical, electrical, and optical properties. Compared with other nanoparticles, the main advantage of copper nanoparticles is their low cost and desirable physicochemical stability. Consequently, copper nanoparticles have received much attention from scientists, and they have been widely used in wound dressing and biocidal properties. Copper nanoparticles can be developed through different routes, such as physical, chemical, and biological. However, due to its environment-friendly nature, the biological route's simplicity and non-toxic nature are more applicable for synthesizing copper nanoparticles [30–31].

Amer and co-worker [32] developed copper nanoparticles from *Citrus limon* fruits extract and examined its antimicrobial activity against gram-negative (*E. coli*) and gram-positive (*S. aureus*) bacteria. The antibacterial test revealed that the copper nanoparticle exhibits high antibacterial activity against *E. coli* than *S. aureus*. This is due to the difference in the cell wall of bacteria. The nanoparticle could have

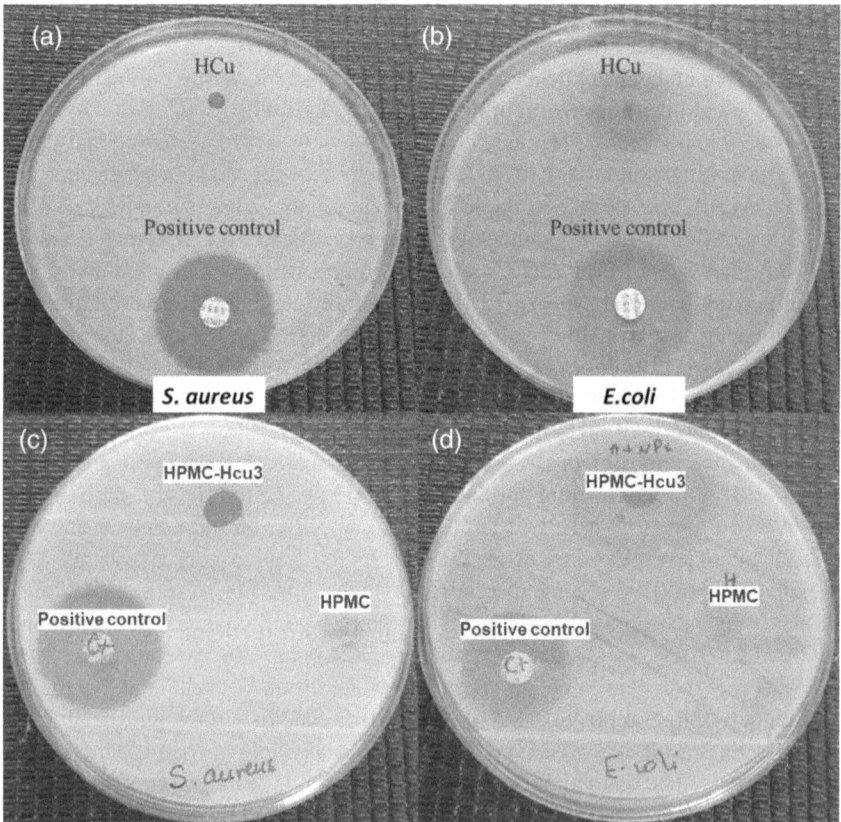

FIGURE 2.2 Inhibition zone of hydroxypropyl methylcellulose—copper nanoparticles against (a, c) *S. aureus* and (b, d) *E. coli* in terms of zone of inhibition.

Source: Reproduced with permission from Elsevier, License Number: 5101381090852

cause rapid destruction of gram-negative bacteria and deactivate the cytochromes. The antibacterial mechanism of copper nanoparticles on *E. coli* is explained by [33]. The copper nanoparticles can destroy the cell wall and cytoplasm of bacteria and are attributed to copper's reducing solid ability. The copper nanoparticle's interaction with bacteria causes its denaturation of bacterial protein. It also has a greater affinity to interact with the genetic material of bacteria (DNA). Eventually, the bacterial cell is wholly destroyed. Jayaramudu et al. [34] fabricated hydroxypropyl methylcellulose—copper nanoparticles by solvent casting techniques and evaluated its antibacterial activity toward gram-positive and gram-negative bacteria. The experimental results show that the prepared nanocomposite is very effective against *E. coli*, and the maximum zone of inhibition comes around 29 mm (Figure 2.2).

2.5 SILVER NANOPARTICLES

Silver nanoparticles have a strong biocidal and inflammatory effect and, therefore, have been widely explored in wound dressing, cosmetics, food packaging, etc. [35–37]. Researchers have employed chemical, physical and biological routes for the synthesis of silver nanoparticles. Compared with the chemical method, reports show that both physical and biological methods require advanced and expensive equipment. Therefore, people focus on a chemical route that is simple and less costly for the synthesis of silver nanoparticle. Owing to its eco-friendly methodology and inexpensive procedure, recently increasing attention is being given to the green synthesis of silver nanoparticles [38–40].

Various theories have been put forward to explain the antimicrobial action of silver particles. Due to their high surface area, silver nanoparticles have a great affinity to anchor the bacterial cell wall and disrupt the DNA replication of the bacterial cell. This eventually leads to cell death. Another mechanism is that silver nanoparticle generates free radical, which adversely affects bacteria's cellular mechanism [41–42]. Singh et al. [43] developed silver nanoparticles through green synthesis using an endophytic fungal *Alternaria* sp. isolated from *Raphanus sativas*. The biogenic silver nanoparticles show high antibacterial activity against gram-positive and gram-negative bacteria. The inhibition zones formed around *B. subtilis*, *S. aureus*, *E. coli*, and *Serratia marcescens* are 23, 12, 26, and 24 mm, respectively (Figure 2.3).

Kim et al. [44] studies indicate that silver's antibacterial activity depends on the bacterial species. They observed a strong inhibitory effect against *E. coli* and yeast. However, only a mild activity was observed for *S. aureus*. This was attributed to the difference in the thickness and structure of the peptidoglycan layer present in bacteria. A similar hypothesis was put forward previously by many researchers. The other possible mechanism is the electrostatic attraction between the positively charged silver ions and negatively charged cell membrane. The silver-induced free-radical formation is another reason for bacterial death. The electron paramagnetic resonance (EPR) studies revealed free-radical formation and thus supported the hypothesis.

Respiratory syncytial virus (RSV) generally attaches to the bronchial epithelium cells and causes severe respiratory problems in children and adults. Curcumin is found to be very effective against (RSV). However, the low water solubility of curcumin restricts its clinical application. Yang, Li, and Huang [45] functionalized

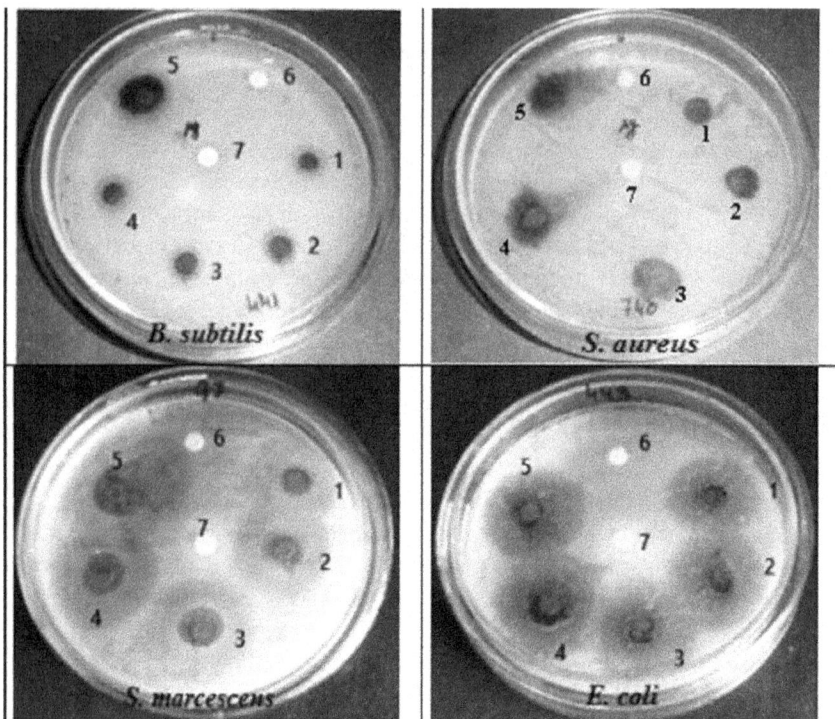

FIGURE 2.3 Antibacterial activity of (1) 5 mg ml^{-1} AgNP, (2) 10 mg ml^{-1} AgNP, (3) 15 mg ml^{-1} AgNP, (4) 20 mg ml^{-1} AgNP, (5) 25 mg ml^{-1} AgNP, (6) 5 mg ml^{-1} fungal supernatant, and (7) 5 mg ml^{-1} AgNO$_3$ [40].

silver nanoparticles with curcumin and proposed it be a virucide against RSV. Curcumin-loaded silver nanoparticles (cAgNPs) are highly stable and possess low toxicity. The experimental results show that he cAgNPs could interact directly with the glycoproteins of RSV and thereby inactivate the virus before it enters into the cell. Gene expression studies well supported this. Al-Dhabi et al. [46] synthesized silver nanoparticles through a green method. The nanoparticle exhibit superior antimicrobial activity against drug-resistant bacteria such as *E. coli*, *K. pneumoniae*, and *P. aeruginosa*.

2.6   ZINC OXIDE NANOPARTICLES

Zinc oxide is commonly used in rubber, paints, textiles, pharmaceuticals, and food packaging. The essential properties of zinc oxide, which increases its usage in biomedical fields, are antibacterial, antimicrobial, UV blocking properties, and photocatalytic disinfecting agents [47–48]. When compared to silver nanoparticles, zinc oxide nanoparticles are less toxic and safe to use in humans as well as animals. Zinc oxide nanoparticles have been incorporated into polymers to generate antibacterial materials [49]. For instance, Silvestre et al. [50] developed a nanocomposite by incorporating ZnO into isotactic polypropylene (iPP) and investigate its biocide effect. The antibacterial study revealed that nanoparticles' exposure time and concentration play an important role in the retardation of bacterial growth. The composite loaded with 95% iPP and 5% zinc nanoparticle exhibit maximum reduction of bacteria (99.9%) when the exposure time was 48 h.

Yamamoto [47] varied the particle size of ZnO from 0.1 to 0.8 μm and investigated its effect on its biocidal property. They reported that with a decrease in particle size, the antibacterial activity increases. The previous report suggests that the hydrogen peroxide generated from the surface of the ZnO nanoparticle is responsible for its antibacterial activity. In the light of the aforementioned work, the authors suggested that with a decrease in particle size, the density of zinc oxide increases and thus leads to a significant increase in the concentration of H_2O_2. The H_2O_2 on interaction with the bacterial cell causes its destruction. A similar result was reported by Stankovic and his team [51]. However, apart from the particle size, the authors also investigate the effect of the morphology of zinc nanoparticles on antibacterial activity. Their experimental result suggests that nanoparticle morphology and the surface area also play a pivotal role in reducing the bacterial population.

Tyagi et al. [52] synthesized zinc oxide nanoparticles through a chemical method and compared their antibacterial activity with the standard antibiotic ciprofloxacin. Their study indicates that the antibacterial activity of zinc oxide nanoparticles is less than that of ciprofloxacin. The zinc nanoparticle–ciprofloxacin conjugate possesses good antibacterial activity, attributed to the synergistic effect of nanoparticles and antibiotics. The antibacterial activity of nanoparticle–ciprofloxacin conjugate against *E. coli* and *S. aureus* increases by 2.9-fold and 2.8-fold, respectively. Recently, there is an increase in the use of eco-friendly routes such as ultrasonic-assisted synthesis, microwave-assisted synthesis, and biological methods for the development of zinc nanoparticles. Pillai et al. [53] adopted the green approach to synthesize zinc nanoparticles. Here, they employed four different plant extracts (*Beta vulgaris, Cinnamomum tamala, Cinnamomum verum,* and *Brassica oleracea* var. *italica*), which act as a reducing agent and assists the development of nanoparticles. The antibacterial assay shows that the nanoparticles possess a good biocidal effect against *E. coli* (gram-negative), *S. aureus* (gram-positive), and *C. albanicans* (fungus) (Figure 2.4). Rekha et al. [54] reported the antibacterial and photocatalytic activity of Mn-doped ZnO. The material is found to exhibit an excellent antibacterial effect. The zone of inhibition around the bacteria such as *E. coli, K. pneumoniae, Shigella dysenteriae, S. typhi, P. aeruginosa, B. subtilis,* and *S. aureus* are, respectively, 2.3, 3.7, 2.3, 10.5, 2.5, 2.3, and 2.6 mm, respectively.

2.7 GRAPHENE NANOPARTICLES

Graphene is an allotrope of carbon with monolayer thickness. The carbon in grapheme is sp^2 hybridized and is linked to the neighbor carbons through an π-conjugated bond. Thus, graphene has a two-dimensional hexagonal honeycomb structure [55]. Graphene is extracted from graphite using methods such as mechanical or chemical exfoliation, chemical vapor deposition (CVD), and graphitization of silicon carbide

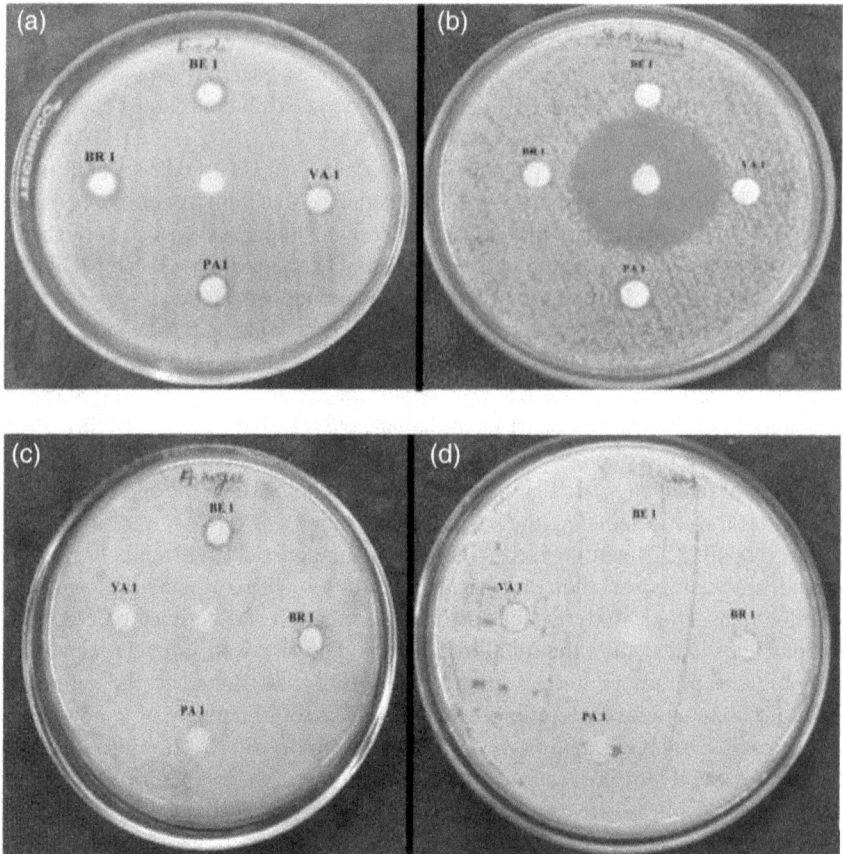

FIGURE 2.4 Inhibition zone of different ZnO-NPs on (a) *E. coli*, (b) *S. aureus*, (c) *Aspergillus niger*, and (d) *Candida albicans*.

Source: Reproduced with permission from Elsevier, License Number: 5101410442622

(SiC) surfaces; CVD and SiC method is commonly employed for the production of a large scale of graphene [56–58].

Graphene is a fascinating material with excellent mechanical, thermal, and electrical properties (Young's modulus: 1 TPa, thermal conductivity: 5000 W m^{-1} K^{-1}, and electrical conductivity: 1738 siemens m^{-1}). It also possesses a high specific surface area (~2630 m^2 g^{-1}) and high electron mobility (~250,000 cm^2 v^l s^{-1}). Moreover, the structural features of graphene enable it to have pi-pi stacking and electrostatic interaction with aromatic molecules. Thus, graphene-based materials revolutionized the industries like biotechnology, optical, nanoelectronics, electrical, and so on [59].

The essential properties of graphene which make it a promising candidate for biomedical applications include high surface area, high stability, good optical properties, non-covalent interaction, good biocompatibility, and the ability to undergo surface fictionalization. Moreover, earlier reports show that graphene-based systems displayed controlled drug release, which is advantageous for drug delivery applications [60–61]. Graphene oxide (GO) and reduced graphene oxide (rGO) are widely used in drug delivery applications. Sima et al. [62] successfully functionalized GO nanocolloids (GONs) with bovine serum albumin (BSA) protein and anticancer drug and was later assembled it on a solid substrate. The authors tested this bio platform for melanoma cells which is a type of skin cancer cell. Thus, this type of bio platform finds application in drug screening, especially cancerous cells. One of the unique features of nano-graphene oxide (NGO) is photoluminescent. The functionalized NGO (pegylated) also displayed good photoluminescence in visible and NIR, and this was explored for imaging biological cells. The functionalized NGO was loaded with drugs and successfully transported into specific cancer cells [63]. The drug-controlled property of GO could be further increased by different functionalizations. For instance, β-CD and cross-linkable FA were introduced onto GO sheets and were later loaded with the anticancer drug, Camptothecin (CPT). The modified GO displayed better-controlled drug release [64]. Temozolomide-loaded GO-FA composite exhibits good biocompatibility. The composite shows sustained drug release and were adequate to kill the rat glioma cells. Therefore, it is suggested as a candidate for cancer therapy [65]. Functionalization of graphene oxide with hyaluronic acid improved the drug delivery efficiency of GO. The *in vitro* cytocompatibility of the modified GO was tested for two cells lines, namely MDA-MB-231 and BT-474. The drug-loaded ([Doxorubicin Dox] and paclitaxel [Ptx]) HA GO was highly efficient in destroying tumor cells. The cancer cell-killing efficacy of the HA GO was further improved by loading the GO with iron oxide particles. Thus, the multifunctionalization of GO leads to high cell death [66]. A pH-sensitive drug delivery system was developed by modifying GO with CMC (carboxymethyl cellulose). The cytotoxicity results revealed that the GO CMC complex is safe for drug delivery. It is non-toxic for tested cells (normal cells NIH-3T3 and HeLa cells) even at high concentrations.

Furthermore, the complex has a good drug loading capacity for DOX and displayed anticancer activity (Figure 2.5) [67]. rGO (reduced graphene oxide) has excellent NIR absorption and photothermal conversion efficiency; therefore, it has been used as a photothermal agent for cancer treatment. Liu et al. [68] develop a novel sandwich structure of reduced graphene oxide and mesoporous silica. The synergistic effect of rGO and silica is responsible for the photothermal effect and pH-responsive drug properties. The cell viability studies further revealed that DOX-loaded rGO/silica nanocarrier destroy more cancerous cell. The simulation and in vivo/in vitro study conducted by Shi et al. [69] revealed that Heparin-reduced graphene oxide nanocomposites displayed good photothermal property and also release the loaded curcumin in a sustainable fashion. In another study, Justin and Chen [70] develop a transdermal drug delivery vehicle using chitosan-reduced GO. Recently Sandhya et al. reported the antibacterial activity of rGO and ZnO decorated rGO [71].

2.8 CONCLUSION

Infectious diseases, if not treated properly, will adversely affect the global human population. COVID, Ebola, smallpox, malaria, AIDS, tuberculosis, etc. are some of the deadly ID which increases the global mortality rate. Nanomaterials have been

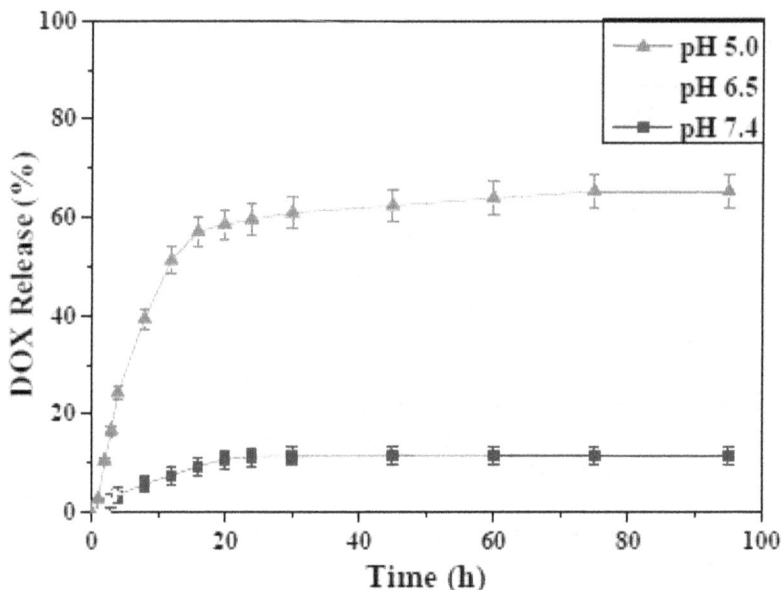

FIGURE 2.5 The in vitro release study of GO-CMC with different pH values.

Source: Reproduced with permission from Elsevier, License Number: 5101390555462

successfully used for the treatment of several infectious diseases. Owing to the excellent antibacterial, antiviral, and antioxidant properties, metal nanoparticles have received global attention and have been used in different pharmaceutical formulations. Metal nanoparticles have been incorporated into polymers to generate antibacterial and antiviral materials. The previous study indicates that the exposure time, concentration, morphology, and surface area of nanoparticles play a pivotal role in retarding the growth of pathogens. The antibacterial property of nanoparticles could be improved by modifying them with different additives such as chitosan. Modified nanoparticle offers excellent antibacterial activity and is advantageous for treating wounds and several infectious diseases.

ACKNOWLEDGMENTS

Authors gratefully thanks for financial support by the King Mongkut's University of Technology North Bangkok (KMUTNB), Thailand through the Post-Doctoral Program (Grant No. KMUTNB-63-Post-03 and KMUTNB-64-Post-03 to SR) and (Grant No. KMUTNB-BasicR-64–16).

REFERENCES

1. Díez-Pascual, Ana. 2018. "Antibacterial Activity of Nanomaterials." *Nanomaterials* 8 (6). doi:10.3390/nano8060359.

2. Nikaeen, Ghazal, Sepideh Abbaszadeh, and Saeed Yousefinejad. 2020. "Application of Nanomaterials in Treatment, Anti-Infection and Detection of Coronaviruses." *Nanomedicine* 15 (15):1501–1512. doi:10.2217/nnm-2020-0117.

3. Kalashnikova, Irina, Soumen Das, and Sudipta Seal. 2015. "Nanomaterials for Wound Healing: Scope and Advancement." *Nanomedicine* 10 (16):2593–2612. doi:10.2217/nnm.15.82.

4. Fujishima, Akira, Tata N. Rao, and Donald A. Tryk. 2000. "Titanium Dioxide Photocatalysis." *Journal of Photochemistry and Photobiology C: Photochemistry Reviews* 1 (1):1–21. doi:10.1016/s1389-5567(00)00002-2.

5. Seisenbaeva, Gulaim A., Karin Fromell, Vasiliy V. Vinogradov, Aleksey N. Terekhov, Andrey V. Pakhomov, Bo Nilsson, Kristina Nilsson Ekdahl, Vladimir V. Vinogradov, and Vadim G. Kessler. 2017. "Dispersion of TiO_2 Nanoparticles Improves Burn Wound Healing and Tissue Regeneration Through Specific Interaction with Blood Serum Proteins." *Scientific Reports* 7 (1). doi:10.1038/s41598-017-15792-w.

6. Esthappan, Saisy Kudilil, Suma Kumbamala Kuttappan, and Rani Joseph. 2012. "Thermal and Mechanical Properties of Polypropylene/Titanium Dioxide Nanocomposite Fibers." *Materials & Design* 37:537–542. doi:10.1016/j.matdes.2012.01.038.

7. Zhang, Yun-Xiang, Yi-hu Song, and Qiang Zheng. 2012. "Mechanical and Thermal Properties of Nanosized Titanium Dioxide Filled Rigid Poly(Vinyl Chloride)." *Chinese Journal of Polymer Science* 31 (2):325–332. doi:10.1007/s10118-013-1219-6.

8. Ansari, Mohd Omaish, and Faiz Mohammad. 2011. "Thermal Stability, Electrical Conductivity and Ammonia Sensing Studies on p-Toluenesulfonic Acid Doped Polyaniline:Titanium Dioxide (pTSA/Pani:TiO_2) Nanocomposites." *Sensors and Actuators B: Chemical* 157 (1):122–129. doi:10.1016/j.snb.2011.03.036.

9. Sankar, Renu, Ravishankar Dhivya, Kanchi Subramanian Shivashangari, and Vilwanathan Ravikumar. 2014. "Wound Healing Activity of Origanum Vulgare Engineered Titanium Dioxide Nanoparticles in Wistar Albino Rats." *Journal of Materials Science: Materials in Medicine* 25 (7):1701–1708. doi:10.1007/s10856-014-5193-5.

10. Ismail, Nur Arifah, Khairul Anuar Mat Amin, Fadzillah Adibah Abdul Majid, and Mohd Hasmizam Razali. 2019. "Gellan Gum Incorporating Titanium Dioxide Nanoparticles Biofilm as Wound Dressing: Physicochemical, Mechanical, Antibacterial Properties and Wound Healing Studies." *Materials Science and Engineering: C* 103. doi:10.1016/j.msec.2019.109770.

11. Sivaranjani, V., and P. Philominathan. 2016. "Synthesize of Titanium Dioxide Nanoparticles Using *Moringa oleifera* Leaves and Evaluation of Wound Healing Activity." *Wound Medicine* 12:1–5. doi:10.1016/j.wndm.2015.11.002.

12. Santhoshkumar, Thirunavukkarasu, Abdul Rahuman, Chidambaram Jayaseelan, Govindasamy Rajakumar, Sampath Marimuthu, Arivarasan Vishnu Kirthi, Kanayairam Velayutham, John Thomas, Jayachandran Venkatesan, and Se-Kwon Kim. 2014. "Green Synthesis of Titanium Dioxide Nanoparticles Using Psidium Guajava Extract and Its Antibacterial and Antioxidant Properties." *Asian Pacific Journal of Tropical Medicine* 7 (12):968–976. doi:10.1016/s1995-7645(14)60171-1.

13. Seydi, Niloofar, Sania Saneei, Ali R. Jalalvand, Mohammad Mahdi Zangeneh, Akram Zangeneh, Reza Tahvilian, and Elham Pirabbasi. 2019. "Synthesis of Titanium Nanoparticles Using *Allium eriophyllum* Boiss Aqueous Extract by Green Synthesis Method and evaluation of Their Remedial Properties." *Applied Organometallic Chemistry* 33 (11). doi:10.1002/aoc.5191.

14. Thakur, B. K., A. Kumar, and D. Kumar. 2019. "Green Synthesis of Titanium Dioxide Nanoparticles Using *Azadirachta indica* Leaf Extract and Evaluation of Their Antibacterial Activity." *South African Journal of Botany* 124:223–227. doi:10.1016/j.sajb.2019.05.024.

15. Akhtar, Sara, Khuram Shahzad, Sadaf Mushtaq, Iftikhar Ali, Muhammad Hassan Rafe, and Syed Muhammad Fazal-ul-Karim. 2019. "Antibacterial and Antiviral Potential of Colloidal Titanium Dioxide (TiO$_2$) Nanoparticles Suitable for Biological Applications." *Materials Research Express* 6 (10). doi:10.1088/2053-1591/ab3b27.

16. Rajakumar, G., A. Abdul Rahuman, S. Mohana Roopan, V. Gopiesh Khanna, G. Elango, C. Kamaraj, A. Abduz Zahir, and K. Velayutham. 2012. "Fungus-Mediated Biosynthesis and Characterization of TiO$_2$ Nanoparticles and Their Activity Against Pathogenic Bacteria." *Spectrochimica Acta Part A: Molecular and Biomolecular Spectroscopy* 91:23–29. doi:10.1016/j.saa.2012.01.011.

17. Hassan, M. Shamshi, Touseef Amna, Amrita Mishra, Soon-Il Yun, Hyun-Chel Kim, Hak-Yong Kim, and Myung-Seob Khil. 2012. "Fabrication, Characterization and Antibacterial Effect of Novel Electrospun TiO$_2$ Nanorods on a Panel of Pathogenic Bacteria." *Journal of Biomedical Nanotechnology* 8 (3):394–404. doi:10.1166/jbn.2012.1393.

18. Guo, Feng, Saman Aryana, Yinghui Han, and Yunpeng Jiao. 2018. "A Review of the Synthesis and Applications of Polymer – Nanoclay Composites." *Applied Sciences* 8 (9). doi:10.3390/app8091696.

19. Rafiee, Roham, and Reza Shahzadi. 2018. "Mechanical Properties of Nanoclay and Nanoclay Reinforced Polymers: A Review." *Polymer Composites* 40 (2):431–445. doi:10.1002/pc.24725.

20. Gabr, Mohamed H., Nguyen T. Phong, Mohammad Ali Abdelkareem, Kazuya Okubo, Kiyoshi Uzawa, Isao Kimpara, and Toru Fujii. 2013. "Mechanical, Thermal, and Moisture Absorption Properties of Nano-Clay Reinforced Nano-Cellulose Biocomposites." *Cellulose* 20 (2):819–826. doi:10.1007/s10570-013-9876-8.

21. John, Bibin, C. P. Reghunadhan Nair, and K. N. Ninan. 2010. "Effect of Nanoclay on the Mechanical, Dynamic Mechanical and Thermal Properties of Cyanate Ester Syntactic Foams." *Materials Science and Engineering: A* 527 (21–22):5435–5443. doi:10.1016/j.msea.2010.05.016.

22. Gaharwar, Akhilesh K., Lauren M. Cross, Charles W. Peak, Karli Gold, James K. Carrow, Anna Brokesh, and Kanwar Abhay Singh. 2019. "2D Nanoclay for Biomedical Applications: Regenerative Medicine, Therapeutic Delivery, and Additive Manufacturing." *Advanced Materials* 31 (23). doi:10.1002/adma.201900332.

23. Liu, Mingxian, Rawil Fakhrullin, Andrei Novikov, Abhishek Panchal, and Yuri Lvov. 2018. "Tubule Nanoclay-Organic Heterostructures for Biomedical Applications." *Macromolecular Bioscience* 19 (4). doi:10.1002/mabi.201800419.

24. Shojaee-Aliabadi, Saeedeh, Mohammad Amin Mohammadifar, Hedayat Hosseini, Abdorreza Mohammadi, Mehran Ghasemlou, Seyede Marzieh Hosseini, Mehrdad Haghshenas, and Ramin Khaksar. 2014. "Characterization of Nanobiocomposite Kappa-Carrageenan Film with Zataria Multiflora Essential Oil and Nanoclay." *International Journal of Biological Macromolecules* 69:282–289. doi:10.1016/j.ijbiomac.2014.05.015.

25. Entezam, Mehdi, Ashkan Ehghaghiyan, Negar Naghdi Sedeh, Seyed Hassan Jafari, and Hossein Ali Khonakdar. 2019. "Physicomechanical and Antimicrobial Characteristics of Hydrogel Based on Poly(Vinyl Alcohol): Performance Improvement via Inclusion of Chitosan-Modified Nanoclay." *Journal of Applied Polymer Science*. doi:10.1002/app.47444.

26. Heydary, H. Amiri, E. Karamian, E. Poorazizi, A. Khandan, and J. Heydaripour. 2015. "A Novel Nano-Fiber of Iranian Gum Tragacanth-Polyvinyl Alcohol/Nanoclay Composite for Wound Healing Applications." *Procedia Materials Science* 11:176–182. doi:10.1016/j.mspro.2015.11.079.

27. Noori, S., M. Kokabi, and Z. M. Hassan. 2015. "Nanoclay Enhanced the Mechanical Properties of Poly(Vinyl Alcohol)/Chitosan/Montmorillonite Nanocomposite Hydrogel as Wound Dressing." *Procedia Materials Science* 11:152–156. doi:10.1016/j.mspro.2015.11.023.

28. Chatterjee, Arijit Kumar, Ruchira Chakraborty, and Tarakdas Basu. 2014. "Mechanism of Antibacterial Activity of Copper Nanoparticles." *Nanotechnology* 25 (13). doi:10.1088/0957-4484/25/13/135101.
29. Longano, D., N. Ditaranto, N. Cioffi, F. Di Niso, T. Sibillano, A. Ancona, A. Conte, M. A. Del Nobile, L. Sabbatini, and L. Torsi. 2012. "Analytical Characterization of Laser-Generated Copper Nanoparticles for Antibacterial Composite Food Packaging." *Analytical and Bioanalytical Chemistry* 403 (4):1179–1186. doi:10.1007/s00216-011-5689-5.
30. Jayaramudu, Tippabattini, Kokkarachedu Varaprasad, Radha D. Pyarasani, K. Koteshwara Reddy, Kanderi Dileep Kumar, A. Akbari-Fakhrabadi, R. V. Mangalaraja, and John Amalraj. 2019. "Chitosan Capped Copper Oxide/Copper Nanoparticles Encapsulated Microbial Resistant Nanocomposite Films." *International Journal of Biological Macromolecules* 128:499–508. doi:10.1016/j.ijbiomac.2019.01.145.
31. Tang, Liangzhen, Li Zhu, Fu Tang, Chuang Yao, Jie Wang, and Lidong Li. 2018. "Mild Synthesis of Copper Nanoparticles with Enhanced Oxidative Stability and Their Application in Antibacterial Films." *Langmuir* 34 (48):14570–14576. doi:10.1021/acs.langmuir.8b02470.
32. Chemistry International. "Green Synthesis of Copper Nanoparticles by *Citrus limon* Fruits Extract, Characterization and Antibacterial Activity." *OSF Preprints.* doi:10.31219/osf.io/76k8r.
33. Raffi, Muhammad, Saba Mehrwan, Tariq Mahmood Bhatti, Javed Iqbal Akhter, Abdul Hameed, Wasim Yawar, and M. Masood ul Hasan. 2010. "Investigations into the Antibacterial Behavior of Copper Nanoparticles Against *Escherichia coli.*" *Annals of Microbiology* 60 (1):75–80. doi:10.1007/s13213-010-0015-6.
34. Jayaramudu, Tippabattini, Kokkarachedu Varaprasad, Radha D. Pyarasani, K. Koteshwara Reddy, A. Akbari-Fakhrabadi, Verónica Carrasco-Sánchez, and John Amalraj. 2021. "Hydroxypropyl Methylcellulose-Copper Nanoparticle and Its Nanocomposite Hydrogel Films for Antibacterial Application." *Carbohydrate Polymers* 254. doi:10.1016/j.carbpol.2020.117302.
35. Franci, Gianluigi, Annarita Falanga, Stefania Galdiero, Luciana Palomba, Mahendra Rai, Giancarlo Morelli, and Massimiliano Galdiero. 2015. "Silver Nanoparticles as Potential Antibacterial Agents." *Molecules* 20 (5):8856–8874. doi:10.3390/molecules20058856.
36. Paladini, Federica, and Mauro Pollini. 2019. "Antimicrobial Silver Nanoparticles for Wound Healing Application: Progress and Future Trends." *Materials* 12 (16). doi:10.3390/ma12162540.
37. Kokura, Satoshi, Osamu Handa, Tomohisa Takagi, Takeshi Ishikawa, Yuji Naito, and Toshikazu Yoshikawa. 2010. "Silver Nanoparticles as a Safe Preservative for Use in Cosmetics." *Nanomedicine: Nanotechnology, Biology and Medicine* 6 (4):570–574. doi:10.1016/j.nano.2009.12.002.
38. Wang, Hongshui, Xueliang Qiao, Jianguo Chen, and Shiyuan Ding. 2005. "Preparation of Silver Nanoparticles by Chemical Reduction Method." *Colloids and Surfaces A: Physicochemical and Engineering Aspects* 256 (2–3):111–115. doi:10.1016/j.colsurfa.2004.12.058.
39. Bankar, Ashok, Bhagyashree Joshi, Ameeta Ravi Kumar, and Smita Zinjarde. 2010. "Banana Peel Extract Mediated Novel Route for the Synthesis of Silver Nanoparticles." *Colloids and Surfaces A: Physicochemical and Engineering Aspects* 368 (1–3):58–63. doi:10.1016/j.colsurfa.2010.07.024.
40. Lin, Hung-Wen, Wen-Hwa Hwu, and Ming-Der Ger. 2008. "The Dispersion of Silver Nanoparticles with Physical Dispersal Procedures." *Journal of Materials Processing Technology* 206 (1–3):56–61. doi:10.1016/j.jmatprotec.2007.12.025.
41. Haider, Adnan, and Inn-Kyu Kang. 2015. "Preparation of Silver Nanoparticles and Their Industrial and Biomedical Applications: A Comprehensive Review." *Advances in Materials Science and Engineering* 1–16. doi:10.1155/2015/165257.

42. García-Barrasa, Jorge, José López-de-Luzuriaga, and Miguel Monge. 2011. "Silver Nanoparticles: Synthesis Through Chemical Methods in Solution and Biomedical Applications." *Open Chemistry* 9 (1):7–19. doi:10.2478/s11532-010-0124-x.
43. Singh, Tej, Kumari Jyoti, Amar Patnaik, Ajeet Singh, Ranchan Chauhan, and S. S. Chandel. 2017. "Biosynthesis, Characterization and Antibacterial Activity of Silver Nanoparticles Using an Endophytic Fungal Supernatant of *Raphanus sativus.*" *Journal of Genetic Engineering and Biotechnology* 15 (1):31–39. doi:10.1016/j.jgeb.2017.04.005.
44. Kim, Jun Sung, Eunye Kuk, Kyeong Nam Yu, Jong-Ho Kim, Sung Jin Park, Hu Jang Lee, So Hyun Kim, Young Kyung Park, Yong Ho Park, Cheol-Yong Hwang, Yong-Kwon Kim, Yoon-Sik Lee, Dae Hong Jeong, and Myung-Haing Cho. 2007. "Antimicrobial Effects of Silver Nanoparticles." *Nanomedicine: Nanotechnology, Biology and Medicine* 3 (1):95–101. doi:10.1016/j.nano.2006.12.001.
45. Yang, Xiao Xi, Chun Mei Li, and Cheng Zhi Huang. 2016. "Curcumin Modified Silver Nanoparticles for Highly Efficient Inhibition of Respiratory Syncytial Virus Infection." *Nanoscale* 8 (5):3040–3048. doi:10.1039/c5nr07918g.
46. Al-Dhabi, Naif Abdullah, Abdul-Kareem Mohammed Ghilan, Mariadhas Valan Arasu, and Veeramuthu Duraipandiyan. 2018. "Green Biosynthesis of Silver Nanoparticles Produced from Marine Streptomyces sp. Al-Dhabi-89 and Their Potential Applications Against Wound Infection and Drug Resistant Clinical Pathogens." *Journal of Photochemistry and Photobiology B: Biology* 189:176–184. doi:10.1016/j.jphotobiol.2018.09.012.
47. Yamamoto, Osamu. 2001. "Influence of Particle Size on the Antibacterial Activity of Zinc Oxide." *International Journal of Inorganic Materials* 3 (7):643–646. doi:10.1016/s1466-6049(01)00197-0.
48. Söderberg, Thor A., Bo Sunzel, Stig Holm, Theodor Elmros, Göran Hallmans, and Staffan Sjöberg. 2009. "Antibacterial Effect of Zinc Oxide in Vitro." *Scandinavian Journal of Plastic and Reconstructive Surgery and Hand Surgery* 24 (3):193–197. doi:10.3109/02844319009041278.
49. Ågren, Magnus S., Lennart Franzén, and Milos Chvapil. 1993. "Effects on Wound Healing of Zinc Oxide in a Hydrocolloid Dressing." *Journal of the American Academy of Dermatology* 29 (2):221–227. doi:10.1016/0190-9622(93)70172-p.
50. Silvestre, Clara, Sossio Cimmino, Marilena Pezzuto, Antonella Marra, Veronica Ambrogi, Jeannette Dexpert-Ghys, Marc Verelst, Sylvain Augier, Ida Romano, and Donatella Duraccio. 2013. "Preparation and Characterization of Isotactic Polypropylene/Zinc Oxide Microcomposites with Antibacterial Activity." *Polymer Journal* 45 (9):938–945. doi:10.1038/pj.2013.8.
51. Stanković, A., S. Dimitrijević, and D. Uskoković. 2013. "Influence of Size Scale and Morphology on Antibacterial Properties of ZnO Powders Hydrothemally Synthesized Using Different Surface Stabilizing Agents." *Colloids and Surfaces B: Biointerfaces* 102:21–28. doi:10.1016/j.colsurfb.2012.07.033.
52. Tyagi, Pankaj Kumar, Deepak Gola, Shruti Tyagi, Ankit Kumar Mishra, Arvind Kumar, Nitin Chauhan, Anami Ahuja, and Sandeep Sirohi. 2020. "Synthesis of Zinc Oxide Nanoparticles and Its Conjugation with Antibiotic: Antibacterial and Morphological Characterization." *Environmental Nanotechnology, Monitoring & Management* 14. doi:10.1016/j.enmm.2020.100391.
53. Pillai, Akhilash Mohanan, Vishnu Sankar Sivasankarapillai, Abbas Rahdar, Jithu Joseph, Fardin Sadeghfar, Ronaldo Anuf A, K. Rajesh, and George Z. Kyzas. 2020. "Green Synthesis and Characterization of Zinc Oxide Nanoparticles with Antibacterial and Antifungal Activity." *Journal of Molecular Structure* 1211. doi:10.1016/j.molstruc.2020.128107.
54. Rekha, K., M. Nirmala, Manjula G. Nair, and A. Anukaliani. 2010. "Structural, Optical, Photocatalytic and Antibacterial Activity of Zinc Oxide and Manganese Doped Zinc

Oxide Nanoparticles." *Physica B: Condensed Matter* 405 (15):3180–3185. doi:10.1016/j.physb.2010.04.042.

55. Yu, Wang, Li Sisi, Yang Haiyan, and Luo Jie. 2020. "Progress in the Functional Modification of Graphene/Graphene Oxide: A Review." *RSC Advances* 10 (26):15328–15345. doi:10.1039/d0ra01068e.

56. López, Vicente, Ravi S. Sundaram, Cristina Gómez-Navarro, David Olea, Marko Burghard, Julio Gómez-Herrero, Félix Zamora, and Klaus Kern. 2009. "Chemical Vapor Deposition Repair of Graphene Oxide: A Route to Highly-Conductive Graphene Monolayers." *Advanced Materials* 21 (46):4683–4686. doi:10.1002/adma.200901582.

57. Chung, Chul, Young-Kwan Kim, Dolly Shin, Soo-Ryoon Ryoo, Byung Hee Hong, and Dal-Hee Min. 2013. "Biomedical Applications of Graphene and Graphene Oxide." *Accounts of Chemical Research* 46 (10):2211–2224. doi:10.1021/ar300159f.

58. Singh, Subhash, Keerti Rathi, and Kaushik Pal. 2018. "Synthesis, Characterization of Graphene Oxide Wrapped Silicon Carbide for Excellent Mechanical and Damping Performance for Aerospace Application." *Journal of Alloys and Compounds* 740:436–445. doi:10.1016/j.jallcom.2017.12.069.

59. Sreenivasulu, B., B. R. Ramji, and Madeva Nagaral. 2018. "A Review on Graphene Reinforced Polymer Matrix Composites." *Materials Today: Proceedings* 5 (1):2419–2428. doi:10.1016/j.matpr.2017.11.021.

60. Lu, Bingan, Ting Li, Haitao Zhao, Xiaodong Li, Caitian Gao, Shengxiang Zhang, and Erqing Xie. 2012. "Graphene-Based Composite Materials Beneficial to Wound Healing." *Nanoscale* 4 (9). doi:10.1039/c2nr11958g.

61. Fan, Zengjie, Bin Liu, Jinqing Wang, Songying Zhang, Qianqian Lin, Peiwei Gong, Limin Ma, and Shengrong Yang. 2014. "A Novel Wound Dressing Based on Ag/Graphene Polymer Hydrogel: Effectively Kill Bacteria and Accelerate Wound Healing." *Advanced Functional Materials* 24 (25):3933–3943. doi:10.1002/adfm.201304202.

62. Sima, Livia E., Gabriela Chiritoiu, Irina Negut, Valentina Grumezescu, Stefana Orobeti, Cristian V. A. Munteanu, Felix Sima, and Emanuel Axente. 2020. "Functionalized Graphene Oxide Thin Films for Anti-Tumor Drug Delivery to Melanoma Cells." *Frontiers in Chemistry* 8. doi:10.3389/fchem.2020.00184.

63. Sun, Xiaoming, Zhuang Liu, Kevin Welsher, Joshua Tucker Robinson, Andrew Goodwin, Sasa Zaric, and Hongjie Dai. 2008. "Nano-Graphene Oxide for Cellular Imaging and Drug Delivery." *Nano Research* 1 (3):203–212. doi:10.1007/s12274-008-8021-8.

64. Ye, Yuanfeng, Xincheng Mao, Jialing Xu, Jingyang Kong, and Xiaohong Hu. 2019. "Functional Graphene Oxide Nanocarriers for Drug Delivery." *International Journal of Polymer Science* 1–7. doi:10.1155/2019/8453493.

65. Wang, Li-Hua, Jia-Yuan Liu, Lin Sui, Peng-Hui Zhao, Hai-Di Ma, Zhen Wei, and Yong-Li Wang. 2020. "Folate-Modified Graphene Oxide as the Drug Delivery System to Load Temozolomide." *Current Pharmaceutical Biotechnology* 21 (11):1088–1098. doi:10.2174/1389201021666200226122742.

66. Pramanik, Nilkamal, Santhalakshmi Ranganathan, Sunaina Rao, Kaushik Suneet, Shilpee Jain, Annapoorni Rangarajan, and Siddharth Jhunjhunwala. 2019. "A Composite of Hyaluronic Acid-Modified Graphene Oxide and Iron Oxide Nanoparticles for Targeted Drug Delivery and Magnetothermal Therapy." *ACS Omega* 4 (5):9284–9293. doi:10.1021/acsomega.9b00870.

67. Rao, Ziqie, Hongyu Ge, Liangling Liu, Chen Zhu, Lian Min, Meng Liu, Lihong Fan, and Dan Li. 2018. "Carboxymethyl Cellulose Modified Graphene Oxide as pH-Sensitive Drug Delivery System." *International Journal of Biological Macromolecules* 107:1184–1192. doi:10.1016/j.ijbiomac.2017.09.096.

68. Liu, Xiao, Xu Wu, Yuqian Xing, Ying Zhang, Xuefei Zhang, Qinqin Pu, Min Wu, and Julia Xiaojun Zhao. 2020. "Reduced Graphene Oxide/Mesoporous Silica Nanocarriers

for pH-Triggered Drug Release and Photothermal Therapy." *ACS Applied Bio Materials* 3 (5):2577–2587. doi:10.1021/acsabm.9b01108.

69.   Shi, Xiaoqun, Yang Wang, Haiyan Sun, Yujuan Chen, Xingzhen Zhang, Jiangkang Xu, and Guangxi Zhai. 2019. "Heparin-Reduced Graphene Oxide Nanocomposites for Curcumin Delivery: In Vitro, in Vivo and Molecular Dynamics Simulation Study." *Biomaterials Science* 7 (3):1011–1027. doi:10.1039/c8bm00907d.

70.   Justin, Richard, and Biqiong Chen. 2014. "Strong and Conductive Chitosan – Reduced Graphene Oxide Nanocomposites for Transdermal Drug Delivery." *Journal of Materials Chemistry B* 2:3759. doi:10.1039/c4tb00390j.

71.   Sandhya, P. K., Jiya Jose, M. S. Sreekala, M. Padmanabhan, Nandakumar Kalarikkal, and Sabu Thomas. 2018. "Reduced Graphene Oxide and ZnO Decorated Graphene for Biomedical Applications." *Ceramics International* 44 (13):15092–15098. doi:10.1016/j.ceramint.2018.05.143.

3 Larvicidal and Antimicrobial Activities of Green-Synthesized Ag Nanoparticles

Lakshmanan Muthulakshmi, Velmurugan Sundarapandian, D. Nagapriyadarshini, Jamespandi Annaraj, M. T. Mathew, H. Nellaiah

CONTENTS

DOI: 10.1201/9781003143093-3

3.1   INTRODUCTION

Nanotechnology is important for advances in several fields, including medicine, pharmaceuticals, textiles, chemicals, paper conservation, removal of dyes and other wastes from water and photocatalytic degradation [1]. Diverse metals like magnesium zinc copper titanium, gold, platinum, and silver, as well as their oxides, are used for the synthesis of nanoparticles [2]. The exceptional functional properties of nanoscale level silver particles (AgNPs) like high surface plasmon resonance (SPR), high stability, good conductivity, photoelectrochemical activity and potent antimicrobial activity provide for more biological applications such as in diagnostics and therapeutics [3].

Though several synthetic processes for AgNPs exist, these involve the use of toxic compounds and excess energy [4]. Therefore, researchers recently are more interested in non-toxic, eco-friendly and cost-effective synthetic routes using plant extracts and substances produced by bacteria, actinomycetes, fungi, yeasts, and algae [5]. Synthesis of AgNPs may be extracellular or intracellular manner, with the former process being carried out through the reduction of metal ions by enzymes or biomolecules on the outer surface of the cell, while intracellular synthesis is accomplished entirely within the cell. However, the simple, quick, and economic extracellular mechanism is more convenient than, and preferable to, the intracellular mechanism, since it is amenable to large-scale production

Several normal strategies for both extracellular and intracellular processes have been addressed till date utilizing microorganisms like bacteria and plants [6]. The use of medicinal plants and bioactive phytocompounds has seen more growing interest. The importance of sources rich in polyphenols has long been underscored because of their radical-scavenging action and anticarcinogenetic properties. Among these, naturally available traditional plant extracts yield better results than others in the synthesis of nanoparticles without toxicity [7]. Furthermore, they can also be utilized in several biological applications, including antimicrobial and larvicidal. Mosquitos act as carriers for several vector-borne diseases. They infect considerable number individuals across the world with lethal pathogens through their bite, thereby causing the deaths of millions of people. Most importantly, the mosquito has been declared "number one public enemy" by the WHO as it was found to infect over 700,000,000 people and 40,000,000 people worldwide and in the Indian population, respectively, every year [8]. Mosquitoes are vectors for the majority of unsafe afflictions like intestinal issues, yellow fever, dengue fever, chikungunya, filariasis, and encephalitis [9]. Therefore, it is very essential to control mosquito-borne diseases and, at the same time, safeguard environmental quality and public health by developing insecticides that are non-toxic or negligibly toxic. The currently used synthetic insecticides for mosquito control such as organochlorine and organophosphate compounds are useless to humans because of their particular, utilitarian, regular, and monetary components [10].

Considering these scenarios, the green/biosynthesis of eco-friendly, cost-effective, and non-toxic metal nanoparticles from several plant-derived metabolites has recently been developed with a surge in interest in nanotechnology. Such nanoparticles have been found to possess catalytic, optical, electronic, antimicrobial, antiviral, antiplasmodial, insecticidal, magnetic, and mosquito larvicidal properties [11]

Nanoparticles from green synthesis displayed greater advantages than their chemically prepared counterparts. Consequently, a large number of plant extracts have been utilized for synthesizing nanoparticles active against mosquitos [12]. Some earlier reports stated that silver and nickel-palladium nanoparticles prepared from *Pedalium murex* seed extract *Melia dubia* leaf extract [13] and *Citrus sinensis* peel extract [14], respectively, had satisfactory activities against larvae, pests, and insect ova. In line with this, we intended to synthesize silver nanoparticles using ethanolic extracts of four medicinal plants (*Vitex nigunda, Azadirachta indica, Mangifera indica*, and *Ocimum basilicum* that are distributed throughout India.

Vitex negundo is a well-known medicinal herb used in the Indian system of medicine. It is commonly known as the Five-Leaved Chaste Tree or Monk's pepper. In India, it is known as *Punjgusht, Nirgundu, Sambhalu,* or *Sephali. V. negundo* extracts have been used in the Unani system of medicine as anti-inflammatory agents, expectorants, tranquilizers, antispasmodics, anticonvulsants, rejuvenating agents, antiarthritic agents, anthelminthic agents, antifungals, and antipyretics. In Unani, the seeds of this plant are recommended for controlling premature ejaculation and enhancing male libido. *V. negundo* relieves muscle aches and joint pains [15]. The Ayurvedic and Unani Pharmacopoeias of India have documented the uses of the leaf, seed and root of this plant to treat excessive vaginal discharge, edema, skin diseases, pruritus, helminthiasis, rheumatism and puerperal fever. *V. negundo* is also used as a constituent of many herbal preparations. Chrysosplenol D has antihistamine and muscle relaxant properties and is a compound found in the Five-Leaved Chaste Tree. Neem (*A. indica*) is a member of the family Meliaceae and its health-promoting effects are attributed to its high content of antioxidants. It has been widely used in Chinese, Ayurvedic, and Unani medicines and especially in the Indian subcontinent for the treatment and prevention of various diseases. *A. indica* L. (neem) has an important role in health management due to its being a rich source of various bioactive ingredients. The most important active constituent is azadirachtin and the others are nimbolinin, nimbin, nimbidin, nimbidol, sodium nimbinate, gedunin, salannin, and quercetin. Neem constituents have biological applications as antifungals, antioxidants, and anticancer agents. Earlier findings have confirmed that neem and its constituents play a role in the scavenging of free radicals and prevention of disease [16]. Studies based on animal models established that neem and its chief constituents play pivotal roles in cancer management through their modulation of various molecular pathways, including p53, pTEN, NF-κB, PI3K/Akt, Bcl-2, and VEGF. p53 is an important tumor suppressor gene involved in inhibiting the proliferation of abnormal cells, thereby containing the development and progression of cancer. A recent report confirmed that treatment with an ethanolic fraction of neem leaves effectively upregulates proapoptotic genes and proteins, including p53, Bcl-2-associated X protein (Bax), Bcl-2-associated death promoter protein (Bad), caspases, phosphatase, the tensin homolog gene (pTEN), and c-Jun N-terminal kinase (JNK) It is considered a safe medicinal plant, as it modulates various biological processes without any adverse effects [17].

M. indica L. has been the focus of attention of many researchers in the tropical and subtropical regions for its phytochemical content, which qualified the mango as a super fruit model. Chemical analysis of mango pulp provided evidence that it has a relatively high caloric content (60 kcal/100 g fresh weights) and is an important source of potassium, fiber, and vitamins. Mango is also a particularly rich source of polyphenols, a diverse group of organic micronutrients found in plants which have specific health benefits such as antioxidant, anti-inflammatory, and anticancer activities.

3.2 COMMONLY USED METHODS FOR SILVER NANOPARTICLE SYNTHESIS

3.2.1 PHYSICAL METHOD

Evaporation-condensation and laser ablation are the very essential physical techniques to prepare uniformly distributed NPs without solvent contamination compared with chemical processes. Though physical synthesis of AgNPs using a tube furnace at atmospheric pressure has some disadvantages, as the tube furnace requires a large space and consumes enormous energy while raising the environmental temperature on the source, it needs much time to reach thermal stability and a stable operating temperature. AgNPs could be prepared through a small ceramic heater. Metal nanoparticle generation using a small ceramic heater with a local heating area for evaporating the source materials. The evaporated vapor may cool at an appropriate rate, which results in the generation of highly stable and concentrated small NPs due to the steady temperature rise with time [18].

Laser ablation technique: synthesis of colloidal nanoparticles during fem to second laser ablation of gold in water. Stabilization and size control of gold nanoparticles during laser ablation in aqueous cyclodextrins also used to produce AgNPs as colloids depending on the wavelength of the laser impinging on the metallic target, laser influence, the ablation time and the effective liquid medium, in the absence and presence of surfactants. Catalytic effect of laser ablated Ni nanoparticles in the oxidative addition reaction for a coupling reagent of benzylchloride and bromoacetonitrile. The size of silver nanoparticles prepared by laser ablation in solution is influenced by the laser wavelength. AgNPs of size 20–50 nm can be prepared by this method in water with femtosecond laser pulses at 800 nm preparation of nano-sized particles of silver with femtosecond laser ablation in water.

3.2.2 CHEMICAL REDUCTION METHOD

Chemical reduction is one of the most common approaches to prepare AgNPs using natural, organic and inorganic reducing agents. Various reducing agents such as sodium citrate, elemental hydrogen, polyol process, ascorbate, Tollens' reagent, sodium borohydride ($NaBH_4$), poly (ethylene glycol)-block copolymers, and N,N-dimethylformamide (DMF) are suitable for silver ions (Ag+) in aqueous/non-aqueous solutions. They can reduce Ag+ and lead to form metallic silver (Ag0), followed by agglomeration into oligomeric clusters. Eventually, those clusters lead to metallic colloidal silver nanoparticles [19]. However, it is essential to use stabilizing agents to obtain dispersive NPs during preparation, and protect their surfaces in order to avoid the agglomeration. consequently, sedimentation protects their surface properties. Polymeric compounds such as poly(vinyl alcohol), poly(ethylene glycol), poly(vinylpyrrolidone), polymethylmethacrylate, and poly(methacrylic acid) have been reported to be efficient protective agents to stabilize NPs. These may lead to dramatic modifications in nanoparticle structure, average size, size distribution width, stability and self-assembly patterns.

3.2.3 MICROEMULSION TECHNIQUES

Microemulsion techniques are used to prepare uniform and size-controllable AgNPs in two immiscible aqueous/organic phase systems based on the early spatial separation of reactants (precursor metal and reducing agent). The boundary between these two solvents and the intensity of interphase transport between two phases, facilitated by a quaternary alkyl-ammonium salt, affect the rate of interactions between metal precursors and reducing agents. The developed metal clusters at the interface are stabilized, because of the coating of their surfaces with stabilizing agents (which may occur in the non-polar aqueous medium), and transferred to the organic medium by the interphase transporter. Aggregative stability and polydispersity of silver nanoparticles prepared using two-phase aqueous organic systems. The major drawback of this technique is the use of highly toxic organic solvents. Hence, huge amounts of surfactant and organic solvents should be separated and decanted from the desired final product. Considering this, the use of non-toxic solvents such as dodecane as the oily phase is preferable as there is no need to separate the solvent from the final reaction mixture. Colloidal NPs synthesized in non-aqueous media for conductive inks are evenly dispersed in a low vapor pressure organic solvent to readily wet the polymeric substrate surface without aggregation. Moreover, excellence can also be found in their applications as catalysts in catalyzing most organic reactions conducted in non-polar solvents. It is very important to transfer metal nanoparticles to various physicochemical environments in real applications. The upsides of this miniature emulsion technique are utilized to set up a size-controlled process for obtaining uniform-size (under 100 nm in size) AgNPs. These kinds of AgNPs are thermodynamically consistent and optically straightforward [20].

3.2.4 MICROWAVE-ASSISTED METHOD

Microwave-assisted amalgamation provides a rapid technique for the significant union of AgNPs. This technique has mainly been utilized to deliver nanoscale-level metal oxides. Microwave (MW) chemistry has been extensively used in synthetic organic chemistry in order to enhance the rates of reactions, selectivity, and product yields. It is also useful for the synthesis of high-quality nanomaterials via direct microwave heating of the molecular precursors. A huge variety of mono- and bi-metallic nanostructures have been synthesized by the microwave-assisted route through one-pot synthesis. It generally involves the reduction of metal salts either in organic solvents like methanol, ethanol, and polyols, or in aqueous medium in the presence or absence of surface-directing agents. Various metal nanoparticles may also be prepared using ionic liquids, known for their excellent microwave-absorbing agents owing to their excellent ionic conductivity and polarizability. By changing the precursor and its concentration, the solvent and instrumental parameters like pressure, temperature and microwave power, metallic nanostructures of various sizes and morphologies have been prepared. Several simple/complex metal oxides have also been synthesized using the microwave-assisted method. The microwave hydrothermal method has been used to prepare a large variety of binary and ternary oxides such as ZnO, CuO, PdO, In_2O_3, Tl_2O_3, SnO_2, HfO_2, $BiVO_4$, $ZnAl_2O_4$, $BaTiO_3$, $CaTiO_3$, and $BaZrO_3$. Organic solvents like ethylene glycol or benzyl alcohol are perfect alternatives to an aqueous system owing to their high boiling points and high dielectric loss factors, and because they combine all the advantages of nonhydrolytic/nonaqueous nanoparticle synthesis with microwave chemistry. The microwave-assisted union has been named "microwave-assisted solvothermal blending for the synthesis of AgNPs." The crystals acquired by microwave-mediated methods are crystalline in nature [21].

3.2.5 HYDROTHERMAL/SOLVOTHERMAL METHOD

Solvothermal responses are done in closed vessels under an autogenous pressure factor over the boiling point of the solvents. Different materials can go through much unexpected substance changes under solvothermal conditions, which are frequently joined by the arrangement of nanoscale morphologies that are not attainable by customary techniques. Much of the time, high-bubbling natural solvents have been utilized for solvothermal responses. The most generally utilized natural solvents are those such as dimethyl formamide, diethyl formamide, acetonitrile, $(CH_3)_2CO$, ethanol, and methanol. Combinations of solvents have additionally been utilized to avoid issues of contrasting dissolvability for the distinctive beginning materials. Solvothermal responses can be carried out in various temperature ranges, contingent upon the prerequisites of the response. For the most part, glass vials are utilized for lower temperature responses, while responses performed at temperatures higher than 400 K require Teflon-lined autoclaves. The aqueous strategy has been utilized effectively for the combination of a tremendous number of inorganic mixtures and inorganic natural hybrid materials. The aqueous technique is a quick method of synthesis of nanoparticles utilizing microporous crystal stones, oxides, leading polymers, earthenware oxides, fluorides, and radiance phosphorus [22].

3.2.6 SOL-GEL METHOD

This strategy is utilized for a blend of the liquid phase and solid phase, and the morphological reach from discrete particles to shape polymer organizations. The sol-gel technique is used to obtain metal nanoparticles of uniform sizes. The process consists of the settling of (nm-sized) particles from a colloidal suspension onto a pre-existing surface, resulting in ceramic materials. The desired solid particles (e.g., metal alkoxides) are suspended in a liquid, forming the "sol," which is deposited on a substrate by spinning, dipping, or coating, or transferred to a mold. The particles in the sol are polymerized by partial evaporation of the solvent, or by addition of an initiator, forming the "gel," which is then heated at high temperature to give the final solid product. The normal strategy utilized for nanoparticles conveys the response of hydrolysis, followed by polycondensation measure, in order to obtain homogenous nanoparticles [23].

3.2.7 MECHANOCHEMICAL SYNTHESIS

Mechanochemical process is a solvent-free system for the preparation of metal nanoparticles. Mechanochemistry is the means of playing out a substance from reaction by applying mechanical forces. Since mechanochemical methods cause no harm to the environment, they are of noteworthy interest in present-day science. Mechanochemical method has been efficiently used for the quick synthesis of AgNPs. Using liquid-assisted grinding (LAG), it was possible to obtain 1D, 2D, and 3D coordination polymers from the same reaction mix. This technique was applied further for the combination of some zeolitic imidazolate frameworks [24].

3.2.8 SONOCHEMICAL SYNTHESIS

Sonochemistry is a marvel by which molecules go through compound changes that occur due to concentrated ultrasonic radiation (20 kHz–10 MHz). Ultrasound-induced compound or physical changes on account of cavitation include growth, advancement, and quick breakdown of air bubbles in a liquid, which creates transient local hotspots of high pressure and temperature. These extreme conditions can propel engineered reactions by creating an abundance of crystallization centers. Sonochemical procedures can create homogeneous nucleation networks and cause an amazing decline in crystallization time through differentiated and standard hydrothermal techniques. AgNPs mixed using sonochemical irradiation in 1-methyl-2-pyrrolidinone (NMP) can make 5–25 mm crustal structures in a period of 30 min, resembling AgNPs fused through solvothermal or microwave techniques [25]. The schematic diagram (1) shows the various modes of nanoparticle synthesis.

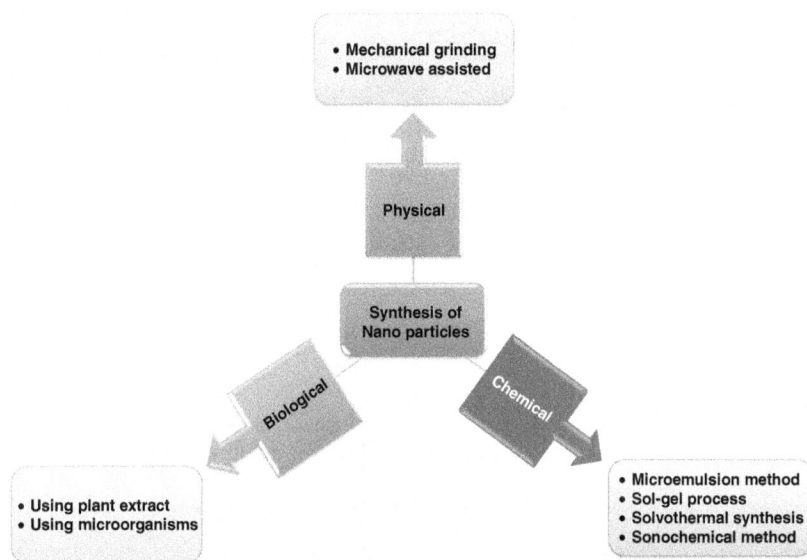

FIGURE 3.1 Different types of methods used for silver nanoparticle synthesis.

3.3 REDUCING AGENTS FOR SYNTHESIS OF SILVER NANOPARTICLES

3.3.1 PLANT EXTRACTS AS REDUCING AGENTS

In recent years, biosynthesis is being used as a green tool for synthesizing silver nanoparticles. In particular, plant extracts are being used as reducing agents for synthesizing many functional materials. Various kinds of lessening and covering specialists are utilized for nanoparticles in combination with accessible decreasing specialists to control the size and state of the incorporated nanomaterials. A few diminishing and settling specialists are utilized for combining nanoparticles including NaBH$_4$, ascorbic corrosive, PVP, and DMF. An attempt was made to use a biopolymer as a reducing agent for preparation of silver nanoparticles [26]. A high level of antibacterial activity was noted with nanoparticles synthesized from natural sources. On account of their high antimicrobial activity, silver nanoparticles are considered to be potent materials for controlling bacterial diseases. Nanoparticles are not restricted to particular fields in their applications, since they are widely used in catalysis, solar cells, bioremediation, electronics, biomedicine, drug delivery, and agricultural research [27]. Numerous diseases are caused by clinical pathogens in humans. Among all properties, antimicrobial activity is a crucial one for the control of pathogens [28]. Figure 3.2 depicts the synthesis of silver nanoparticles from medicinal plants.

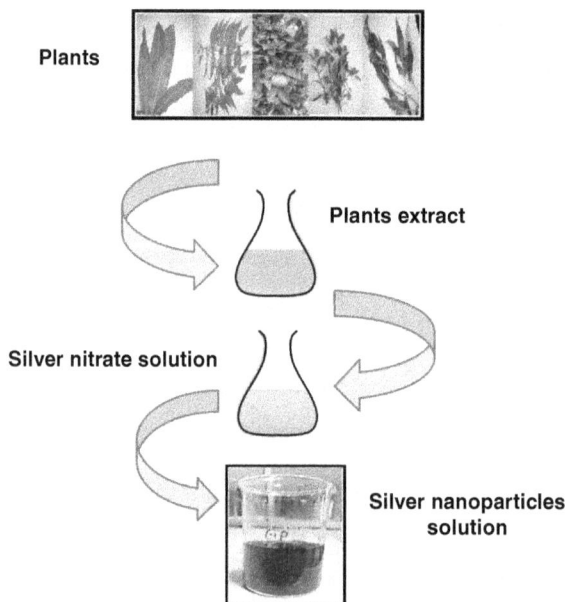

FIGURE 3.2   Green synthesis of silver nanoparticles.

3.3.2 Microbial Polymer as a Reducing Agents

Biopolymers are advantageous mixtures discharged from microorganisms during their growth period. On account of their biodegradable nature, biopolymers are broadly utilized for biomedical applications. Biopolymers were inferred to be materials for natural and scientific applications [29]. The polysaccharide bioflocculant-based nanoparticles are very stable and have great potential for controlling the growth of pathogens. Generally, bioflocculant polymers are used for dye degradation, metal removal, and wastewater treatment, and as reducing agents for nanoparticle production, generating a highly stable controlled size. Existing antibiotics developed from different sources are ineffective in controlling food-borne and urinary tract infection pathogens. Chitosan polymers have a dynamic aldehyde and ketone bunch that firmly bind harmful metals. The vast majority of biopolymers having viable functional groups are considered to be effective in chelating bio-sorbent materials for color removal. Biodegradable polymers like poly(dioxanone), poly(trimethylenecarbonate) copolymers, poly(e-caprolactone) homopolymers and copolymers, and polyanhydrides are used for planting of muscular inserts and manufacturing biodegradable sutures. Recently, the biopolymers most utilized as bundling material include chitosan, sodium alginate, carrageenan, and polylactic corrosive [30]. For preparation of nanoparticles of controlled size, researchers mostly use top-down approaches, with the nanoparticles being prepared by homogenization, ball milling and extrusion methods. In other methods, researchers are studying the effect of changes in the environment like pH, temperature, ionic strength and concentration of reducing agents on the preparation of nanoparticles [31]. Biopolymers possess potential antimicrobial properties by virtue of their having various functional groups. The peptidoglycan layer in the cell walls of pathogens provides strength and rigidity to the cell wall. Biopolymer-based nanoparticles induce cell wall damage and cause damage to cell organelles, leading to the loss of cellular integrity. Polysaccharides in the cell walls of pathogens interact electrostatically with the functional groups of antimicrobial compounds [32]. For example, silver nanoparticles containing silver ions and biopolymers containing sulfhydryl, amino and glycoprotein groups interact with cell wall components and induce loss of cellular integrity. These associations initiate the depolarization of the cell wall, leading to the loss of cellular organelles and integrity [33]. The main functional groups of bioflocculant containing glycoprotein, glycolipids, and amino compounds act as reducing agents in the synthesis of nanoparticles. Copper nanoparticles synthesized using bioflocculants are used for wastewater treatment. Biopolymers have been considered as suitable agents for the union and adjustment of silver nanoparticles. This sort of union with polymers allows for the dispersion of nanoparticles inside a polymer grid, which impacts the underlying strength and homogeneity of the nanocomposite film. It also promotes the preservation of solid antimicrobial properties in silver nanoparticles synthesized with biopolymers as reducing agents [34]. Figure 3.3 depicts the biosynthesis of silver nanoparticles from a biopolymer as a reducing agent.

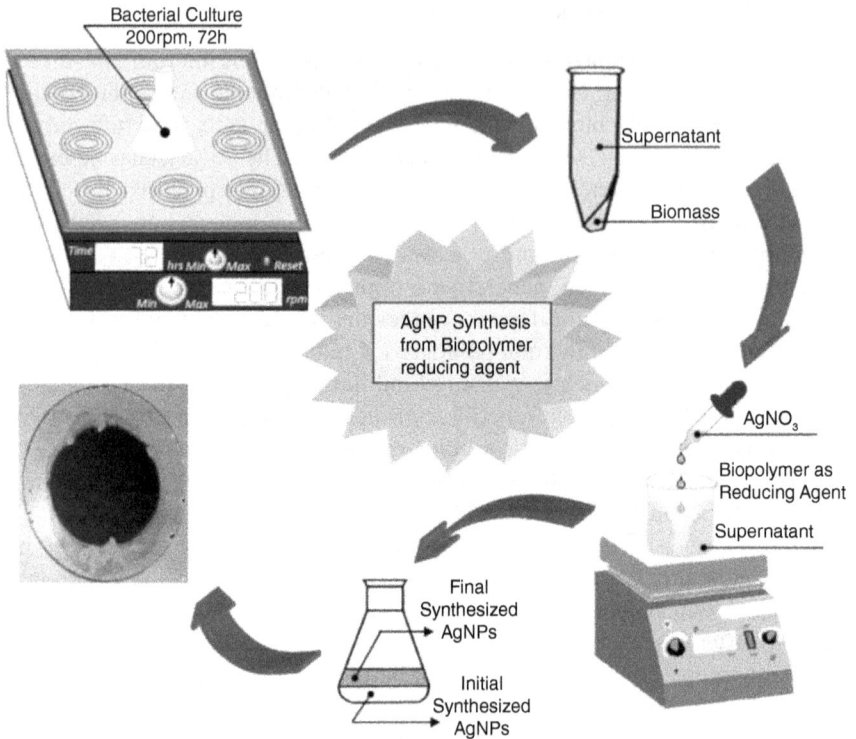

FIGURE 3.3   Synthesis of silver nanoparticles from biopolymer as a reducing agent.

3.4   GENERAL CHARACTERIZATION OF AGNPS

3.4.1   COLOR CHANGES

In the wake of adding 10 ml of a leaf extract to 90 ml of a 1 mM solution of silver nitrate, after the hatching for 1 h, the reaction mixture underwent a color change from pale yellow to brown in color, indicating the generation of AgNPs, which were separated and analyzed by surface Plasmon resonance spectroscopy [35]. At the same time, the green leaf extract also changed its color to a cherry red as shown in Figure 3.4. This signifies the color changes that accompany the synthesis of AgNPs using a plant extract as a reducing agent.

3.4.2   UV–VISIBLE SPECTROSCOPY

Spectrophotometry provides a way for breaking down fluids, gases, and solids using radiant energy in the far- and near-ultraviolet, visible, and infrared regions of the electromagnetic spectrum. The programmed electromagnetic radiation frequencies for ultraviolet, visible, and near-infrared radiation are characterized as follows: UV radiation: 300–400 nm, visible radiation: 400–765 nm, and NIR radiation:

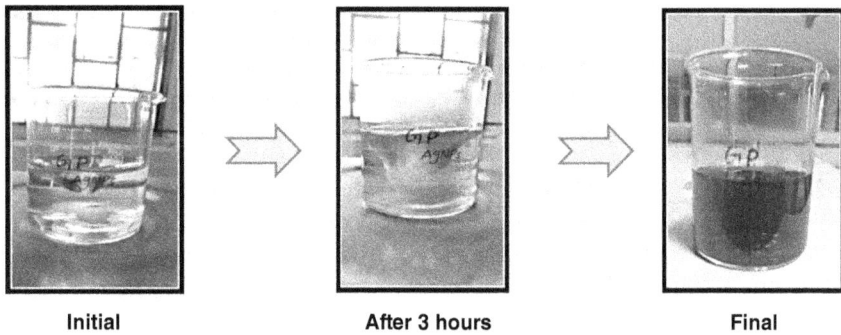

| Initial | After 3 hours | Final |

FIGURE 3.4 Images of color differences in silver nanoparticles using plant extract as a reducing agent.

765–3200 nm. The instrument works by passing a beam of light through a sample and estimating the frequency of the light arriving at an indicator. Insightful data can be obtained in terms of conveyance, absorbance or reflectance of energy in the frequency range 400–450 nm [36]. The presence of AgNPs is reflected in their optical and electromagnetic property of showing absorption bands in the range 400–450 nm. Das et al. [37] have reported data on AgNPs from *Euphorbia hirta* L. in terms of UV spectra and surface plasmon resonance (SPR) bands [36]. On account of their optical resonance, the silver nanoparticles were found to exhibit strong absorption of electromagnetic radiation in the 400–450 nm range. The oscillating electrons are collectively influenced by surface plasmon resonance and control the size and shape of the AgNPs. The secondary metabolites in the plant played a vital role in the reduction/conversion of silver nitrate to silver nanoparticles during the preparation process. Free electrons in metal nanoparticles led to SPR absorption band at 451 nm, suggesting that joint vibrations of electrons occurred between metal nanoparticles in resonance with light waves. The UV–Vis spectroscopy examination of silver nanoparticles was performed as a component of bioreduction time at ambient temperature. The UV–Vis spectrometric readings were recorded at a checking pace of 200–800 nm, as illustrated in Figure 3.5, with silver nanoparticles obtained using plant extract as the reducing agent. The flow examination showed the advancement of silver nanoparticles by the decline of the watery silver metal particles during receptiveness to the concentrate [38].

3.4.3 FTIR ANALYSIS

It is suggested that biological molecules in plant extracts play a dual role in the synthesis of metal nanoparticles. They act as reducing and stabilizing or capping agents. These roles of plant extracts are recognized by comparing FTIR spectra of pure plant extracts and extracts mediated by Ag nanoparticles. FTIR analysis is one of the appropriate methods for the identification of the possible functional groups of biomolecules that confer stabilizing factors during the formation of AgNPs. IR spectra provide information on the local molecular environment of

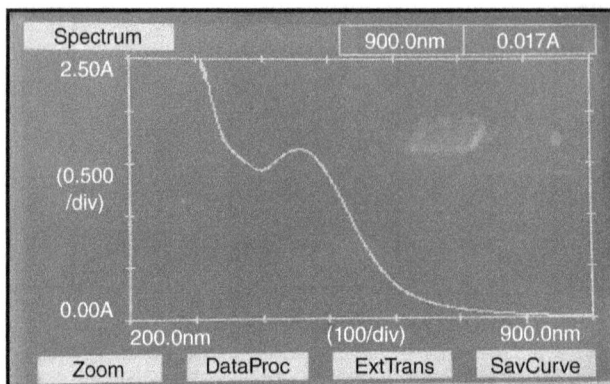

FIGURE 3.5   UV–visible spectra showing absorbance of silver nanoparticles.

the organic molecules on the surface of nanoparticles. In this study, FTIR spectral measurements were performed to identify the potential biomolecules in the *Terminalia catappa* leaf extract, which is responsible for reducing and capping the bioreduced silver nanoparticles. This technique is used to analyze the chemical composition of many organic chemicals, paints, coatings, adhesives, semiconductor materials, coolants, gases, polymers, lubricants, biological samples, minerals, and inorganics [39]. It can be used to analyze a wide range of materials in bulk or thin films, liquids, solids, pastes, powders, fibers, and other forms. FTIR analysis can not only provide qualitative (identification) analysis of materials, but, with relevant standards, can also be used for quantitative (amount) analysis. This technique can be used to analyze samples up to ~11 millimeters in diameter and either measure in bulk or the top ~1 μm layer. FTIR measurements were carried out to identify the possible biomolecules responsible for capping and efficient stabilization of the metal nanoparticles synthesized by *T. catappa* leaf extract. Typically, a range is characteristic of strong samples. Solids might be inspected as an alkali blend, and potassium bromide fills the need. The substance being scrutinized ought to be totally dry as water assimilates firmly at 3710 cm^{-1} and furthermore close to 1630 cm^{-1}. The range 1500–500 cm^{-1} is known as the finger impression region, which is exceptionally helpful in deciphering the practical gatherings of nanoparticles. FTIR evaluations were done to see the biomolecules for covering and fit difference in the metal nanoparticles united. The FTIR extent of silver nanoparticles, both of 60:1 and 120:1, showed that the band between 3490 and 3500 cm^{-1} relates to O-H growing H-developed alcohols and phenols. The summit found around 1500–1550 cm^{-1} showed a stretch for the C–H bond, and the top around 1450–1500 cm^{-1} showed the bond stretch for N–H. However, the stretch for silver nanoparticles was found around 500–550 cm^{-1}. Figure 3.6 shows the utilitarian gathering present in silver nanoparticles. In this way, the joined nanoparticles were circumnavigated by proteins and metabolites, for example, terpenoids having functional groups [40].

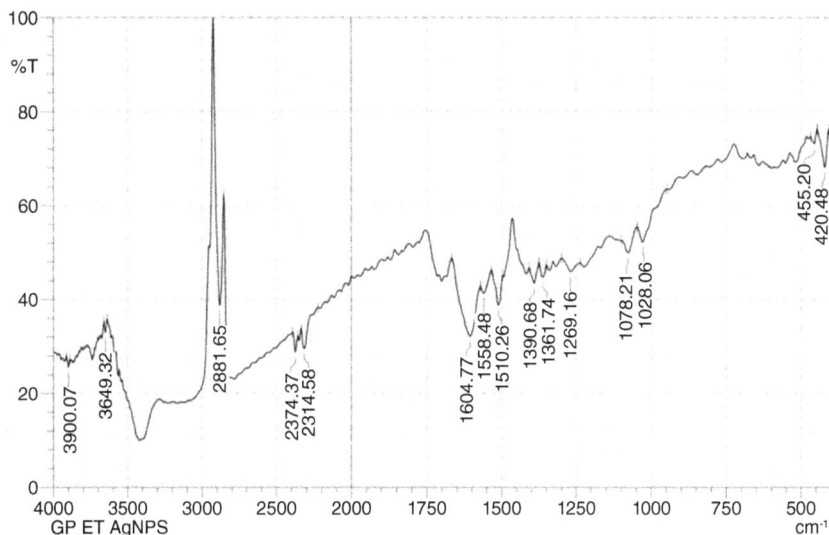

FIGURE 3.6   FTIR spectra of synthesized silver nanoparticles.

3.4.4   XRD ANALYSIS

X-ray diffraction (XRD) is a non-destructive analytical technique, which provides valuable insight into the lattice structure of a crystalline substance, like information on unit cell dimensions, bond angles, chemical composition, and the crystallographic structure of natural and synthetic materials [41]. It is based on the principle of constructive interference of X-rays and the sample concerned, which should be crystalline. The X-rays which are generated by a cathode ray tube (CRT) are filtered, collimated, and then directed toward the sample. The interaction yields a constructive interference based on Bragg's law, which relates wavelength of the incident radiation to the diffraction angle and lattice spacing. X-ray powder diffraction (XRD) is a rapid analytical technique primarily used for phase identification of the crystalline material and can provide information on unit cell dimension and atomic spacing. The X-rays are generated by a cathode ray tube, filtered to produce monochromatic radiation, collimated to concentrate, and directed toward the sample. The interaction of the incident monochromatic rays with the sample produces constructive interference (and diffracted ray) when conditions satisfy Bragg's law $n\lambda = 2d\sin\theta$ [42]. This equation relates the wavelength (λ) of electro-magnetic radiation to the diffraction angle (θ) and the lattice spacing (d) in a crystalline sample by scanning the sample through the arrangement of 2θ angles. All the possible diffraction directions of the lattice are attained due to the random orientation of the powdered materials. The modern X-ray diffractor comprises an X-beam tube, identifier, graphite monochromator, channel, and cut. The copper X-beam tube used in XRD has a frequency of Cu radiation at 1.54 Å. The associations between the X-beam and the translucent material assist to distinguish its design. A variety of diffraction forces is acquired against the point (2θ) of diffraction. The blended AuNP XRD designs showed that the AuNPs were cubic in nature, and this was affirmed by the JCPDS database (PDF no. 652870) and by comparison with the cross-section planes filed to (111), (200), (220), and (311). The size of the AuNPs was determined to be 36.35 nm using XRD information according to the line width of the greatest power [43].

3.4.5 ELECTRON MICROSCOPY OF SILVER NANOPARTICLES

The size of the silver nanoparticles was confirmed by microscopic imaging techniques, the electron beam associated with silver ions, signals received, and the different directions of the images.

3.4.5.1 Scanning Electron Microscopy

A scanning electron microscope (SEM) is a type of electron microscope that provides images of a sample by scanning it with a high-energy beam of electrons in a raster scan pattern. The electrons interact with the atoms which induce the sample to produce signals that contain information about the sample's surface topography, composition, and other properties such as electrical conductivity. SEM can produce very high-resolution images of a sample surface, revealing details about less than 1 to 5 nm in size. Due to the very narrow electron beam, SEM micrographs have a large depth of field yielding a characteristic three-dimensional appearance useful for understanding the surface structure of a sample. Under vacuum, electrons generated by a source are accelerated in a field gradient. The beam passes through electromagnetic lenses, focusing onto the specimen. As result of this bombardment, different types of electrons are emitted from the specimen. A detector catches the secondary electrons and an image of the sample surface is constructed by comparing the intensity of these secondary electrons with the scanning primary electron beam. Finally, the image is displayed on a monitor. In most of the applications, the data collected is over a pre-selected area of the sample surface and following this, a 2D image is generated that shows the various spatial variations. Conventional SEMs with a magnification range of 20x–30,000x with a spatial resolution of 50–100 nm can scan areas which vary from 1 cm to 5 μm in width [44]. SEM also has the ability to analyze particular points as can be seen during EDX operations, which help in determining the chemical composition of the sample concerned. In SEM, a wellspring of electrons is engaged into a shaft, with an exceptionally fine spot size of 5 nm and having energy going from 200 or 300 eV to 50 KeV that is re-established over the outside of the specimen by deflection coils. As the electrons strike and enter the surface, various connections happen that outcomes in the outflow of electrons and photons from the sample and SEM pictures are created by gathering the transmitted electrons on a cathode beam tube. The chief pictures created in SEM are of three kinds: auxiliary electron pictures, backscattered electron pictures and basic X-beam maps. At the point when a high-energy essential electron interfaces with a molecule, it goes through either inelastic dispersing with nuclear electrons or flexible dissipating with the nuclear core. In an inelastic crash with an electron, the essential electron moves part of its energy to the next electron. In the event that the discharged electron has energy under 50 eV, it is alluded to as a secondary electron. Backscattered electrons are the high-energy electrons that are flexibly dispersed and basically have similar energy as the occurrence or essential electrons. The likelihood of backscattering increments with the nuclear number of the sample material. Despite the fact that backscattering pictures cannot be utilized for essential distinguishing proof, valuable differentiation can be created between areas of the sample. The excited atom will decay to its ground state by radiating either a trademark X-beam photon or an Auger electron, the two of which have been utilized for synthetic portrayal. Consolidating with chemical logical abilities, SEM provides not just the picture of the morphology and microstructures of mass and nanostructured materials and gadgets, but also definite data on synthetic creation and appropriation. If the samples are conducting, they could be directly measured, while less conducting samples are to be gold sputtered before taking them onto the specimen stage of the SEM. SEM images may confirm the size and the distribution of nanoparticles and capture individual and aggregated nanoparticles. Furthermore, the surface morphology and nanometric resolution was measured by atomic force microscopic images. The sample surface and probe create repulsive forces and the images were recorded by AFM images. These microscopic studies give information related to the aggregation and distribution of nanoparticles.

From the scanning electron microscopic images, AgNPs were seen to show a self-assembled flower-like structure whose size varied between 20 and 25 nm [45].

3.4.5.2 Transmission Electron Microscopy

A transmission electron microscope constitutes: (a) two or three condenser lenses to focus the electron beam on the sample, (b) an objective lens to form the diffraction in the back focal plane and the image of the sample in the image plane, and (c) intermediate lenses to magnify the image or the diffraction pattern on the screen. If the sample is thin (<200 nm) and constituted of light chemical elements, the image presents a very low contrast when it is focused. To obtain an amplitude contrasted image, an objective diaphragm is inserted in the back focal plane to select the transmitted beam along with a few diffracted beams. The crystalline parts in the Bragg orientation appear dark and the amorphous or non-Bragg oriented parts appear bright. This imaging mode is called bright field mode (BF). In the diffraction mode, another intermediate lens is inserted to image the diffraction pattern of the back focal plane on the screen. If the diffraction is constituted OF many diffracting phases, each of them can be differentiated by selecting one of its diffracted beams with the objective diaphragm. To do this, the incident beam must be tilted so that the diffracted beam is put on the objective lens axis to avoid off-axis aberrations. This mode may be referred to as dark field (DF). The two (BF and DF) modes are used for imaging materials at the nanoscale level. The selected area electron diffraction (SAED) and microdiffraction patterns of a crystal permit obtaining the symmetry of its lattice and calculation of its interplanar distances (with the Bragg law). This is useful to confirm the identification of a phase, after making assumptions based on the literature of the system studied and on chemical analyses. HR-SEM generates electron beams of diameter less than 1 nm. The powerful microscope uses a Schottky-type field emission source with voltage ranging from 200 V to 30 kV. Resolutions of 1.5 nm at >10 kV and 2.5 nm at 1 kV were achieved. The microscope provides detectors for secondary imagining and backscattered electrons imaging. HRSEM is an advanced tool for analysis in the areas of materials science, semiconductors and electronics and life sciences [46].

This powerful tool is used for detecting the sizes of nanoparticles by transmission electron microscopy and images can be observed in two-/three-dimensional directions. In this study, the morphology of AgNPs, as analyzed by TEM images reveals the nanoparticles to be spherical in shape, with their size ranging from 20 nm to 80 nm. The results obtained agree with earlier reports [47].

3.5   APPLICATIONS OF SILVER NANOPARTICLES

3.5.1   ANTIMICROBIAL ACTIVITY

The association of silver nanoparticles with the cell layer caused the synthesis of envelope proteins that facilitate the quick dispersal of proton power. AgNPs caused destabilization of the outside cell divider and exhaustion of ATP in the cell [48–49]. Though the exact mechanism of the antibacterial effects of silver nanoparticles has yet to be elucidated, various explanations have been proposed for this. The consecutive release of silver ions from silver nanoparticles may be considered to be means of killing microbes. Because of their electrostatic attraction to, and affinity for, sulfur proteins, silver ions can cohere to the cell wall and cytoplasmic membrane. The permeability of the cytoplasmic membrane may consequently be enhanced by these attached ions, leading to the disruption of the bacterial envelope. Later, the uptake of free silver ions by the cells may lead to the deactivation of respiratory enzymes, resulting in the generation reactive oxygen species along with the interruption of adenosine triphosphate synthesis. The reactive oxygen species may act as the principal agent for the provocation of cell membrane disruption and deoxyribonucleic acid (DNA) modification. As sulfur and phosphorus are important components of DNA, the interaction of silver ions with these atoms in DNA could disturb DNA replication and cellular reproduction, or even cause the death of microorganisms. Moreover, silver ions can inhibit the synthesis of proteins by denaturing ribosomes in the cytoplasm. Besides releasing silver ions, silver nanoparticles can themselves kill bacteria. Silver nanoparticles can accumulate in the pits that form on the cell wall after they anchor to the cell surface, which causes the denaturation of cell membranes. Silver nanoparticles also have the ability to penetrate bacterial cell walls and subsequently change the structure of the cell membrane because of their nanoscale size. The denaturation of the cytoplasmic membrane can lead to the rupture of organelles and even cell lysis. Additionally, silver nanoparticles can be involved in bacterial signal transduction. Bacterial signal transduction is affected by phosphorylation of protein substrates, and nanoparticles can dephosphorylate tyrosine residues on the peptide substrates. Disruption of signal transduction can lead to cell apoptosis and termination of cell multiplication.

Figure 3.7 illustrates the antimicrobial mechanism of silver nanoparticles obtained using plant extract as a reducing agent. Chemically synthesized AuNPs have excellent antimicrobial activity (shown by the sizes of the zones of clearance in parentheses following each organism) against *Pseudomonas aeruginosa* (24 mm), *Staphylococcus aureus* (15 mm), *Escherichia coli* (18 mm), *Vibrio cholerae* (14 mm), *Salmonella* sp. (15 mm), and *Klebsiella pneumoniae* (21 mm), as shown in Figure 3.8. Upon comparison with the standard antibiotic ampicillin, it was concluded that chemically

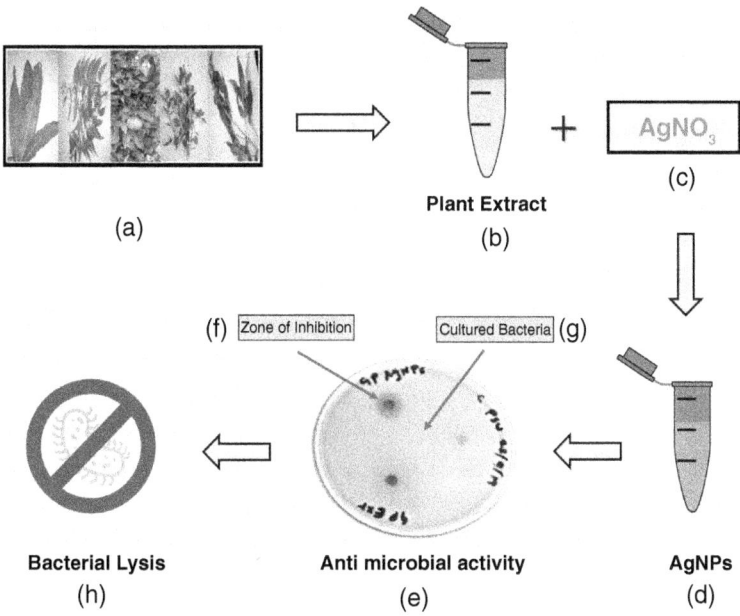

FIGURE 3.7   Antimicrobial mechanism of silver nanoparticles.

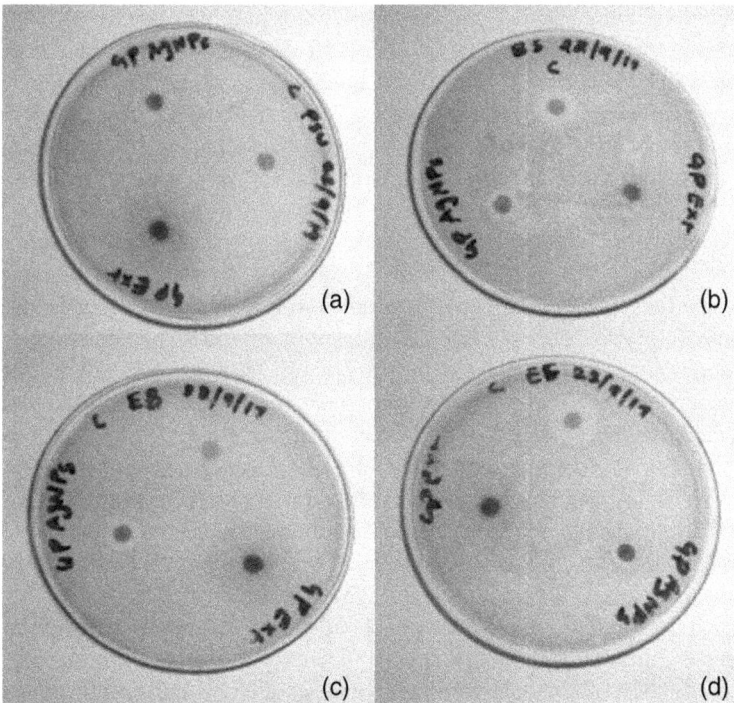

FIGURE 3.8   Antimicrobial activity of silver nanoparticles.

synthesized AuNPs can act as a potential antimicrobial agent. The antimicrobial effect of silver nanoparticles synthesized from a group of medicinal plants and their crude extracts was evaluated against human pathogens such as *Bacillus subtilis, Pseudomonas* sp., *E. coli*, and *Enterobacter* sp.by the disc diffusion method shown in Figure 3.8. The concentration of nanoparticles was directly proportional to the size of the zone of clearance for each bacterial strain [50].

3.5.2 Mosquito-Borne Diseases

Mosquitoes cause more human suffering than any other organism and WHO has declared it "number one public enemy. Every year, over one million people world-wide die from mosquito-borne diseases. Mosquitoes can not only carry diseases that afflict humans, they also transmit several diseases and parasites that dogs and horses are very susceptible to, including dog heartworm, West Nile virus (WNV), and eastern equine encephalitis (EEE). Additionally, mosquito bites can cause severe skin irritation through an allergic reaction to the mosquito's saliva, whose symptoms are a red bump and itching. Mosquito-vectored diseases include proto-zoan diseases such as malaria, filarial diseases such as dog heartworm, and virus diseases such as dengue, encephalitis, and yellow fever. The disease-spreading vectors are: Culex, the mosquito commonly found in houses that is a carrier of encepha-litis and filariasis in tropical, sub-tropical, and humid climates, with a lifecycle of 10–14 days; the female Anopheles mosquito, the carrier of malaria with an average lifespan of two months; and the *Aedes aegypti* mosquito, the carrier of yellow fever, dengue fever, encephalitis, and so on, with a lifecycle of around 10 days to a month, infecting a large number of individuals around the world (WHO, 1996). Yellow fever is typically for a short duration whose symptoms include fever, chills, loss of appetite, nausea, muscle pain (particularly in the back), and headache in most cases. Symptoms tend to improve within five days; however, approximately 30,000 people around the world die from yellow fever every year. The "yellow" in its name refers to the jaundice that affects several patients. Dengue fever can develop into dengue hemorrhagic fever, a more severe form of the disease, which includes symptoms such as bleeding under the skin and constant vomiting. In recent decades, the global incidence of dengue has grown dramatically, with around 40 per cent of the world's population now at risk. Every year, approximately 25,000 people around the world die from dengue fever. Chikungunya is another viral disease transmitted to humans via infected mosquitoes; its typical symptoms include fever, joint pain, headache, muscle pain, joint swelling, and rash. In most cases, a patient's condition will improve within a week; but occasionally the joint pain may last for months or even years. Chikungunya shares some clinical signs with Zika and dengue, leading to potential misdiagnosis in areas where these diseases are prevalent. Mosquitoes can communicate a larger number of ailments than any other get-together of arthropods and impact an immense number of people all through the world. Mosquito-borne infections are unavoidable in more than 100 countries across the world, infecting in excess of 700,000,000 people worldwide and 40,000,000 Indians. In order to pre-vent the development of mosquito-borne disease, and ensure environmental health and general prosperity, mosquito control is essential. The critical instrument in the mosquito control movement is the utilization of fabricated bug harms like organochlorine and organophosphorus compounds. Nonetheless, this has not been particularly effective on account of human, specific, utilitarian, normal, and financial components. Plants are considered to be a rich wellspring of bioactive engineered materials and may well be an effective resource for mosquito control according to subject matter experts [51].

3.5.3 TRADITIONAL PLANTS AGAINST THE MOSQUITO

Overall, biological sources are favored in consideration of their less destructive nature toward non-target living organisms and on account of their inalienable biodegradability. Various studies on the action of plant isolates against mosquito hatchlings have been coordinated throughout the planet. The entire plant is used for the treatment of wilderness fever, leishmaniasis, vaginitis, loose bowels, and gastrointestinal issues. Notwithstanding that larvicides play a primary role in controlling mosquitoes, the fact that these have an unfriendly outcome in spaces of important and nontarget living things is raising objections against their widespread use. Considering extending revenue in making plant starting bug showers as an alternative rather than substance bug splash, this assessment was endeavored to assess the larvicidal capacity of concentrates obtained from remedial plants against two restoratively critical sorts of vector: *Anopheles subpictus* for wilderness fever and *Culex tritaeniorhynchus* for Japanese encephalitis (JE). One of the philosophies for control of these mosquito-borne diseases is the impedance of contamination transmission by killing mosquitoes, thwarting them from biting people (by using enemies of specialists), or causing larval mortality in a huge extension at the breeding grounds of these vectors. This assessment is focused on the use of suitable plant sources against the larvae of mosquitoes. Extracts from different plants contain useful compounds like flavonoids, alkaloids, and number of secondary metabolites. The medicinal plants *O. basilicum*, *M. indica*, *Videx nigundo*, and *A. indica* possess different pharmacological activities. Of these, *V. nigundo* and *O. basilicum* have good larvicidal activities [52]. *M. indica* and *Citrus limon* have been used as larvicides as they have a pleasant odor coupled with antimicrobial activity. Furthermore, these plants do not have any unwanted side effects, as they are natural medicines for many diseases. The technique for preparing antimosquito agents from therapeutic plants involves the gathering of the desired plants, followed by their conceal drying for around 15 days at 28 °C ±2 °C. After drying, the leaves are powdered and utilized for blending with silver nanoparticles. The totally dried leaves are ground and sieved to get a fine powder from which the concentrates are prepared [53–54]. The leaf powder of each plant was tested independently for its effectiveness in controlling mosquitoes.

The rapid natural blend of AgNPs with the leaves of *A. indica* provides for a combination with potent antimicrobial and larvicidal properties. A sheet-shaped appearance is seen with an increase in the concentration of nanoparticles. From the commercial perspective, the AgNPs obtained have likely applications in the biomedical field coupled with advantages like economy, comparability for clinical and drug applications, and the potential for creating a lucrative business opportunity.

TABLE 3.1
List of Medicinal Plants Used for Biosynthesis of Silver Nanoparticles

Plants	Plant parts used	Nanoparticle	Shape	Size in nm	Reference
A. indica	Leaf	Ag and Au nanoparticle	Spherical	50–100 nm	[55]
Hibiscus	Peel	Ag nanoparticle	Spherical	20 nm	[56]
Aloe vera	Leaf	Ag and Au nanoparticle	Spherical	15.2 nm	[57]
Citrus sinensis	Peel	Ag nanoparticle	Spherical	28.4 nm	[58]
Chenopodium album	Leaf	Ag and Au nanoparticle	Spherical	13 nm	[59]
Moringa oleifera	Leaves, stem bark	Ag nanoparticle	Spherical	40 nm	[60]
Nelumbo nucifera	Leaf, root	Ag nanoparticle	Spherical, Polydispersed	25–80 nm	[61]
V. negundo	Leaf	Ag nanoparticle	Spherical	5–47 nm	[62]

3.6 CONCLUSION

Silver nanoparticles were synthesized using medicinal plant extracts as reducing agents and examined for their enhanced antimicrobial and larvicidal activities. The coordinated nanoparticles were spherical and sheet-shaped, with their sizes evaluated to be in the range 160–180 nm. The size of the nanoparticles was more prominent, as these were surrounded by a shaky layer of proteins and metabolites, for instance, terpenoids, amines, alcohols, ketones, and aldehydes, which was evident from spectrophotometric and FTIR data. The techniques for preparing silver nanoparticles from plant extracts underscore the central role of these extracts in determining the shape of the nanoparticles synthesized. Table 3.1 provides information on the utility of various medicinal plants for the biosynthesis of silver nanoparticles.

REFERENCES

1. Hossain A, Abdallah Y, Ali M, Masum M, Islam M, Li B, An Q. Lemon-fruit-based green synthesis of zinc oxide nanoparticles and titanium dioxide nanoparticles against soft rot bacterial pathogen *Dickeya dadantii*. *Biomolecules*, 2019;9(12):863.
2. Nasrollahzadeh M, Atarod M, Sajjadi M, Sajadi SM, Issaabadi Z. Plant-mediated green synthesis of nanostructures: Mechanisms, characterization, and applications. *Interface Science and Technology*, 2019;28:199–322.
3. Wang Y. Nanometer-sized semiconductor clusters: Materials synthesis, quantum size effects, and photophysical properties. *Journal of Physical Chemistry A*, 1991;95:525–532.
4. Xu L, Wang YY, Huang J, Chen CY, Wang ZX, Xie H. Silver nanoparticles: Synthesis, medical applications and biosafety. *Theranostics*. 2020;10:8996–9031.
5. Md. Ali A A, Ahmed T, Wu W, Hossain A, Hafeez R, Md. Masum MI, Wang Y, An Q, Sun G, Li B. Advancements in plant and microbe-based synthesis of metallic nanoparticles and their antimicrobial activity against plant pathogens. *Nanomaterials*, 2020;10:1146.

6. Hossain A, Hong X, Ibrahim E, Li B, Sun G, Meng Y, Wang Y, An Q. Green synthesis of silver nanoparticles with culture supernatant of a bacterium Pseudomonas rhodesiae and their antibacterial activity against soft rot pathogen Dickeya dadantii. *Molecules*, 2019;24:2303.

7. Ogunyemi SO, Abdallah Y, Zhang M, Fouad H, Hong X, Ibrahim E, Masum MMI, Hossain A, Mo J, Li, B. Green synthesis of zinc oxide nanoparticles using different plant extracts and their antibacterial activity against Xanthomonas oryzae pv. oryzae. *Artificial Cells Nanomedicine and Biotechnology*, 2019;47:341–352.

8. Keiser J, Maltese MF, Erlanger TE, Bos R, Tanner M, Singer BH, et al. Effect of irrigated rice agriculture on Japanese encephalitis, including challenges and opportunities integrated vector management. *Acta Tropica*, 2005;95:40–57.

9. Senthilkumar N, Varma P, Gurusubramanian G. Larvicidal and adulticidal activities of some medicinal plants against the malarial vector, *Anopheles stephensi* Liston. *Parasitology Research*, 2009;1042:237–244.

10. Santhoshkumar T, Rahuman AA, Rajakumar G, Marimuthu S, Bagavan A, Jayaseelan C, Kamaraj C. Synthesis of silver nanoparticles using *Nelumbo nucifera* leaf extract and its larvicidal activity against malaria and filariasis vectors. *Parasitology Research*, 2011;108:693–702.

11. Ramalingam V, Revathidevi S, Shanmuganayagam T, Muthulakshmi L, Rajaram, R Biogenic gold nanoparticles induce cell cycle arrest through oxidative stress and sensitize mitochondrial membranes in A549 lung cancer cells. *RSC Advances*, 2016;6:20598.

12. Worrall EA, Hamid A, Mody KT, Mitter N, Pappu HR. Nanotechnology for plant disease management. *Agronomy*, 2018;8:285.

13. Kaviya S, Santhanalakshmi J, Viswanathan B, Muthumary J, Srinivasan K. Biosynthesis of silver nanoparticles using Citrussinensis peel extract and its antibacterial activity. *Spectrochimica Acta Part A: Molecular and Biomolecular Spectroscopy*, 2011;79:594–598.

14. Kathiravan V, Ravi S, Ashokkumar S. Synthesis of silver nanoparticles from Meliadubia leaf extract and their in vitro anticancer activity. *Spectrochimica Acta Part A: Molecular and Biomolecular Spectroscopy*, 2014;130:116–121.

15. Mittal AK, Chisti Y, Banerjee UC. Synthesis of metallic nanoparticles using plant extracts. *Biotechnology Advances*, 2013;31,346–356.

16. Shankar SS, Rai A, Ahmad A, Sastry M. Rapid synthesis of Au, Ag, and bimetallic Au core – Ag shell nanoparticles using neem (*Azadirachta indica*) leaf broth. *Journal of Colloid and Interface Science*, 2004;275:496–502.

17. Huy Tran Q, Nguyen VQ, Le AT. Silver nanoparticles: Synthesis, properties, toxicology, applications and perspectives. *Natural Sciences: Nanoscience and Nanotechnology*, 2003;4:033001.

18. Pourzahedi L, Eckelman MJ. Comparative life cycle assessment of silver nanoparticle synthesis routes. *Environmental Science: Nano*, 2015;2:361–369.

19. Wang Y. Nanometer-sized semiconductor clusters: Materials synthesis, quantum size effects, and photophysical properties. *Journal of Physical Chemistry A*, 1991;95:525–532.

20. Ji M, Chen X, Wai CM. Synthesizing and dispersing silver nanoparticles in a water-in supercritical carbon dioxide microemulsion. *Journal of the American Chemical Society*, 1999;121:2631.

21. Navaladian S, Viswanathan B, Varadarajan TK, Viswanath RP. Microwave-assisted rapid synthesis of anisotropic Ag nanoparticles by solid state transformation. *Nanotechnology*, 2008;19:045603.

22. Mahltig B, Gutmann E, Reibold M, Meyer DC, Bottcher H. Synthesis of Ag and Ag/SiO_2 sols by solvothermal method and their bactericidal activity. *Journal of Sol-Gel Science and Technology*, 2009;51:204–214.

23.   Li H, Wang J, Liu H, Yang C, Xu H, Li X, Cui H. Sol-gel preparation of transparent zinc oxide films with highly preferential crystal orientation. *Vacuum*, 2004;77:57–62.
24.   de Oliveira, Paulo FM, et al. Challenges and opportunities in the bottom-up mechano-chemical synthesis of noble metal nanoparticles. *Journal of Materials Chemistry A*, 2020;8(32):16114–16141.
25.   Socol Y, Abramson O, Gedanken A, Meshorer Y, Berenstein L, Zaban A. Suspensive electrode formation in pulsed sonoelectrochemical synthesis of silver nanoparticles. *Langmuir*, 2002;18:4736–4740.
26.   Muthulakshmi L, Mathangi JB, Suryasankar RP, Padmanaban VC, Helen Kalavathy M, Sanjay MR, Siengchin S. Extraction of polymeric bioflocculant from *Enterobacter*sp. and adsorptive kinetic studies on industrial dye removal applications. *Journal of Polymers and the Environment*, 2020. doi:10.1007/s10924-020-01871-z.
27.   Muthulakshmi L, Annaraj J, Ramakrishna S, Ranjan S, Dasgupta N, Rangappa SM, Siengchin S. A sustainable solution for enhanced food packaging via a science-based composite blend of natural-sourced chitosan and microbial extracellular polymeric substances. *Journal of Food Processing and Preservation*, 2020:e15031.
28.   Wei D, et al. The synthesis of chitosan-based silver nanoparticles and their antibacterial activity. *Carbohydrate Research*, 2009;344(17):2375–2382.
29.   Muthulakshmi L, Rajini N, Varada Rajalu A, Siengchin S, Kathiresan T. Synthesis and characterization of cellulose/silver nanocomposites from bioflocculant reducing agent. *International Journal of Biological Macromolecules*, 2017;103:1113–1120.
30.   Muthulakshmi L, Varada Rajalu A, Kaliaraj GS, Siengchin S, Parameswaranpillai J, Saraswathi R. Preparation of cellulose/copper nanoparticles bionanocomposite films using a bioflocculant polymer as reducing agent for antibacterial and anticorrosion applications. *Composites Part B*, 2019;175:107177.
31.   Huang J, Li Q, Sun D, Lu Y, Su Y, Yang X, Chen C. Biosynthesis of silver and gold nanoparticles by novel sundried *Cinnamomum camphora* leaf. *Nanotechnology*, 2007; 18(10):105104.
32.   Chen J, Wang K, Xin J, Jin Y. Microwave-assisted green synthesis of silver nanoparticles by carboxymethyl cellulose sodium and silver nitrate. *Materials Chemistry and Physics*, 2008;108:421–424.
33.   Medina-Ramirez I, Bashir S, Luo Z, Liu JL. Green synthesis and characterization of polymer-stabilized silver nanoparticles. *Colloids and Surfaces B*, 2009;73:185–191.
34.   Muthulakshmi L, Rajini N, Nellaiah H, Kathiresan T, Jawaid M, Varada Rajalu A. *Terminalia catappa* plant based copper nanoparticle embedded composite films and its characterization studies. *International Journal of Biological Macromolecules*, 2017;95:1064–1071.
35.   Selvam P, Vijayakumar T, Wadhwani A, Muthulakshmi L. Bioreduction of silver nanoparticles from aerial parts of *Euphorbia hirta* L. (EH-ET) and its potent anti-cancer activities against neuroblastoma cell lines. *Indian Journal of Biochemistry & Biophysics*, 2019;56:132–136.
36.   Singh V, Shrivastava A, Wahi N. Biosynthesis of silver nanoparticles by plants crude extracts and their characterization using UV, XRD, TEM and EDX. *African Journal of Biotechnology*, 2015;14:2554–2567.
37.   Das VL, Thomas R, Varghese RT, et al. Extracellular synthesis of silver nanoparticles by the *Bacillus* strain CS 11 isolated from industrialized area. *3 Biotech*, 2014;4:121–126. doi:10.1007/s13205-013-0130-8.
38.   Logeswari P, Silambarasan S, Abraham J. Synthesis of silver nanoparticles using plants extract and analysis of their antimicrobial property. *Journal of Saudi Chemical Society*, 2015;19(3):311–317.
39.   Muthulakshmi L, Rajini N, Varada Rajalu A, Siengchin S, Kathiresan, T. Synthesis and characterization of cellulose/silver nanocomposites from bioflocculant reducing agent. *International Journal of Biological Macromolecules*, 2017;103:1113–1120.

40. Alpert, NL, Keiser WE, Szymanski HA. *Theory and Practice of InfraredSpectroscopy*, Plenum Press, New York, 1970.
41. Cullity BD. *Elements of X-Ray Diffraction*, second edition. Addison-Wesley Publishing Co., Inc., Reading, MA, 1978, 99.
42. Muthulakshmi L, Rajini N, Nellaiah H, Kathiresan T, Jawaid M, Varada Rajulu A. Experimental investigation of cellulose/silver nanocomposites using *in situ* generation method. *Journal of Polymers and the Environment*, 2016;24(3):1–12.
43. Muthulakshmi L, Vijayakumar T, Selvam P, Annaraj J, Ranjan S, Dasgupta N. Strong and nonspecific synergistic antibacterial/antibiofilm impact of nano-silver biosynthesized and decorated with active ingredients of *Oscimum basilicum*L. *3 Biotech*, 2021;11:153.
44. Shervani Z, Ikushima Y, Sato M, Kawanami H, Hakuta Y, Yokoyama T, et al. Morphology and size-controlled synthesis of silver nanoparticles in aqueous surfactant polymer solutions. *Colloid and Polymer Science*, 2008;286:403–410.
45. Harvey D. *Modern Analytical Chemistry*, McGraw-Hill, New York, 2001.
46. Chatwal GR, Anand SK. *Instrumental Methods of Chemical Analysis*, Himalaya Publishing House, New Delhi, 1979.
47. Brundle CR, Evans CA, Wilson S. (Eds.) *Encyclopaedia of Materials Characterization*, Butterworth-Heinemann, London, 1992.
48. Venkatpurwar V, Pokharkar V. Green synthesis of silver nanoparticles using marine polysaccharide: Study of *in-vitro* antibacterial activity. *Materials Letters*, 2011;65:999–1002.
49. Shahverdi AR, Minaeian S, Shahverdi HR, Jamalifar H, Nohi A. Rapid synthesis of silver nanoparticles using culture supernatants of enterobacteria: A novel biological approach *Process Biochemistry*, 2007;42:919–923.
50. Satyavani K, Ramanathan T, Gurudeeban S. Plant mediated synthesis of biomedical silver nanoparticles by using leaf extract of *Citrullus colocynthis*. *Research Journal of Nanoscience and Nanotechnology*, 2011;1(2):95–101.
51. Chandrasekaran T, Thyagarajan A, Santhakumari PG, Pillai AKB, Krishnan UM. Larvicidal activity of essential oil from *Vitex negundo* and *Vitex trifolia* on dengue vector mosquito *Aedes aegypti*. *Revista da Sociedade Brasileira de Medicina Tropical*, 2019;20180459. doi:10.1590/0037-8682-0459-2018.
52. Sundar A, Arunachalam S, Jayavel S, Muthulakshmi L. Encapsulation of amphotericin B into quercetin based silver nanoparticles: Preparation, characterization and preliminary investigation of antiparasitic activity. *Springer Nature Springer Proceedings in Materials, ICON*, 2019:1–9.
53. Roopan SM, Rohit Madhumitha G. Low-cost and ecofriendly phyto-synthesis of silver nanoparticles using *Cocos nucifera* coir extract and its larvicidal activity. *Industrial Crops and Products*, 2013;43:631–635.
54. Luz TRSA, de Mesquita LSS, Amaral FMMD, Coutinho DF. Essential oils and their chemical constituents against *Aedes aegypti* L. (Diptera: Culicidae) larvae. *Acta Tropica*, 2020 December;212:105705. doi:10.1016/j.actatropica.2020.105705. Epub 2020.
55. Shankar SS, Rai A, Ahmad A, Sastry M. Rapid synthesis of Au, Ag, and bimetallic Au core – Ag shell nanoparticles using neem (*Azadirachta indica*) leaf broth. *Journal of Colloid and Interface Science*, 2004;275:496–502.
56. Philip D. Green synthesis of gold and silver nanoparticles using *Hibiscus rosa-sinensis*. *Physica E: Low-Dimensional Systems and Nanostructures*, 2010;42(5):1417–1424.
57. Chandran SP, Chaudhary M, Pasricha R, Ahmad A, Sastry M. Synthesis of gold nanotriangles and silver nanoparticles using *Aloe vera* plant extract. *Biotechnology Progress*, 2006;22:577–583.
58. Huang J, Li Q, Sun D, Lu Y, Su Y, Yang X, Chen C. Biosynthesis of silver and gold nanoparticles by novel sundried *Cinnamomum camphora* leaf. *Nanotechnology*, 2007; 18(10):105104.

59.   Dwivedi, A.D.; Gopal, K. Biosynthesis of silver and gold nanoparticles using Chenopodium album leaf extract. Colloids Surf. A Physicochem. Eng. Asp. **2010**, 369, 27–33.
60.   Vasanth K, Ilango K, MohanKumar R, Agrawal A, Dubey GP. Anticancer activity of *Moringa oleifera* mediated silver nanoparticles on human cervical carcinoma cells by apoptosis induction. *Colloids and Surfaces B: Biointerfaces*, 2014;117:354–359.
61.   Santhoshkumar T, Rahuman AA, Rajakumar G, Marimuthu S, Bagavan A, Jayaseelan C, Kamaraj C. Synthesis of silver nanoparticles using *Nelumbo nucifera* leaf extract and its larvicidal activity against malaria and filariasis vectors. *Parasitology Research*, 2011;108(3):693–702.
62.   Prabhu D, Arulvasu C, Babu G, Manikandan R, Srinivasan P. Biologically synthe sized green silver nanoparticles from leaf extract of *Vitex negundo* L. induce growth-inhibitory effect on human colon cancer cell line HCT15. *Process Biochemistry*, 2013;48:317–324.

4 Biofilms and Materials' Infectivity

Hideyuki Kanematsu, Dana M. Barry,
Risa Kawai, Takeshi Kogo, Akiko Ogawa,
Paul McGrath, and Toshihiro Tanaka

CONTENTS

4.1 INTRODUCTION

Infection has attracted global concern, since the pandemic caused by COVID-19 occurred at the end of 2019. Infection is generally defined as the phenomenon that microorganisms and viruses as pathogens attach to cell surfaces and enter organisms, which serve as their hosts. However, infection is not restricted to the phenomenon where bacteria and viruses move from human to human. For example, in the case of COVID-19, viruses seem to move from human to human through materials. If this is true for other infections, then the role of materials, the force between materials and microorganisms/viruses, and their attachments must be studied in detail.

In this chapter, we focus on bacteria and viruses, and discuss their structures, the general mechanisms of infection in humans, and the interaction with materials' surfaces. When we discuss the interaction between materials' surfaces and microorganisms/viruses, biofilms must be mentioned. They are produced by bacterial activities and appear as unique structures on materials' surfaces [1–8]. Biofilms are mainly composed of water, proteins, nucleic acids (DNA and RNA), and lipids at the initial stage. They cause materials' surfaces to be sticky and a "hot bed" for bacteria resisting biocides, antibiotics, etc.

Biofilms seem to play an important role for infections spread from human to human. They are strongly related to materials too. In this chapter, an outline is provided about

DOI: 10.1201/9781003143093-4

biofilms in terms of infectivity of materials, the appropriate quantitative evaluation methods, and potential countermeasures from the viewpoint of materials science.

4.2 BACTERIA, VIRUSES, AND INFECTION

Bacteria are classified into two biological domains. One of them is the Bacteria Domain and consists of many eubacteria. The other is the Archaea domain and consists of archaebacteria. Long ago, the two domains were mixed and confused. However, they have been classified by using gene analyses. The bacteria in the latter domain tend to live in extreme conditions of climates.

From the viewpoint of appearance (shape, size, etc.), they are usually classified into the coccus (cocci) which are round bacteria, the rod-shaped bacillus (bacilli), the spiral spirochaete, etc. The size is usually 0.2–10 μm and many of them can be observed by using optical microscopes.

Figure 4.1 shows a simple schematic diagram for general rod-shaped bacteria [9]. The inner structure of bacteria is generally occupied by cytoplasm. It is composed of water, proteins, carbohydrates, lipids, and salts. The water content is 80% or more. The nuclear area contains deoxyribonucleic acid (DNA) and it is not enclosed in a nucleus. This is a big difference between prokaryotic organisms and eukaryotic ones. For the latter organism, DNA carrying the genetic information is basically enclosed by a double layer nuclear membrane (nuclear envelope). Bacteria often contain one or more extra pieces of DNA. They are called plasmids. The synthesis of proteins takes place dispersedly in the ribosomes.

These inner contents are surrounded by a glycocalyx, a sticky polysaccharide/polypeptide containing layer, called a capsule, and plasma membranes. Outside of these outer structures of bacteria, is the cell wall. Also, flagella (which make bacterial motile), pili, and fimbriae are observed on the surface of many bacteria.

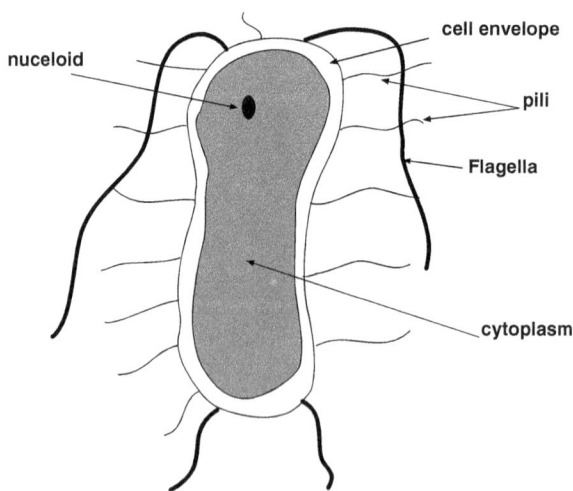

FIGURE 4.1   Schematic structure of a rod-shaped bacterium.

Cell walls are unique structures that are divided into two categories: gram-positive cell walls and gram-negative cell walls, depending on their structures.

Figure 4.2 shows the schematic illustration of cross-sectional cell walls [9]. In Figure 4.2(a), the surface structure of a gram-positive cell wall is shown schematically. Peptidoglycan layers have network structures composed of parallel *N*-acetylglucosamine (NAG) and *N*-acetylmuramic acids (NAM) to cell membranes and perpendicular peptides. Teichoic acid protrudes perpendicularly through peptidoglycan layers. For gram-positive bacteria, the peptidoglycan layers are generally much thicker than those of gram-negative bacteria. In the outer gram-negative bacterial structure, outer membranes exist on the few, thin peptidoglycan layers. Outer membranes are composed of phospholipids, lipoprotein, porin protein, lipopolysaccharides, etc. (see Figure 4.2[b]).

According to the difference of cell wall structures, bacteria could be differentiated by using gram stain. Figure 4.3 shows the general process for using gram

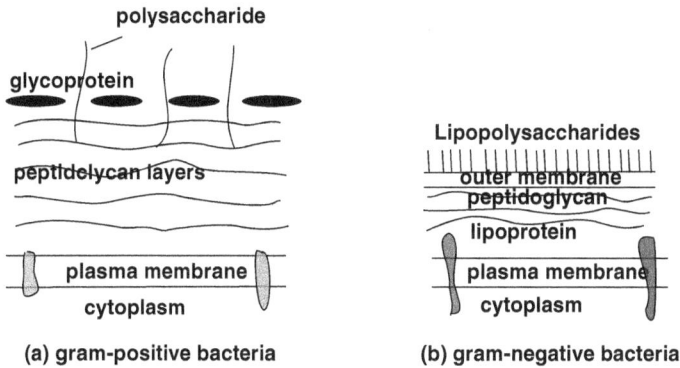

FIGURE 4.2 Schematic outer structure of bacterial cells (a) gram-positive bacteria (b) gram-negative bacteria.

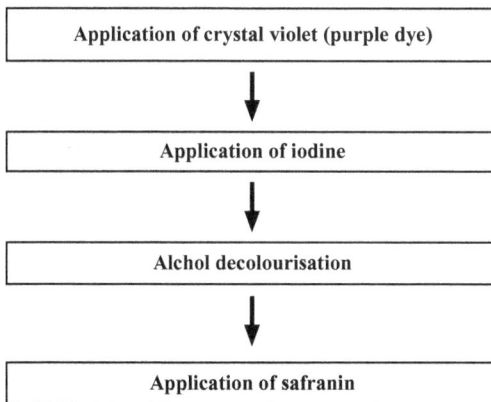

FIGURE 4.3 The general procedure of gram staining.

stain [10]. For the first step, crystal violet is applied. After the dye is washed off with water, all bacteria are stained in a purple color. Next, an iodine solution is added to firmly fix the purple color. Then, alcohol is applied to remove the purple color. In the case of gram-positive bacteria, the purple dye is retained, while it is removed for gram-negative bacteria. Finally, safranin or neutral red is applied to those bacteria to be stained. For gram-positive bacteria, the purple color remains. On the other hand, gram-negative bacteria are stained with a red color.

It is well known that bacteria grow by cell division, as shown in Figure 4.4 schematically. When a cell divides, DNA also divides. Then, the cell wall and membrane form a transverse septum and the daughter cells separate. In this way, the bacterial number increases with time [10].

On the other hand, viruses also bring about infections. Viruses are not living organisms, strictly speaking. Usually, living organisms must fulfill all of the following conditions [9].

1. A high degree of chemical complexity and microscopic organization.
2. Systems for extracting, transforming, and using energy from the environment.
3. Defined functions for each of an organism's components and regulated interactions among them.
4. Mechanisms for sensing and responding to alterations in their surroundings.
5. A capacity for precise self-replication and self-assembly.
6. A capacity to change over time by gradual evolution.

Viruses seem to fulfill most of the requirements for organisms. However, the fifth rule (self-replication) is obviously lacking. Viruses need host cells to replicate.

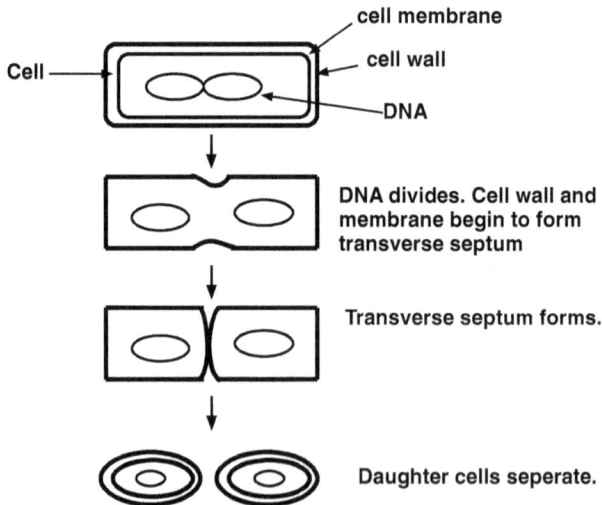

FIGURE 4.4 Schematic illustration for cell fission and growth.

Viruses can be classified into many types from the structural viewpoint. Figure 4.5 shows some simple forms of viruses schematically [10–15]. As shown in Figure 4.5(a), virus is composed of one type of nucleic acid that is enclosed by a protein capsomere. The protein capsomeres are called capsids. On the other hand, Figure 4.5(b) shows a more complicated structure for another virus. In this case, the core nucleic acid and the capsid are enclosed by an envelope that is a lipid bilayer derived from the membrane of the host cell. The glycoproteins are called spikes that protrude from the envelope. Table 4.1 shows various types of viruses, their sizes, and characteristics.

Viruses enter the human body to find host cells so they can replicate. Usually, such a "foreign matter" (including viruses) is detected by T-cells or macrophages and killed. However, viruses try to hide from those T-cells and macrophages and to survive in host cells. Also, they can mutate to escape from the immune system.

When viruses enter the human body and attach to host cells, they penetrate cells and the core nucleic acids are uncoated. At this point, genes and proteins have different pathways to be replicated. Replicated virions are released from their host cells.

When bacteria and viruses enter the human body, the person's defense systems become active [10, 43–44]. Usually, the defense systems for humans involves three steps. The first one to act is the skin and the mucous membranes that exist in the skin layers. The skin is composed of two layers: the epidermis and the dermis. The epidermis is composed of epithelial cells. They are made of keratin which has high resistance to enzymes and toxins. Therefore, the epidermis can provide a strong defense against bacteria. The dermis has sebaceous glands that secrete oily substances called sebum. These substances have high resistance to many bacteria because they are capable of lowering pH. A mucous membrane (which is epithelium derived from the ectoderm) is always wet with mucosal fluids. Therefore, it can easily trap foreign particles including bacteria.

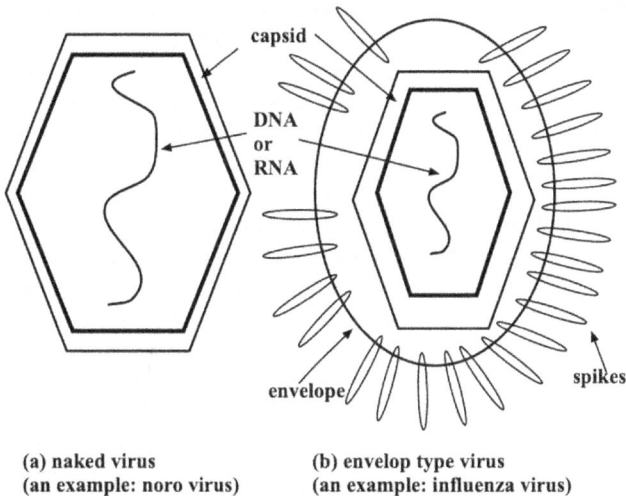

FIGURE 4.5 Schematic illustration of viral structures. (a) naked virus (an example: noro virus), (b) envelop type virus (an example: influenza virus)

TABLE 4.1
Various Viruses, Sizes, and Structures

Type of nucleic acids	Name of virus	Envelope	size
DNA	Parvovirus [16–18]	No	20 nm
	Papovavirus [19–20]	No	40–50 nm
	Adenovirus [21–24]	No	90–100 nm
	Bacteriophage [25–30]	No	25–200 nm
	Herpesvirus [31–32]	Yes	155–240 nm
	Poxivirus [33]	Yes	220–450 nm
RNA	Picoronavirus [34]	Yes	30 nm
	Reovirus [35]	No	60–80 nm
	Togavirus [36]	Yes	40–70 nm
	Coronavirus [37]	Yes	80–120 nm
	Myxovirus [38]	Yes	60–300 nm
	Tobacco-mosaic virus [39]	Yes	300 nm
	Rhabdovirus [40–41]	Yes	180 nm
	Paramyxovirus [42]	Yes	150–300 nm

Bacteria escaping from the first line of defense meet the second one. This is called natural immunity, which is an inherent immunity in our lives. For this process, the defense system is grouped into two types. One is a direct attack to microbes by antibacterial molecules. Peptides, lysozyme, lectin, their complements, etc. make pathogens collapse. The other type is called phagocytes (examples: macrophage, neutrophil, and dendritic cell). They are activated by signal deduction processes and threaten entering pathogens.

The final line of defense is acquired immunity. In this process T-cells and B-cells (kinds of lymph corpuscles) play important roles to threaten pathogens. Those cells could differentiate the previous pathogens from the new ones and threaten/attack them.

Our immune systems always protect us. However, pathogenic bacteria and viruses sometimes pass through our immune systems. In such a case, we need medication.

Antibiotics are usually used to kill bacteria within our bodies. Biocides have been used to treat bacteria on the outside of our body. However, bacteria inside biofilms have strong tolerance and resistance to biocides and antibiotics.

The immunity processes apply to both bacteria and viruses. However, as already mentioned, bacteria produce biofilms to protect themselves from detergents, antibiotics, etc.

4.3 BIOFILMS, MATERIALS' SURFACES, AND INFECTION

Biofilms form at the interface between gas/liquid, liquid/liquid, gas/solid, and liquid/solid. It means that biofilms generally form on interfaces between an arbitrary phase and a condensed phase (in this case, liquid phases are included in the category, since the cohesion power works for a restricted short range too). Biofilms cause many material-related problems [45–46]. Figure 4.6 shows the schematic illustration to explain how biofilms form at such an interface. Generally, planktonic bacteria exist and float in environments alone to seek nutrition. Their nutrition is generally carbon compounds. Since materials' surfaces are unstable in the light of energy, carbon compounds tend to adsorb to them. As a result, the very thin films composed of carbon compounds generally form on materials' surfaces. They are called "conditioning films." Bacteria generally move toward nutrition. This feature of bacteria is called chemotaxis. The absorbed bacteria also have the tendency to aggregate on materials' surfaces. When the number of bacteria increases to a certain threshold value, then they are signaled (by quorum sensing) to excrete polysaccharides (almost simultaneously) as a result [47–57]. The surface area of the material becomes sticky. This is due to the initial biofilms, which are composed of water, external polymeric substances (EPSs) including polysaccharides, and bacteria themselves. When biofilms grow, they incorporate inorganic and organic matters from various environments or from the substrate material itself. Many chemical/electrochemical reactions occur inside biofilms. Those reactions make the appearance, structures, and components of biofilms, different with time. Finally, biofilms can break apart due to the lack of nutrition in biofilms or shear stresses against biofilms generated by flow. After biofilms break down, bacteria inside the biofilms are liberated and seek other materials' surfaces. In such a way, biofilms are propagated and prevail to cover more surface areas [57–67].

When we look at the biofilm formation and growth process, we can immediately realize that the phenomena (called "biofouling") could be treated from the viewpoint of surface science and engineering. Something relating to "forces" or "interaction" must happen between bacteria and materials' surfaces.

Usually, materials exist through cohesion forces (coagulation power). Therefore, materials could be classified into some categories, according to the cohesion forces:

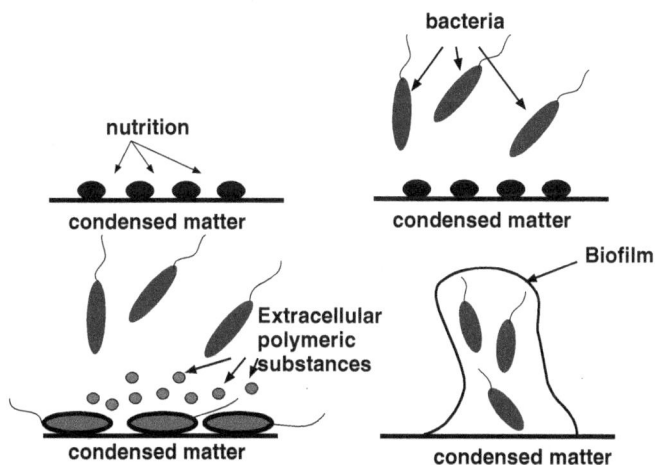

FIGURE 4.6 Schematic illustration of biofilm formation.

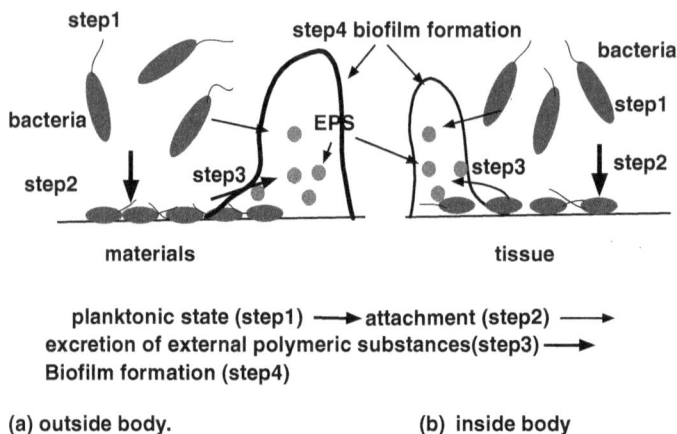

FIGURE 4.7 The comparison of biofilm formation process outside bodies (a) and inside bodies (b).

metallic materials, ceramics, and organics. Metallic materials' cohesion forces are metallic binding. In the case of ceramics, intermolecular forces and ionic bonding work for the cohesion. In the case of polymeric substances, intermolecular force is the main one. According to the main cohesion force of materials, the interaction between materials and biofilms is affected.

People often say that biofilms are almost equivalent to infection. The statement has a meaning. Figure 4.7 shows biofilm growth inside and outside of the human body. In both the cases, the same and typical characteristics can be seen. For example, bacteria seek nutrition on condensed substrates and attach to them at the initial stage. In the case of inside the body, bacteria attach to a tissue due to the same reason. In both cases, the number of attached bacteria increases to a threshold value. Then, polysaccharides are excreted from the bacterial cells through quorum sensing. (This involves a signal deduction system and biofilms form at this point.) Since infection is defined as the growth of pathogens inside bodies, biofilms are equivalent to infection itself.

Since biofilms are a sort of reservoir to keep bacteria alive against the natural immune system of human beings, antibiotics, and biocides, it is very important to remove them. Biofilms could spread infections between humans through materials. As for viruses, clear evidence of their relationship with biofilms is still lacking. However, viruses could keep the infectivity longer with humidity. From that viewpoint, viruses could keep their infectivity in biofilms. Further experiments and investigations are needed to confirm this presumption.

4.4   QUANTITATIVE EVALUATION OF BIOFILMS AND THE DEVELOPMENT OF ANTIBIOFILM MATERIALS

How could we evaluate biofilms? There are many methods to evaluate biofilms. One method is the use of microscopes such as the confocal laser microscope, optical

TABLE 4.2
Analytical Methods for Biofilms on Materials

Name of instrument	Qualitative/quantitative	References
Optical microscope	Qualitative	[68–70]
Confocal laser microscope	Semi-quantitative	[71–80]
SEM-EDX & FIB-SEM	Qualitative	[81–89]
TEM	Qualitative	[90–92]
FTIR	Semi-quantitative	[93–97]
Raman spectroscopy	Semi-quantitative	[98–108]
Mass spectroscopy	Semi-quantitative	[109–116]
NMR	Semi-quantitative	[117–121]
Fluorescent microscopy	Semi-qualitative	[122–126]
Gene analyses	Qualitative	[127–136]
Staining	Qualitative	[137–146]

microscopes, SEM-EDX, TEM, Raman spectroscopy, FTIR, and other expensive equipment (each with its own merits and demerits) [45–46]. Table 4.2 summarizes some analyses used for biofilm research.

However, most of those methods are qualitative or semi-quantitative. "Semi-quantitative" corresponds to the situations where quantitative results could be obtained, but the values would not always mean any absolute values. Industries and practical applications always need the absolute figures showing the amounts of biofilms. To achieve the purpose, the staining method is favorable. Crystal violet is very often used to evaluate biofilms. Figure 4.8 shows an example of the process schematically.

Biofilms form on materials. Then, the biofilms are stained by crystal violet solution [147–156]. Usually, 0.1% crystal violet is used. Crystal violet is composed of a cationic triphenylmethane group and chloride ion (ionized in the solution). Biofilms are composed of external polymeric substances, bacteria, and 80% or more of water. Polymeric substances are polarized and charged locally. Therefore, triphenylmethane cations absorb the negatively charged parts and stain them in violet color. Stained biofilms are extracted in an appropriate surfactant or ethanol. Crystal violet absorbs the light of 570 nm specifically. Therefore, using a plate reader, one could get the absorbance value of extracted crystal violet. The value corresponds to the amount of biofilm. In this way, one can evaluate biofilms quantitatively.

Using the quantitative method, we will get a chance to develop the countermeasures. There are already many proposals for drugs and antibiofilm agents. However, there are only a few for antibiofilm materials. At this point, most of the antibiofilm materials are the same as the antibacterial materials. The differences between the two characteristics need to be studied more.

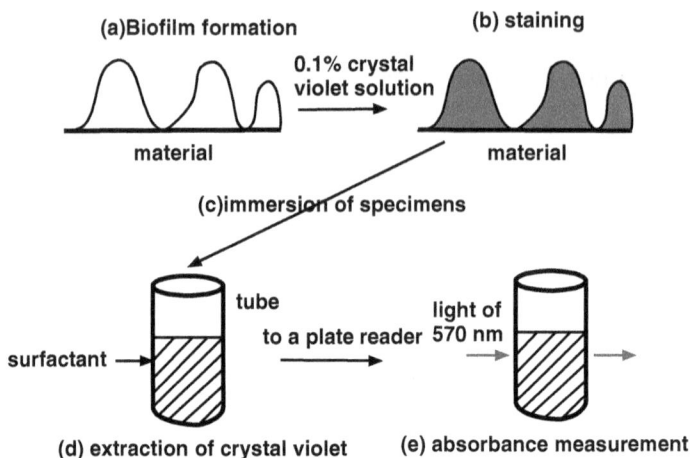

FIGURE 4.8 Quantitative measurements of biofilms using crystal violet staining.

The antibacterial effect is just a phenomenon at a certain time, within the whole process of biofouling, where biofilms are produced. Biofilm formation, growth, etc. involve multi-steps, as already described. Included are the formation of conditioning films, the attachment process of bacteria on materials' surfaces, the quorum sensing process, the growth stage, the rupture stage, etc. Therefore, we must confirm cautiously, if the antibacterial effect would really control biofilms or not. The antibacterial effect might be cancelled by other factors.

The antibacterial effect is generally evaluated by the number of viable bacteria. Therefore, the proper quantitative evaluation very often utilizes the counting methods of viable bacteria. However, such an evaluation might not always lead to the number of biofilms. This is because dead and collapsed bacteria (due to lysis, etc.) would be added to biofilm growth. Bacteria are main components of biofilms. Therefore, the antibacterial effect might be equivalent to the antibiofilm property.

In the light of those differences, the countermeasures should be established in the future. For example, the conditioning films could be controlled for this purpose. New materials and chemicals could be proposed, so that the formed biofilms would be detached easily from materials. Countermeasures focusing on the other stages of biofilm formation could be proposed and investigated.

4.5   CONCLUSIONS AND FUTURE PERSPECTIVE

In this chapter, we provided outlines for general infections inside the human body and compared them with cases outside of the human body. We discussed how biofilm is involved with infection and explained the importance of controlling biofilms to prevent infections. Biofilms usually form on materials. Therefore, anti-infectivity problems would be equivalent to antibiofilm problems. In the light of that, the research and development of antibiofilm materials is very important to control infections. At this point, the differences between antibacterial effect and antibiofilm characteristics are obscure. In addition, the involvement of viruses is not so clear. The research is still at the cradle stage. Hopefully, more information will be available in the future. Then, infections from human–materials–human will be controlled well and infection problems will be solved easily.

ACKNOWLEDGMENTS

A part of this work was supported by the GEAR 5.0 Project of the National Institute of Technology (KOSEN) in Japan as well as JSPS KAKENHI (Grants-in-Aid for Scientific Research from the Japan Society for the Promotion of Science, Grant Number 20K05185 and 21K12739. We also appreciate SIAA (The Society of International Sustaining Growth for Antimicrobial Articles) for their useful advice. And we also appreciate Prof. Peerawatt Nunthavarawong for his well-timed advices, kind consideration, encouragements, and patience.

REFERENCES

1. Costerton, J. W., Cheng, K. J., Geesey, G. G., Timothy, I., Ladd, J., Nckel, C., . . . Marrie, T. J. (1987). Bacterial biofilms in nature and disease. *Annual Reviews in Microbiology, 41*(1), 435–464.
2. Stewart, P. S., & Costerton, J. W. (2001). Antibiotic resistance of bacteria in biofilms. *The Lancet, 358*, 135–138.
3. Donlan, R. M. (2002). Biofilms: Microbial life on surfaces. *Emerging Infectious Diseases, 8*(9), 881–890.
4. Stoodley, P., Sauer, K., Davies, D. G., & Costerton, J. W. (2002). Biofilms as complex differentiated communities. *Annual Review of Microbiology, 56*, 187–209. doi:10.1146/annurev.micro.56.012302.160705.
5. Hall-Stoodley, L., Costerton, J. W., & Stoodley, P. (2004). Bacterial biofilms: From the natural environment to infectious diseases. *Nature Reviews Microbiology, 2*, 95–108.
6. Flemming, H. C., Murthy, S. P., Venkatesan, R., & Cooksey, K. E. (2009). *Marine and industrial biofouling*. Berlin: Springer.
7. Lewandowski, Z., & Beyenal, H. (2007). *Fundamentals of biofilm research*. Boca Raton, London and New York: CRC Press, 1st ed.
8. Lewandowski, Z., & Beyenal, H. (2014). *Fundamentals of biofilm research*. Boca Raton, London and New York: CRC Press.
9. Nelson, D. L., & Cox, M. M. (2008). *Lehninger principles of biochemistry*. New York: W. H. Freeman, 5th ed., p. 1100.
10. Lee, G., & Bishop, P. (2015). *Microbiology – and infection control for health professional*, 6th ed, London, UK: Pearson.
11. Wigginton, K. R., & Kohn, T. (2012). Virus disinfection mechanisms: The role of virus composition, structure, and function. *Current Opinion in Virology, 2*(1), 84–89.
12. Graziano, V. R., Wei, J., & Wilen, C. B. (2019). Norovirus attachment and entry. *Viruses, 11*, 495.
13. Smith, K. O. (1964). Relationship between the envelope and the infectivity of herpes simplex virus. *Proceedings of the Society for Experimental Biology and Medicine, 115*, 814–816.
14. Harrap, K. (1972). The structure of nuclear polyhedrosis viruses: II. The virus particle. *Virology, 50*, 124–132.

15. Klenk, H. D., Rott, R., & Becht, H. (1972). On the structure of the influenza virus envelope. *Virology*, *47*, 579–591.
16. Goddard, A., & Leisewitz, A. L. (2010). Canine parvovirus. *Veterinary Clinics: Small Animal Practice*, *40*, 1041–1053.
17. Pollock, R. V. H., & Parrish, C. R. (2019). Canine parvovirus. *Comparative Pathobiology of Viral Diseases*, 145–177.
18. Nandi, S., & Kumar, M. (2010). Canine parvovirus: Current perspective. *Indian Journal of Virology*, *21*(1), 31–44.
19. Takemoto, K. K., Mattern, C. F. T., & Murakami, W. T. (1971). The papovavirus group. In *Comparative virology*. Cambridge, MA: Academic Press, pp. 81–104.
20. Mattern, C. F. T., Allison, A. C., & Rowe, W. P. (1963). Structure and composition of K virus, and its relation to the "papovavirus" group. *Virology*, *20*(3), 413–419.
21. Rux, J. J., & Burnett, R. M. (2004). Adenovirus structure. *Human Gene Therapy*, *15*(12), 1167–1176.
22. San Martín, C. (2012). Latest insights on adenovirus structure and assembly. *Viruses*, *4*(5), 847–877.
23. Stewart, P. L. (2016). Adenovirus structure. In *Adenoviral vectors for gene therapy*. Cambridge, MA: Academic Press, pp. 1–26.
24. Nemerow, G. R., Stewart, P. L., & Reddy, V. S. (2012). Structure of human adenovirus. *Current Opinion in Virology*, *2*(2), 115–121.
25. Leiman, P. G., Kanamaru, S., Mesyanzhinov, V. V., Arisaka, F., & Rossmann, M. G. (2003). Structure and morphogenesis of bacteriophage T4. *Cellular and Molecular Life Sciences CMLS*, *60*(11), 2356–2370.
26. Mueser, T. C., Hinerman, J. M., Devos, J. M., Boyer, R. A., & Williams, K. J. (2010). Structural analysis of bacteriophage T4 DNA replication: A review in the virology journal series on bacteriophage T4 and its relatives. *Virology Journal*, *7*(1), 1–16.
27. Abrescia, N. G. A., Cockburn, J. J. B., Grimes, J. M., Sutton, G. C, Diprose, J. M., Butcher, S. J., . . . Fuller S. D. (2004). Insights into assembly from structural analysis of bacteriophage PRD1. *Nature*, *432*(7013), 68–74.
28. Goldbourt, A. (2019). Structural characterization of bacteriophage viruses by NMR. *Progress in Nuclear Magnetic Resonance Spectroscopy*, *114*, 192–210.
29. Van Belleghem, J. D., Dąbrowska, K., Vaneechoutte, M., Barr, J. J., & Bollyky, P. L. (2019). Interactions between bacteriophage, bacteria, and the mammalian immune system. *Viruses*, *11*(1), 10.
30. Young, R., & Bläsi, U. (1995). Holins: Form and function in bacteriophage lysis. *FEMS Microbiology Reviews*, *17*(1–2), 191–205.
31. McGeoch, D. J., Rixon, F. J., & Davison, A. J. (2009). Topics in herpesvirus genomics and evolution. *Virus Research*, *117*(1), 90–104.
32. Davison, A. J. (2010). Herpesvirus systematics. *Veterinary Microbiology*, *143*(1), 52–69.
33. Buller, R. M., & Palumbo, G. J. (1991). Poxvirus pathogenesis. *Microbiological Reviews*, *55*(1), 80–122.
34. Jiang, P., Liu, Y., Ma, H. C., Paul, A. V., & Wimmer, E. (2014). Picornavirus morphogenesis. *Microbiology and Molecular Biology Reviews*, *78*(3), 418–437.
35. Clements, D., Helson, E., Gujar, S. A., & Lee, P. W. K. (2014). Reovirus in cancer therapy: An evidence-based review. *Oncolytic Virotherapy*, *3*, 69.
36. Horzinek, M., Maess, J., & Laufs, R. (1971). Studies on the substructure of togaviruses. *Archiv für die gesamte Virusforschung*, *33*(3), 306–318.
37. Dhama, K., Pawaiya, R. V. S., Chakraborty, S., Tiwari, R., Saminathan, M., & Verma, A. K. (2014). Coronavirus infection in equines: A review. *Asian Journal of Animal and Veterinary Advances*, *9*(3), 164–176.
38. Horne, R. W., Waterson, A. P., Wildy, P., & Farnham, A. E. (1960). The structure and composition of the myxoviruses: I. Electron microscope studies of the structure of myxovirus particles by negative staining techniques. *Virology*, *11*(1), 79–98.

39. Klug, A. (1999). The tobacco mosaic virus particle: Structure and assembly. *Philosophical Transactions of the Royal Society of London. Series B: Biological Sciences, 354*(1383), 531–535.

40. Albertini, A. A. V., Baquero, E., Ferlin, A., & Gaudin, Y. (2012). Molecular and cellular aspects of rhabdovirus entry. *Viruses, 4*(1), 117–139.

41. Wagner, R. R. (1987). Rhabdovirus biology and infection. In *The rhabdoviruses.* Boston, MA: Springer, pp. 9–74.

42. Cox, R. M., & Plemper, R. K. (2017). Structure and organization of paramyxovirus particles. *Current Opinion in Virology, 24*, 105–114.

43. Tiwari, S., & Talreja, S. (2010). Human immune system and importance of immunity boosters on human body: A review. *Journal of Global Trends in Pharmaceutical Sciences*, 8641–8649.

44. Arleevskaya, M. I., Aminov, R., Brooks, W. H., Manukyan, G., & Renaudineau, Y. (2019). Shaping of human immune system and metabolic processes by viruses and microorganisms. *Frontiers in Microbiology, 10*, 816.

45. Kanematsu, H., & Barry, D. M. (2015). *Biofilm and materials science.* New York: Springer, p. 196.

46. Kanematsu, H., & Barry, D. M. (2020). *Formation and control of biofilm in various environments.* Singapore: Springer, 2020.

47. Characklis, W. G., & Cooksey, K. E. (1983). Biofilms and microbial fouling. *Advances in Applied Microbiology, 29*, 93–138.

48. Characklis, W. G., & Marshall, K. C. (1990). *Biofilms.* New York: John Wiley & Sons, Inc.

49. Lappin-Scott, H. M. J. J., & Costerton, J. W. (1993). Microbial biofilm formation and characterisation. *Society for Applied Bacteriology Technical Series, Society for Applied Bacteriology Symposium, 30.*

50. Costerton, J. W., & Lappin-Scott, H. M. (1995). Introduction to microbial biofilms. In *Microbial biofilms*, Lappin-Scott, H. M., & Costerton, J. W., Eds. Cambridge: Cambridge University Press, pp. 1–11.

51. Costerton, J. W. (1999). Introduction to biofilm. *International Journal of Antimicrobial Agents, 11*, 217–221; discussion 237–239.

52. Flemming, H. C., Szewzyk, U., & Griebe, T. (2000). *Biofilms – investigative methods & applications.* Boca Raton, FL: CRC Press.

53. Fux, C., Costerton, J. W., Stewart, P. S., & Stoodley, P. (2005). Survival strategies of infectious biofilms. *Trends in Microbiology, 13*, 34–40.

54. Costerton, J. W. (2007). The biofilm primer. In *Springer series on biofilms.* Berlin and New York: Springer, pp. viii, 199.

55. Flemming, H. C., Neu, T. R., Wozniak, D. J. (2007). The EPS matrix: The "house of biofilm cells". *Journal of Bacteriology, 189*(22), 7945–7947. doi:10.1128/JB.00858-07.

56. Kanematsu, H., & Barry, D. M. (2020). *Formation and control of biofilm in various environments.* Singapore: Springer, p. 249.

57. Kanematsu, H., Barry, D. M. (2020). Biofilm on materials' surface in marine environments. In *Marine ecology: Current and future developments-monitoring artificial materials and microbes in marine ecosystems: Interactions and assessment methods*, Takahashi, T., Ed. Sharjah: Bentham Science Publishers, volume 2, pp. 177–187.

58. Yeon, K. M., Cheong, W. S., Oh, H. S., Lee, W. N., Hwang, B. K., Lee, C. H., Beyenal, H., Lewandowski, Z. (2009). Quorum sensing: A new biofouling control paradigm in a membrane bioreactor for advanced wastewater treatment. *Environmental Science & Technology, 43*, 380–385.

59. Costerton, J. W., & Balaban, N. (2010). *Control of biofilm infections by signal manipulation.* Berlin and Heidelberg: Springer, p. 191.

60. Sato, M., & Nakayama, J. (2010). Quorum sensing of gram-positive bacteria and its inhibitors. *Japan Society for Lactic Acid Bacteria, 21*, 95–106.

61. Kim, M., Lee, S., Park, H. D., Choi, S. I., & Hong, S. (2012). Biofouling control by quorum sensing inhibition and its dependence on membrane surface. *Water Science & Technology, 66,* 1424–1430. doi:10.2166/wst.2012.307.

62. Olson, M. E., Todd, D. A., Schaeffer, C. R., Paharik, A. E., Dyke, M. J. V., Büttner, H., ... Fey, P. D. (2014). *Stapylococcus epidermidis* agr quorum-sensing system: Signal identification, cross talk, and importance in colonization. *Journal of Bacteriology, 196,* 3482–3493. doi:10.1128/JB.01882-14.

63. Le, K. Y., & Otto, M. (2015). Quorum-sensing regulation in staphylococci-an overview. *Frontier Microbiology, 6,* 1174. doi:10.3389/fmicb.2015.01174.

64. Kim, M. K., Zhao, A., Wang, A., Brown, Z. Z., Muir, T. W., Stone, H. A., & Bassler, B. L. (2017). Surface-attached molecules control *Staphylococcus aureus* quorum sensing and biofilm development. *Nature Microbiology, 2,* 17080. doi:10.1038/nmicrobiol.2017.80.

65. Abisado, R. G., Benomar, S., Klaus, J. R., Dandekar, A. A., & Chandler, J. R. (2018). Bacterial quorum sensing and microbial community interactions. *MBio, 9.* doi:10.1128/mBio.02331-17.

66. Remy, B., Mion, S., Plener, L., Elias, M., Chabriere, E., & Daude, D. (2018). Interference in bacterial quorum sensing: A biopharmaceutical perspective. *Frontier Pharmacology, 9,* 203. doi:10.3389/fphar.2018.00203.

67. Sharma, A., Singh, P., Sarmah, B. K., & Nandi, S. P. (2020). Quorum sensing: Its role in microbial social networking. *Research Microbiology.* doi:10.1016/j.resmic.2020.06.003.

68. de Carvalho, C. C. C. R., & Manuela R. da Fonseca, M. (2007). Assessment of three-dimensional biofilm structure using an optical microscope. *BioTechniques, 42*(5), 616–620.

69. Larimer, C., Suter, J. D., Bonheyo, G., & Addleman, R. S. (2016). In situ non-destructive measurement of biofilm thickness and topology in an interferometric optical microscope. *Journal of Biophotonics, 9*(6), 656–666.

70. Bakke, R., & Olsson, P. Q. (1986). Biofilm thickness measurements by light microscopy. *Journal of Microbiological Methods, 5*(2), 93–98.

71. Kuehn, M., Hausner, M., Bungartz, H. J., Wagner, M., Wilderer, P. A., & Wuertz, S. (1998). Automated confocal laser scanning microscopy and semiautomated image processing for analysis of biofilms. *Applied and Environmental Microbiology, 64*(11), 4115–4127.

72. Lawrence, J. R., Wolfaardt, G. M., & Korber, D. R. (1994). Determination of diffusion coefficients in biofilms by confocal laser microscopy. *Applied and Environmental Microbiology, 60*(4), 1166–1173.

73. Wood, S. R., Kirkham, J., Marsh, P. D., Shore, R. C., Nattress, B., & Robinson, C. (2000). Architecture of intact natural human plaque biofilms studied by confocal laser scanning microscopy. *Journal of Dental Research, 79*(1), 21–27.

74. Neu, T. R., & Lawrence, J. R. (1997). Development and structure of microbial biofilms in river water studied by confocal laser scanning microscopy. *FEMS Microbiology Ecology, 24*(1), 11–25.

75. Manz, W., Wendt-Potthoff, K., Neu, T. R., Szewzyk, U., & Lawrence, J. R. (1999). Phylogenetic composition, spatial structure, and dynamics of lotic bacterial biofilms investigated by fluorescent in situ hybridization and confocal laser scanning microscopy. *Microbial Ecology, 37*(4), 225–237.

76. Zhang, T., & Fang, H. H. P. (2001). Quantification of extracellular polymeric substances in biofilms by confocal laser scanning microscopy. *Biotechnology Letters, 23*(5), 405–409.

77. Surman, S. B., Walker, J. T., Goddard, D. T., Morton, L. H. G., Keevil, C. W., Weaver, W., Skinner, A., Hanson, K., Caldwell, D., & Kurtz, J. (1996). Comparison of microscope techniques for the examination of biofilms. *Journal of Microbiological Methods, 25*(1), 57–70.

78. Möhle, R. B., Langemann, T., Haesner, M., Augustin, W., Scholl, S., Neu, T. R., Hempel, D. C., & Horn, H. (2007). Structure and shear strength of microbial biofilms as determined with confocal laser scanning microscopy and fluid dynamic gauging using a novel rotating disc biofilm reactor. *Biotechnology and Bioengineering*, *98*(4), 747–755.
79. Villena, G. K., Fujikawa, T., Tsuyumu, S., & Gutiérrez-Correa, M. (2010). Structural analysis of biofilms and pellets of *Aspergillus niger* by confocal laser scanning microscopy and cryo scanning electron microscopy. *Bioresource Technology*, *101*(6), 1920–1926.
80. Hu, H., Johani, K., Gosbell, I. B., Jacombs, A. S. W., Almatroudi, A., Whiteley, G. S., Deva, A. K., Jensen, S., & Vickery, K. (2015). Intensive care unit environmental surfaces are contaminated by multidrug-resistant bacteria in biofilms: Combined results of conventional culture, pyrosequencing, scanning electron microscopy, and confocal laser microscopy. *Journal of Hospital Infection*, *91*(1), 35–44.
81. Remoundaki, E., Kousi, P., Joulian, C., Battaglia-Brunet, F., Hatzikioseyian, A., & Tsezos, M. (2008). Characterization, morphology and composition of biofilm and precipitates from a sulphate-reducing fixed-bed reactor. *Journal of Hazardous Materials*, *153*(1–2), 514–524.
82. Osorio, J. H. M., Benettoni, P., Schmidt, M., Stryhanyuk, H., Schmitt-Jansen, M., Pinto, G., . . . Pollio, A. (2019). Investigation of architecture development and phosphate distribution in Chlorella biofilm by complementary microscopy techniques. *FEMS Microbiology Ecology*, *95*(4), fiz029.
83. Milanesi, C., Baldi, F., Borin, S., Vignani, R., Ciampolini, F., Faleri, C., & Cresti, M. (2006). Biodeterioration of a fresco by biofilm forming bacteria. *International Biodeterioration & Biodegradation*, *57*(3), 168–173.
84. Ashrafi, B., Rashidipour, M., Marzban, A., Soroush, S., Azadpour, M., Delfani, S., & Ramak, P. (2019). Mentha piperita essential oils loaded in a chitosan nanogel with inhibitory effect on biofilm formation against *S. mutans* on the dental surface. *Carbohydrate Polymers*, *212*, 142–149.
85. McLean, R. J. C., Jamieson, H. E., & Cullimore, D. R. (1997). Formation of nesquehonite and other minerals as a consequence of biofilm dehydration. *World Journal of Microbiology and Biotechnology*, *13*(1), 25–28.
86. Seiffert, F., Bandow, N., Bouchez, J., Von Blanckenburg, F., & Gorbushina, A. A. (2014). Microbial colonization of bare rocks: Laboratory biofilm enhances mineral weathering. *Procedia Earth and Planetary Science*, *10*, 123–129.
87. Li, Y., Feng, S., Liu, H., Tian, X., Xia, Y., Li, M., Xu, K., Yu, H., Liu, Q., & Chen, C. (2020). Bacterial distribution in SRB biofilm affects MIC pitting of carbon steel studied using FIB-SEM. *Corrosion Science*, *167*, 108512.
88. Bittermann, A. G., Schaer, D., Mitsi, M., Vogel, V., & Wepf, R. (2012). *Thin layer plastification vs. block embedding: Two alternative preparation strategies for 3D-imaging of cultured cells and biofilms by FIB/SEM*. Society European Microscopy Conference, Manchester.
89. Kizilyaprak, C., Bittermann, A. G., Daraspe, J., & Humbel, B. M. (2014). FIB-SEM tomography in biology. In *Electron microscopy*. Totowa, NJ: Humana Press, pp. 541–558.
90. Sangetha, S., Zuraini, Z., Suryani, S., & Sasidharan, S. (2009). In situ TEM and SEM studies on the antimicrobial activity and prevention of *Candida albicans* biofilm by Cassia spectabilis extract. *Micron*, *40*(4), 439–443.
91. McCutcheon, J., & Southam, G. (2018). Advanced biofilm staining techniques for TEM and SEM in geomicrobiology: Implications for visualizing EPS architecture, mineral nucleation, and microfossil generation. *Chemical Geology*, *498*, 115–127.
92. Reese, S., & Guggenheim, B. (2007). A novel TEM contrasting technique for extracellular polysaccharides in in vitro biofilms. *Microscopy Research and Technique*, *70*(9), 816–822.

93. Nivens, D. E., Schmit, J., Sniatecki, J., Anderson, T., Chambers, J. Q., & White, D. C. (1993). Multichannel ATR/FT-IR spectrometer for on-line examination of microbial biofilms. *Applied Spectroscopy*, *47*(5), 668–671.

94. Bosch, A., Serra, D., Prieto, C., Schmitt, J., Naumann, D., & Yantorno, O. (2006). Characterization of Bordetella pertussis growing as biofilm by chemical analysis and FT-IR spectroscopy. *Applied Microbiology and Biotechnology*, *71*(5), 736–747.

95. Gieroba, B., Krysa, M., Wojtowicz, K., Wiater, A., Pleszczyńska, M., Tomczyk, M., & Sroka-Bartnicka, A. (2020). The FT-IR and Raman spectroscopies as tools for biofilm characterization created by cariogenic streptococci. *International Journal of Molecular Sciences*, *21*(11), 3811.

96. Nichols, P. D., Michael Henson, J., Guckert, J. B., Nivens, D. E., & White, D. C. (1985). Fourier transform-infrared spectroscopic methods for microbial ecology: Analysis of bacteria, bacteria-polymer mixtures and biofilms. *Journal of Microbiological Methods*, *4*(2), 79–94.

97. Suci, P. A., Mittelman, M. W., Yu, F. P., & Geesey, G. G. (1994). Investigation of cipro-floxacin penetration into *Pseudomonas aeruginosa* biofilms. *Antimicrobial Agents and Chemotherapy*, *38*(9), 2125–2133.

98. Schmid, T., Messmer, A., Yeo, B. S., Zhang, W., & Zenobi, R. (2008). Towards chemical analysis of nanostructures in biofilms II: Tip-enhanced Raman spectroscopy of algi-nates. *Analytical and Bioanalytical Chemistry*, *391*(5), 1907–1916.

99. Millo, D., Harnisch, F., Patil, S. A., Ly, H. K., Schröder, U., & Hildebrandt, P. (2011). In situ spectroelectrochemical investigation of electrocatalytic microbial biofilms by surface-enhanced resonance Raman spectroscopy. *Angewandte Chemie International Edition*, *50*(11), 2625–2627.

100. Lebedev, N., Strycharz-Glaven, S. M., & Tender, L. M. (2014). High resolution AFM and single-cell resonance Raman spectroscopy of *Geobacter sulfurreducens* biofilms early in growth. *Frontiers in Energy Research*, *2*, 34.

101. Samek, O., Mlynariková, K., Bernatová, S., Ježek, J., Krzyžánek, V., Šiler, M., Zemánek, P., Růžička, F., Holá, V., & Mahelová, M. (2014). *Candida parapsilosis* biofilm identi-fication by Raman spectroscopy. *International Journal of Molecular Sciences*, *15*(12), 23924–23935.

102. Ly, H. K., Harnisch, F., Hong, S. F., Schröder, U., Hildebrandt, P., & Millo, D. (2013). Unraveling the interfacial electron transfer dynamics of electroactive microbial bio-films using surface-enhanced Raman spectroscopy. *ChemSusChem*, *6*(3), 487–492.

103. Samek, O., Al-Marashi, J. F. M., & Telle, H. H. (2010). The potential of Raman spec-troscopy for the identification of biofilm formation by *Staphylococcus epidermidis*. *Laser Physics Letters*, *7*(5), 378–383.

104. Kanematsu, H., Oizumi, A., Sato, T., Kamijo, T., Honma, S., Barry, D. M., . . . Kuroda, D. (2018). Biofilm formation of a polymer brush coating with ionic liquids compared to a polymer brush coating with a non-ionic liquid. *Coatings*, *8*, 398–412. doi:10.3390/coatings8110398.

105. Kanematsu, H., Kudara, H., Kanesaki, S., Kogo, T., Ikegai, H., Ogawa, A., & Hirai, N. (2016). Application of a loop-type laboratory biofilm reactor to the evaluation of biofilm for some metallic materials and polymers such as urinary stents and catheters. *Materials*, *9*, 824–834. doi:10.3390/ma9100824.

106. Kanematsu, H., Sakagami, Y., Barry, D. M., Yoshitake, M., Ogawa, A., Hirai, N. . . . Mizunoe, Y. (2018). *Evaluation for immunity of biomaterials based on Raman spec-troscopy*. Proceedings of the Materials Science and Technology 2018 (MS&T18), Greater Columbus Convention Center, Columbus, Ohio, October 14–18, pp. 1482–1489.

107. Sano, K., Kanematsu, H., Hirai, N., Ogawa, A., Kogo, T., & Tanaka, T. (2017). The development of the anti-biofouling coating agent using metal nanoparticles and analysis by Raman spectroscopy and FIB system. *Surface & Coating Technology*, *325*, 715–721.

108. Kanematsu, H., Kanesaki, S., Kudara, H., Barry, D. M., Ogawa, A., & Mizunoe, Y. (2018). Biofilm formation on titanium alloy surfaces in a laboratory biofilm reactor. In *Ceramic transactions – advances in ceramics for environmental, functional, structural, and energy applications*, Mahmoud, M. M., Sridharan, K., Colorado, H., Bhalla, A. S., J. P. Singh, Gupta, S., Langhorn, J., Jitianu, A., & Manjooran, N. J., Eds. New York: John Wiley & Sons Inc., volume 265, pp. 221–228.

109. Bacon, C. W., Hinton, D. M., & Mitchell, T. R. (2018). Screening of *Bacillus mojavensis* biofilms and biosurfactants using laser ablation electrospray ionization mass spectroscopy. *Journal of Applied Microbiology*, *125*(3), 867–875.

110. Denkhaus, E., Meisen, S., Telgheder, U., & Wingender, J. (2007). Chemical and physical methods for characterisation of biofilms. *Microchimica Acta*, *158*(1), 1–27.

111. Toporski, J. K. W., Steele, A., Westall, F., Avci, R., Martill, D. M., & McKay, D. S. (2002). Morphologic and spectral investigation of exceptionally well-preserved bacterial biofilms from the Oligocene Enspel formation, Germany. *Geochimica et Cosmochimica Acta*, *66*(10), 1773–1791.

112. Wolcott, R., Costerton, J. W., Raoult, D., & Cutler, S. J. (2013). The polymicrobial nature of biofilm infection. *Clinical Microbiology and Infection*, *19*(2), 107–112.

113. Geddes-McAlister, J., Kugadas, A., & Gadjeva, M. (2019). Tasked with a challenging objective: Why do neutrophils fail to battle *Pseudomonas aeruginosa* biofilms. *Pathogens*, *8*(4), 283.

114. Chavez de Paz, L. E., Davies, J. R., Bergenholtz, G., & Svensäter, G. (2015). Strains of Enterococcus faecalis differ in their ability to coexist in biofilms with other root canal bacteria. *International Endodontic Journal*, *48*(10), 916–925.

115. Fernandes, G., Camotti Bastos, M., Mondamert, L., Labanowski, J., Burrow, R. S., & dos Santos Rheinheimer, D. (2021). Organic composition of epilithic biofilms from agricultural and urban watershed in South Brazil. *Environmental Science and Pollution Research*, *28*(22), 28808–28824.

116. Konhauser, K. O., Schultze-Lam, S., Ferris, F. G., Fyfe, W. S., Longstaffe, F. J., & Beveridge, T. J. (1994). Mineral precipitation by epilithic biofilms in the Speed River, Ontario, Canada. *Applied and Environmental Microbiology*, *60*(2), 549–553.

117. Lewandowski, Z., Altobelli, S. A., & Fukushima, E. (1993). NMR and microelectrode studies of hydrodynamics and kinetics in biofilms. *Biotechnology Progress*, *9*(1), 40–45.

118. Hoskins, B. C., Fevang, L., Majors, P. D., Sharma, M. M., & Georgiou, G. (1999). Selective imaging of biofilms in porous media by NMR relaxation. *Journal of Magnetic Resonance*, *139*(1), 67–73.

119. Zhang, B., & Powers, R. (2012). Analysis of bacterial biofilms using NMR-based metabolomics. *Future Medicinal Chemistry*, *4*(10), 1273–1306.

120. Reichhardt, C., & Cegelski, L. (2014). Solid-state NMR for bacterial biofilms. *Molecular Physics*, *112*(7), 887–894.

121. Vogt, M., Flemming, H. C., & Veeman, W. S. (2000). Diffusion in *Pseudomonas aeruginosa* biofilms: A pulsed field gradient NMR study. *Journal of Biotechnology*, *77*(1), 137–146.

122. Surman, S. B., Walker, J. T., Goddard, D. T., Morton, L. H. G., Keevil, C. W., Weaver, W., . . . Kurtz, J. (1996). Comparison of microscope techniques for the examination of biofilms. *Journal of Microbiological Methods*, *25*(1), 57–70.

123. Yawata, Y., Uchiyama, H., & Nomura, N. (2009). Visualizing the effects of biofilm structures on the influx of fluorescent material using combined confocal reflection and fluorescent microscopy. *Microbes and Environments*, 0912220146.

124. Bogachev, M. I., Volkov, V. Y., Markelov, O. A., Trizna, E. Y., Baydamshina, D. R., Melnikov, V., . . . Kayumov, A. R. (2018). Fast and simple tool for the quantification of biofilm-embedded cells sub-populations from fluorescent microscopic images. *PLOS ONE*, *13*(5), e0193267.

125. Diaz, R. R., Picciafuoco, S., Gabriela Paraje, M., Angel Villegas, N., Miranda, J. A., Albesa, I., Cremonezzi, D., Commisso, R., & Paglini-Oliva, P. (2011). Relevance of biofilms in pediatric tonsillar disease. *European Journal of Clinical Microbiology & Infectious Diseases*, *30*(12), 1503–1509.

126. Lawrence, J. R., Korber, D. R., Hoyle, B. D., William Costerton, J., & Caldwell, D. E. (1991). Optical sectioning of microbial biofilms. *Journal of Bacteriology*, *173*(20), 6558–6567.

127. Beloin, C., & Ghigo, J. M. (2005). Finding gene-expression patterns in bacterial biofilms. *Trends in Microbiology*, *13*(1), 16–19.

128. Lazazzera, B. A. (2005). Lessons from DNA microarray analysis: The gene expression profile of biofilms. *Current Opinion in Microbiology*, *8*(2), 222–227.

129. Yao, Y., Sturdevant, D. E., & Otto, M. (2005). Genomewide analysis of gene expression in *Staphylococcus epidermidis* biofilms: Insights into the pathophysiology of S. epidermidis biofilms and the role of phenol-soluble modulins in formation of biofilms. *Journal of Infectious Diseases*, *191*(2), 289–298.

130. Friedman, L., & Kolter, R. (2004). Genes involved in matrix formation in *Pseudomonas aeruginosa* PA14 biofilms. *Molecular Microbiology*, *51*(3), 675–690.

131. Beloin, C., Roux, A., & Ghigo, J. M. (2008). *Escherichia coli* biofilms. *Bacterial Biofilms*, 249–289.

132. Whiteley, M., Gita Bangera, M., Bumgarner, R. E., Parsek, M. R., Teitzel, G. M., Lory, S., & Greenberg, E. P. (2001). Gene expression in *Pseudomonas aeruginosa* biofilms. *Nature*, *413*(6858), 860–864.

133. Kalmbach, S., Manz, W., & Szewzyk, U. (1997). Isolation of new bacterial species from drinking water biofilms and proof of their in situ dominance with highly specific 16S rRNA probes. *Applied and Environmental Microbiology*, *63*(11), 4164–4170.

134. Pérez-Osorio, A. C., Williamson, K. S., & Franklin, M. J. (2010). Heterogeneous rpoS and rhlR mRNA levels and 16S rRNA/rDNA (rRNA gene) ratios within *Pseudomonas aeruginosa* biofilms, sampled by laser capture microdissection. *Journal of Bacteriology*, 2991–3000.

135. Drewes, J. L., White, J. R., Dejea, C. M., Fathi, P., Iyadorai, T., Vadivelu, J., . . . Roslani, A. C. (2017). High-resolution bacterial 16S rRNA gene profile meta-analysis and biofilm status reveal common colorectal cancer consortia. *NPJ Biofilms and Microbiomes*, *3*(1), 1–12.

136. Corcoll, N., Österlund, T., Sinclair, L., Eiler, A., Kristiansson, E., Backhaus, T., & Martin Eriksson, K. (2017). Comparison of four DNA extraction methods for comprehensive assessment of 16S rRNA bacterial diversity in marine biofilms using high-throughput sequencing. *FEMS Microbiology Letters*, *364*(14).

137. Ommen, P., Zobek, N., & Meyer, R. L. (2017). Quantification of biofilm biomass by staining: Non-toxic safranin can replace the popular crystal violet. *Journal of Microbiological Methods*, *141*, 87–89.

138. Kragh, K. N., Alhede, M., Kvich, L., & Bjarnsholt, T. (2019). Into the well – a close look at the complex structures of a microtiter biofilm and the crystal violet assay. *Biofilm*, *1*, 100006.

139. Tram, G., Korolik, V., & Day, C. J. (2013). MBDS solvent: An improved method for assessment of biofilms. *Advances in Microbiology*, *3*(2).

140. Burton, E., Yakandawala, N., LoVetri, K., & Madhyastha, M. S. (2007). A microplate spectrofluorometric assay for bacterial biofilms. *Journal of Industrial Microbiology and Biotechnology*, *34*(1), 1–4.

141. Xu, Z., Liang, Y., Lin, S., Chen, D., Li, B., Li, L., & Deng, Y. (2016). Crystal violet and XTT assays on *Staphylococcus aureus* biofilm quantification. *Current Microbiology*, *73*(4), 474–482.

142. Vieira, H. L. A., Freire, P., & Arraiano, C. M. (2004). Effect of *Escherichia coli* morphogene bolA on biofilms. *Applied and Environmental Microbiology*, *70*(9), 5682–5684.
143. Kerstens, M., Boulet, G., Clais, S., Lanckacker, E., Delputte, P., Maes, L., and Cos, P. (2015). A flow cytometric approach to quantify biofilms. *Folia Microbiologica*, *60*(4), 335–342.
144. Merritt, J. H., Kadouri, D. E., & O'Toole, G. A. (2006). Growing and analyzing static biofilms. *Current Protocols in Microbiology*, *1*, 1B–1.
145. Romanova, N. A., Gawande, P. V., Brovko, L. Y., & Griffiths, M. W. (2007). Rapid methods to assess sanitizing efficacy of benzalkonium chloride to *Listeria monocytogenes* biofilms. *Journal of Microbiological Methods*, *71*(3), 231–237.
146. Sandasi, M., Leonard, C. M., & Viljoen, A. M. (2008). The effect of five common essential oil components on *Listeria monocytogenes* biofilms. *Food Control*, *19*(11), 1070–1075.
147. Xu, Z., Liang, Y., Lin, S., Chen, D, Li, B., Li, L., & Deng, Y. (2016). Crystal violet and XTT assays on *Staphylococcus aureus* biofilm quantification. *Current Microbiology*, *73*(4), 474–482.
148. Shukla, S. K., & Subba Rao, T. (2017). An improved crystal violet assay for biofilm quantification in 96-well microtitre plate. *Biorxiv*, 100214.
149. Adetunji, V. O., & Isola, T. O. (2011). Crystal violet binding assay for assessment of biofilm formation by *Listeria monocytogenes* and *Listeria* spp on wood, steel and glass surfaces. *Global Veterinaria*, *6*(1), 6–10.
150. Ommen, P., Zobek, N., & Meyer, R. L. (2017). Quantification of biofilm biomass by staining: Non-toxic safranin can replace the popular crystal violet. *Journal of Microbiological Methods*, *141*, 87–89.
151. Kragh, K. N., Alhede, M., Kvich, L., & Bjarnsholt, T. (2019). Into the well – a close look at the complex structures of a microtiter biofilm and the crystal violet assay. *Biofilm*, *1*, 100006.
152. Burton, E., Yakandawala, N., LoVetri, K., & Madhyastha, M. S. (2007). A microplate spectrofluorometric assay for bacterial biofilms. *Journal of Industrial Microbiology and Biotechnology*, *34*(1), 1–4.
153. Sun, P., Hui, C., Wang, S., Wan, L., Zhang, X., & Zhao, Y. (2016). *Bacillus amyloliquefaciens* biofilm as a novel biosorbent for the removal of crystal violet from solution. *Colloids and Surfaces B: Biointerfaces*, *139*, 164–170.
154. O'Toole, G. A. (2011). Microtiter dish biofilm formation assay. *Journal of Visualized Experiments: JoVE*, *47*.
155. Chavant, P., Gaillard-Martinie, B., Talon, R., Hébraud, M., & Bernardi, T. (2007). A new device for rapid evaluation of biofilm formation potential by bacteria. *Journal of Microbiological Methods*, *68*(3), 605–612.
156. Stepanović, S., Vuković, D., Dakić, I., Savić, B., & Švabić-Vlahović, M. (2000). A modified microtiter-plate test for quantification of staphylococcal biofilm formation. *Journal of Microbiological Methods*, *40*(2), 175–179.

5 Preparation, Characterization, and Applications of Polymer Nanocomposite Films and Fabrics with *In Situ* Generated Metal Nanoparticles by Bioreduction Method

Basa Ashok, Natarajan Rajini, Paramasivan Sivaranjana, and Anumakonda Varada Rajulu

CONTENTS

DOI: 10.1201/9781003143093-5

5.1   INTRODUCTION

Due to their unique higher surface area to volume ratio, metal nanoparticles (MNPs) exhibit properties different from the micro- and macrodimensional materials [1–2]. Especially, the MNPs have efficient antibacterial activity [3] and hence find many applications in the medical field [4]. Due to the increasing applications of MNPs, many researchers are paying attention to their synthesis, characterization, and identifying their applications. Of the MNPs, gold, silver, and copper nanoparticles are gaining importance due to their excellent antibacterial activity. There are various methods of generating the MNPs, such as physical and chemical methods. The physical methods include plasma method, chemical vapor deposition method, microwave irradiation method, pulsed laser method, sonochemical reduction method, and gamma radiation method. On the other hand, the chemical methods generally used are the polyol method, microemulsions method, thermal decomposition, and electrochemical synthesis. However, most of them are time-consuming, complicated, and expensive. Furthermore, some of the chemical processes are not environmentally friendly. In order to overcome the shortcomings of these methods, recently, an environmentally friendly bioreduction approach involving the leaf extracts is being practiced. In this green method, the inherently present reducing biochemicals in leaf extracts synthesize the MNPs from their corresponding metal salts. Various leaf extracts have been used to generate MNPs effectively. To cite a few, in one study, Satyavathi et al. [5] generated silver nanoparticles (AgNPs) with an average size of 26 nm using the leaf extract of *Coriandrum sativum*. They reported excellent nonlinear properties for the AgNPs developed. In another study, Banerjee et al. [6] used the leaf extracts of *Ocimumtenuiflorum*, *Azadirachta indica*, and *Musa balbisiana* generated AgNPs excellent antibacterial activity. In another study, Kaviya et al. [7] developed the AgNPs using *Citrus sinensis* peel extract to reduce agents. The generated spherical AgNPs were in size range of 10–35 nm. Similarly, Bindhani and Panigrahi [8] used the aqueous extract of *Ocimum sanctum* leaf to prepare AgNPs with a 15–45 nm size range. Some researchers generated copper nanoparticles (CuNPs) using leaf extracts. For instance, Sutradhar et al. [9] developed CuNPs using coffee powder and tea leaves extracts. Similarly, Brumbaugh et al. [10] employed plant tea to generate ultrasmall CuNPs effectively. In some other studies, to create smaller CuNPs, Gebremedhn et al. [11], Kulkarni et al. [12], and Ananda Murthy et al. [13] used the leaf extracts of *Catha edulis*, *Eucalyptus*, and *Hageniaabyssinica (Brace) JF. Gmel*, respectively. In the works cited here, the researchers generated the MNPs separately, which have to be isolated, washed with distilled water several times, and finally centrifuge to get their clusters which can be later used as fillers in suitable matrices nanocomposites. However, when the MNPs are dispersed in polymer matrices, there is every possibility for the particles to agglomerate at many places leading to low properties. To overcome this problem, it is recommended to *in situ* generate the MNPs in the polymer matrices. Our group recently developed AgNPs and CuNPs in a cellulose matrix and successfully made biodegradable nanocomposite films using different leaf extracts. In one study, Sadanand et al. prepared the nanocomposites of cellulose with *in situ* generated AgNPs [14] and CuNPs [15] using *O. sanctum* leaf extract as a reducing agent. The nanocomposite films prepared exhibited excellent antibacterial activity. Sivaranjana et al. prepared cellulose nanocomposite films with *in situ* generated AgNPs [16] and CuNPs [17] using aqueous leaf extract of *Cassia alata* as a reducing agent. Both these materials exhibited good antibacterial activity and hence, can be considered for antibacterial packaging purposes. Similarly, Muthulakshmi et al. using the aqueous leaf extract of *Terminalia catappa* as a reducing agent, prepared the nanocomposite cellulose films with *in situ* generated AgNPs [18] and CuNPs [19]. Since these films exhibited antibacterial activity, they suggested these materials be used as antibacterial packaging films. Muthulakshmi et al. [18–19] recommended these for antibacterial packaging applications.

For medical applications, antibacterial fabrics are more suitable for wound dressing and also as hospital bed materials. Keeping these requirements in mind, our group recently also prepared antibacterial nanocomposite cotton fabrics with *in situ* generated AgNPs [20] and CuNPs [21] using aqueous extract of red sanders powder as a reducing agent and different concentrated respective metal salt solutions as a source of metal nanoparticles. Our group also prepared antibacterial nanocomposite polyester fabrics with *in situ* generated AgNPs [22] and CuNPs [23] using tamarind leaf extract as a reducing agent and suggested these fabrics as antibacterial apparel. Our group also prepared nanocomposite cotton fabrics with *in situ* generated bimetallic silver and copper nanoparticles [24] using *Moringa oleifera* leaf extract as a reducing agent. These nanocomposite fabrics exhibited improved properties when compared to pristine fabrics. Similarly, Venkata Ramanamoorthy et al. [25] used *Tino sporacordiofolia* leaf extract to reduce agent and *in situ* generated silver and silver oxide nanoparticles in cotton fabrics. These fabrics exhibited significant antibacterial properties and so can be used as antibacterial hospital bed materials.

In all these systems, the leaf extracts with hydroxyl groups, polyphenols, flavonoids, etc., reduced the metal salts into their respective MNPs inside the matrices. However, the cotton fabrics themselves have cellulose molecules with OH groups. However, the inherently present hydroxyl groups in the cotton fabrics cannot *in situ* generate the MNPs rapidly at room temperature, as the reduction process is a slow one. In order to hasten up the process, our group prepared the nanocomposite cotton fabrics with *in situ* generated AgNPs [26] and CuNPs [27] by the thermal-assisted (hydrothermal) one-step process at 80 °C without the aid of external leaf extracts.

In the present chapter, as an example, we present the preparation, characterization, and possible applications of two nanocomposite cellulose films with *in situ* generated AgNPs [14] and CuNPs [15] and two nanocomposite cotton fabrics with *in situ* generated AgNPs [26] and CuNPs [27] by one-step thermally assisted method without using any leaf extracts. All these four systems presented in this chapter were characterized by scanning electron microscopy, Fourier-transform infrared (FTIR) spectroscopy, X-ray diffraction, and antibacterial activity tests.

5.2 MATERIALS AND METHODS

5.2.1 MATERIALS

In the nanocomposite cellulose films with *in situ* generated AgNPs [14] and CuNPs [15], cotton linter pup supplied by M/s Hubei Chemical Fiber Company Ltd, P.R. China was used. The leaves of *O. sanctum* procured from the local area were washed with distilled water for making the extraction. The chemicals LiOH, urea, and $CuSO_4 \cdot 5H_2O$ were purchased from S.D. Chemicals, Mumbai, India. M/s Aldrich Chemicals Limited supplied $AgNO_3$. Ethyl alcohol (M/s Jebsen and Jessen Company, Germany) was used for regenerating the cellulose films.

In the case of the nanocomposite cotton fabrics with *in situ* generated AgNPs [26] and CuNPs [27], the white cotton fabric was procured from the local market in Hyderabad, India. These fabrics were washed thoroughly with mild detergent and subsequently washed thoroughly with distilled water to remove impurities and sizing materials and dried before use.

5.2.2 METHODS

For the preparation of the nanocomposite cellulose films [14–15], following methods were adopted.

5.2.2.1 Dissolution of Cellulose

We used the environment-friendly aqueous solution of 8 wt.% LiOH along with 15 wt.% urea that was pre-cooled to −12.7 °C as a solvent as described elsewhere [28]. To the pre-cooled alkali solvent, cotton linters (4 wt.% by weight of the solvent) were added, and using a mechanical stirrer was stirred at a high speed of 1000 rpm (at room temperature). The cellulose solution obtained in this step was centrifuged at a rate of 7200 rpm (maintaining a temperature of 5 °C during centrifugation) to remove the impurities and undissolved cellulose if any. Within 2 minutes, the cellulose solution was obtained as it is a rapid process. The process of cellulose dissolution is illustrated in Figure 5.1.

5.2.2.2 Preparation of the Leaf Extraction

In the present study, *O. sanctum* leaf extract was used as a reducing agent to generate the MNPs in the cellulose matrix. To make the leaf extract, 10 wt.% of the small pieces of the cleaned leaves were added to the hot distilled water (80 °C) and maintained at that temperature for 20 minutes. The container having the leaf extract and the leaves was cooled to room temperature, and then the extract was filtered to get the decant (leaf extract), which was stored at 5 °C till used. The leaf extraction process is illustrated in Figure 5.2.

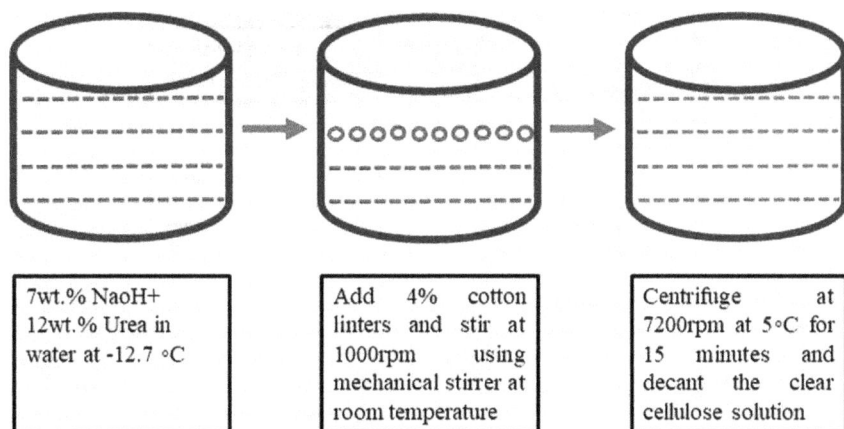

| 7wt.% NaoH+ 12wt.% Urea in water at -12.7 °C | Add 4% cotton linters and stir at 1000rpm using mechanical stirrer at room temperature | Centrifuge at 7200rpm at 5°C for 15 minutes and decant the clear cellulose solution |

FIGURE 5.1 Illustration of the dissolution of cotton linter pulp.

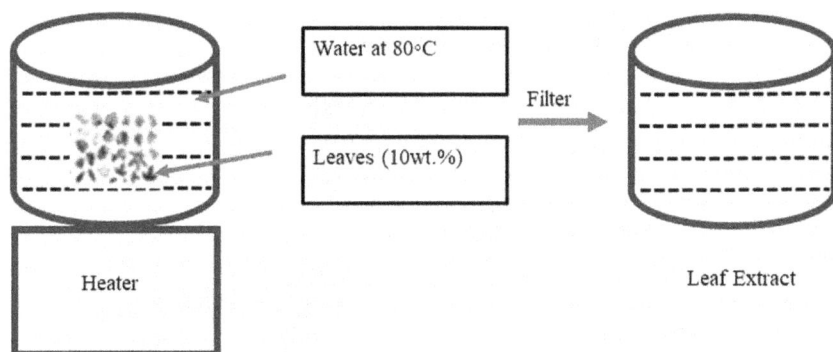

Water at 80°C

Filter

Leaves (10wt.%)

Heater

Leaf Extract

FIGURE 5.2 Illustration of preparation of the *O. sanctum* leaf extract.

5.2.2.3 Preparation of the Matrix

In this process, in the first step, cellulose gel films (wet films) were prepared to employ the regeneration method. In this step, ethyl alcohol was used as a coagulation bath. The prepared clear cellulose solution was poured on glass plates and spread with a glass spreader. The glass plate with spread cellulose solution was kept in the alcohol bath to regenerate the wet cellulose film. The regenerated cellulose films were washed thoroughly with distilled water and then kept in the leaf extract taken in a beaker and stirred on a magnetic stirrer at room temperature at a speed of 500 rpm for about two hours for uniform diffusion of the leaf extract into the wet films. These wet cellulose films with diffused leaf extract formed the matrix. This process is illustrated in Figure 5.3.

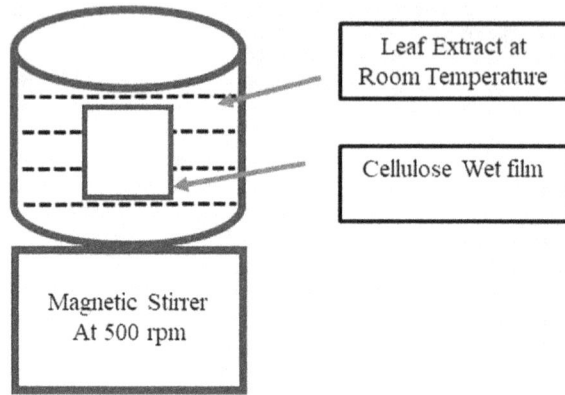

FIGURE 5.3   Illustration of the preparation of cellulose wet films with diffused leaf extract (matrix).

5.2.2.4   Preparation of Nanocomposite Cellulose Films with *In Situ* Generated MNPs

In the present work, to *in situ* generate MNPs, different concentrated respective metal salt solutions were made. Each concentrated metal salt solution (source solution) was taken in separate beakers in the subsequent step. Every two pieces of the matrix wet films were added and kept on a magnetic stirrer at 100–200 rpm at room temperature for 24 hours. During this step, the color of the matrix slowly changed, indicating the *in situ generation* of MNPs in the matrix. At the end of 24 hours, the nanocomposite cellulose films with *in situ* generated MNPs were removed from the beakers, washed thoroughly with distilled water, and dried to get the nanocomposite dry films. This process is illustrated in Figure 5.4.

The entire process of making the nanocomposite cellulose films is illustrated in a nutshell in Figure 5.5.

For making the nanocomposite cotton fabrics with *in situ* generated MNPs, following method was adopted.

5.2.2.5   Preparation of Nanocomposite Cotton Fabrics with *In Situ* Generated MNPs by One-Step Method

In the first step, respective metal salt solutions of different concentrations were prepared in deionized water. Each solution was taken in separate beakers. Two pieces of the cleaned and dried white cotton fabrics (150 mm × 60 mm) were immersed in each beaker. These beakers were kept in a hot air oven at 80 °C for 24 hours. During this period, the color of the white cotton fabric changed, indicating the *in situ generation* of MNPs, thus forming the nanocomposite cotton fabrics. This process is illustrated in Figure 5.6.

The entire process is briefly illustrated in Figure 5.7.

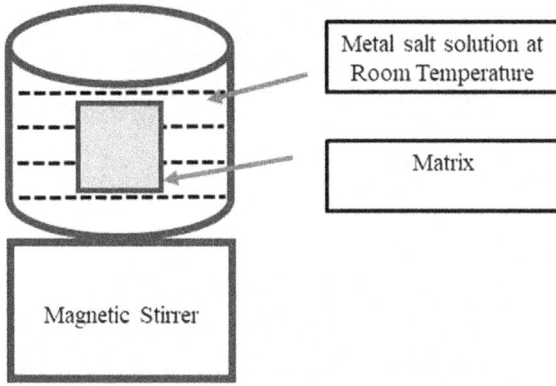

FIGURE 5.4 Illustration of preparation of the nanocomposite cellulose films with *in situ* generated MNPs.

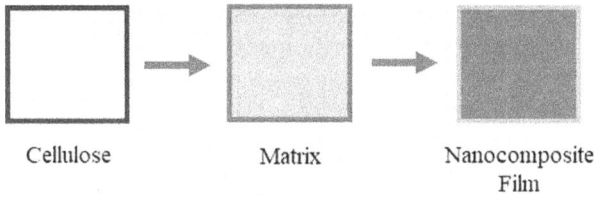

FIGURE 5.5 Illustration of the different steps in a nutshell.

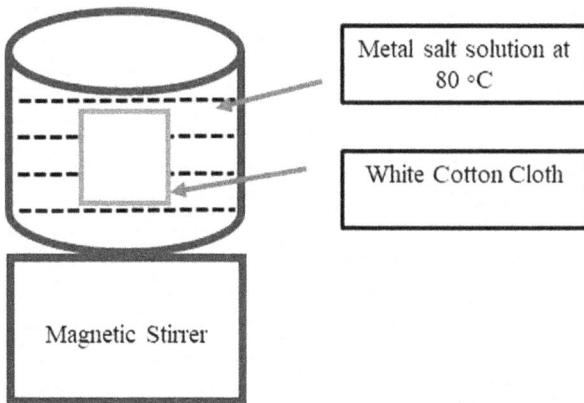

FIGURE 5.6 Illustration of preparation of nanocomposite cotton fabrics with *in situ* generated MNPs in one-step thermal-assisted method.

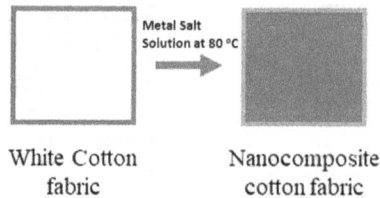

White Cotton   Nanocomposite
fabric   cotton fabric

FIGURE 5.7 Illustration of the preparation of nanocomposite cotton fabric with *in situ* generated MNPs by the one-step thermal-assisted method.

5.2.3 CHARACTERIZATION

The *in situ* generated MNPs in the nanocomposite cellulose films and cotton fabrics were observed using Zeiss 01 scanning electron microscope at an accelerating voltage of 10 kV. The specimens were gold coated before recording the micrographs. Using the same instrument, the dispersive energy X-ray (EDX) spectra were also recorded. The size of the nanoparticles observed in the micrographs was measured using the built-in SmartTiff software of the microscope. The Fourier-transform infrared (FTIR) spectra were recorded employing Smart iTR ATR Nicolet is 10 spectrophotometer. All the spectra were recorded in the range of 4000–500 cm^{-1} at 4 cm^{-1} resolution in each case with 32 scans.

In order to study the effect of generated MNPs on the crystallinity of the nanocomposites understudy, the X-ray diffractograms were recorded employing Bruker Eco D8 X-ray diffractometer. The diffractograms were recorded in the $2\theta = 10°–80°$ range at a rate of 4°/min. The operating conditions maintained were 40 kV and 20 mA.

The antibacterial activity of the nanocomposite films and fabrics was examined by the standard disc method adopting the procedure described elsewhere [29]. The method is described in brief in the following lines. Initially, the nutrient agar medium was made by mixing 5 g of sodium chloride, 5 g of peptone, 3 g beef extract in 1 liter of distilled water. This agar medium was then sterilized and subsequently transferred to Petri dishes, which were then kept in a Laminar air flow chamber. The agar was then allowed to solidify. Then, the bacterial culture (50 µL) was spread on the media and inoculated. Subsequently, circular discs of the nanocomposite films and fabrics with *in situ* generated MNPs were placed on the inoculated medium and incubated at 37 °C for 48 hours in the incubation chamber. The formed clear zones indicating the inhibition of bacteria by the nanocomposite specimens were photographed. In each case, the diameter of the inhibition (clear) zone was measured using ImageJ software.

5.3 RESULTS AND DISCUSSION

In this chapter, as an example, the results and discussion of the following four systems are presented:

1. Nanocomposite cellulose films with *in situ* generated AgNPs [14] using *O. sanctum* leaf extract as a reducing agent.
2. Nanocomposite cellulose films with *in situ* generated CuNPs [15] using *O. sanctum* leaf extract as a reducing agent.
3. Nanocomposite cotton fabrics with *in situ* generated AgNPs [26] by the one-step thermal-assisted method.
4. Nanocomposite cotton fabrics with *in situ* generated AgNPs [27] by the one-step thermal-assisted method.

5.3.1 NANOCOMPOSITE CELLULOSE FILMS WITH *IN SITU* GENERATED AGNPS USING *O. SANCTUM* LEAF EXTRACT AS A REDUCING AGENT

The matrix was light brown while the nanocomposite cellulose films made using *O. sanctum* leaf extract as a reducing agent and 25, 125, and 250 mM aq. $AgNO_3$ as source solutions were black, and the color proportionally increased with source solution concentration [14]. The color change indicates the *in situ generation* of AgNPs in the nanocomposite films. To observe the *in situ* generated AgNPs in the nanocomposite films, the SEM images and EDX spectra of the nanocomposite film made using 250 mM source solution are presented in Figure 5.8.

From Figure 5.8, it is evident that the nanocomposites understudy had roughly spherical nanoparticles with sizes varying between 70 and 100 nm. At the same time, the EDX spectrum had a peak representing the silver element. Hence, these nanocomposite films had *in situ* generated spherical AgNPs.

The FTIR spectral studies indicated similar bands for both the matrix and the nanocomposite films showing similar chemical groups in them [14]. However, in the nanocomposite films, the intensity of the broadband at 3336 cm^{-1} (corresponding to the OH of cellulose) was lower than the matrix. This indicates the involvement of OH groups to generate the AgNPs in the nanocomposite films. The X-ray analysis of the matrix and the nanocomposites exhibited familiar diffraction peaks at $2\theta = 12.8°$, 20.1°, and 21.9°[14], indicating the cellulose-II structure [30]. On the other hand, the

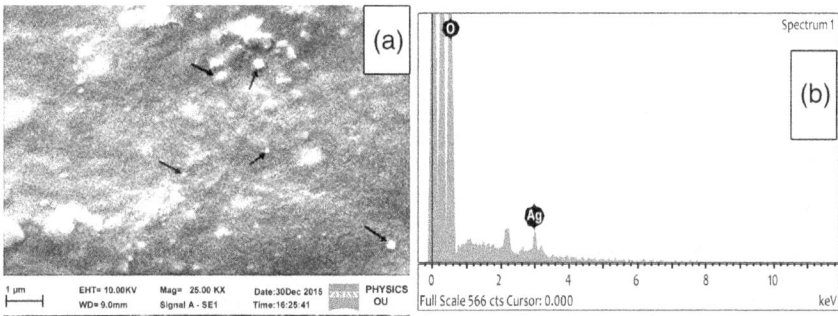

FIGURE 5.8   The SEM image (a) and the EDX spectrum (b) of the nanocomposite cellulose film with *in situ* generated AgNPs using 250 mM source solution. Some of the generated nanoparticles are indicated by arrows.

nanocomposite films had additional low-intensity peaks at $2\theta = 38.6°$, $64.4°$, and $77.4°$, which arose due to the reflections from the (111), (220), and (211) panes of silver [31]. Thus the X-ray analysis further confirmed the generation of AgNPs in the nanocomposite films.

The antibacterial test indicated that though the matrix exhibited little antibacterial activity, the nanocomposite films possessed significant antibacterial activity against *Escherichia coli* bacteria. The diameters of the nanocomposite cellulose films made using 25, 125, and 250 mM source solutions were 16, 20, and 22.5 mm, respectively [14], indicating increasing antibacterial activity with source solution concentration. Thus, the nanocomposite cellulose films with *in situ* generated AgNPs can be considered as antibacterial packaging and wound dressing materials.

5.3.2 NANOCOMPOSITE CELLULOSE FILMS WITH *IN SITU* GENERATED CUNPS USING *O. SANCTUM* LEAF EXTRACT AS A REDUCING AGENT

As silver salts are expensive, to lower the cost, in the present work, the nanocomposite cellulose films were prepared with *in situ* generated CuNPs using *O. sanctum* leaf extract as a reductant and 25, 125, and 250 mM aq.$CuSO_4 \cdot 5H_2O$ as source solutions. It was found that the leaf extract diffused cellulose (matrix) was brown while the nanocomposite films were greenish-blue in color, and the intensity of the color increased with source solution concentration. The color change preliminarily indicates the *in situ generation* of the CuNPs in the nanocomposite films [15]. For confirmation, the SEM analysis was carried out. The SEM image and the corresponding EDX spectrum of the nanocomposite film using 250 mM source solution are presented in Figure 5.9.

From Figure 5.9, it can be visualized that the nanoparticles generated were roughly spherical. The size range for all the nanocomposite films varied between 50 and 60 nm, with an overall average of 60 nm. The EDX spectra had a peak corresponding to the copper element. Thus, the SEM analysis confirmed the *in situ generation* of CuNPs in the nanocomposite films [15]. The FTIR spectral analysis

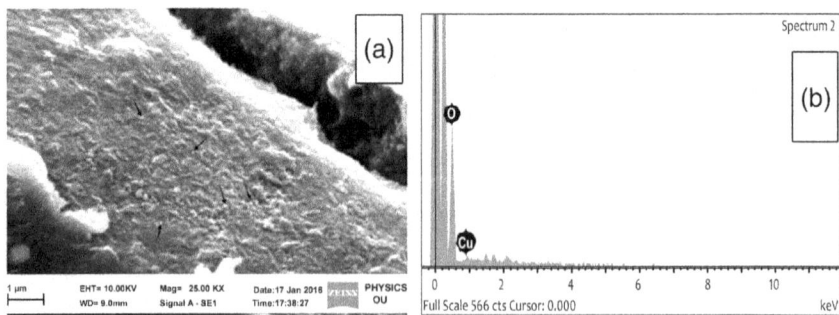

FIGURE 5.9 The SEM image (a) and the EDX spectrum (b) of the nanocomposite cellulose film with *in situ* generated CuNPs using 250 mM source solution. Some of the generated nanoparticles are indicated by arrows.

indicated that both the matrix and the nanocomposite films understudy had typical bands at 3328 cm^{-1} (OH), 2891 cm^{-1} (CH$_2$), 1021 cm^{-1} (C–OH), and 1638 cm^{-1} (crystallization of water), which indicate cellulose-II structure. The intensity of the peak corresponding to the OH group for the nanocomposite films was lower than that of the matrix showing the role of these groups in the generation of the CuNPs.

Furthermore, in nanocomposite films, an additional peak at 1742 cm^{-1} (C=O) was observed. A similar observation was made by Alekseeva et al. [32] in the case of cellulose derivative composites with CuNP. They attributed this to the oxidation of some of the OH groups to C=O groups by the generated CuNPs due to their catalytic activity in the oxidation of organic moieties [15, 32].

X-ray analysis indicated the typical diffraction peaks of cellulose-II structure for both the matrix and the nanocomposite films. However, in nanocomposite cellulose films with *in situ* generated CuNPs, some faint additional peaks were observed at $2\theta = 32.3°$, $36.8°$, $44°$, and $50°$, respectively, for Cu$_2$O, Cu$_2$O, Cu, and Cu [15, 32]. Thus, the nanocomposite films understudy had both copper and copper oxide nanoparticles. The antibacterial test analysis indicated the formation of inhibition (clear) zones in nanocomposite cellulose films showing their antibacterial activity against *E.coli* bacteria [15]. The diameters of the inhibition zones of the nanocomposite films made using 25, 125, and 250 mM source solutions were found to be 8, 14, and 18 mm, respectively, indicating that the activity increased proportionately with source solution concentration. Thus, the nanocomposite cellulose films with *in situ* generated CuNPs using *O. sanctum* leaf extract as a reducing agent can be considered as antibacterial packaging and wound dressing materials.

5.3.3 NANOCOMPOSITE COTTON FABRICS WITH *IN SITU* GENERATED AGNPS BY THE ONE-STEP THERMAL-ASSISTED METHOD

For medical applications, nanocomposite fabrics will be more useful than nanocomposite films. In the present work, the nanocomposite cotton fabrics were prepared with *in situ* generated AgNPs by one-step thermal-assisted (hydrothermal) method exploiting the inherently present OH groups of cellulose molecules in reducing the metal salt solutions to the corresponding metal nanoparticles. It was observed that the color of the white cotton fabrics changed to brown after the *in situ generation* of AgNPs by the one-step hydrothermal method. The color deepened with increasing concentration of the aq.AgNO$_3$ source solutions (1–5 mM). The color change preliminarily indicates the *in situ generation* of AgNPs in the nanocomposite cotton fabrics under study [26]. To confirm the presence of AgNPs in the nanocomposite cotton fabrics, an SEM analysis was carried out. As an example, the SEM image and EDX spectrum of the nanocomposite cotton fabric made using 5 mM source solution are presented in Figure 5.10.

From Figure 5.10, it is evident that the size of the generated roughly spherical nanoparticles varied in the size range of 47 nm to 70 nm. The EDX spectrum had the peak corresponding to the silver element. The SEM analysis thus confirmed the generation of the AgNPs in the system under study [26].

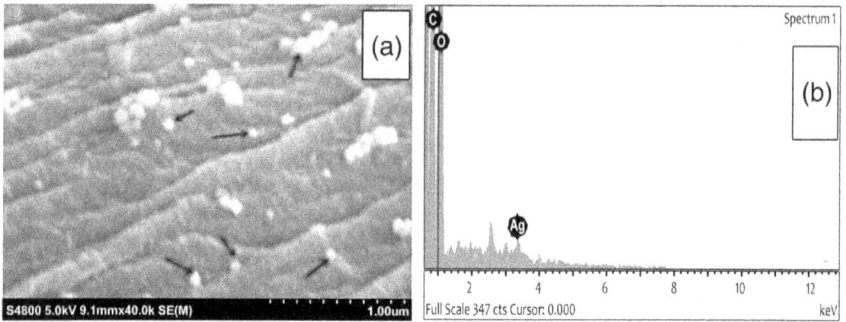

FIGURE 5.10   The SEM image (a) and the EDX spectrum (b) of the nanocomposite cellulose fabrics with *in situ* generated AgNPs using 5 mM source solution. Some of the generated nanoparticles are indicated by arrows.

The FTIR spectral analysis of the matrix and the nanocomposite cotton fabrics indicated the presence of typical bands at 3334 cm^{-1}, 2923 cm^{-1}, 1429 cm^{-1}, 1317 cm^{-1}, 1149 cm^{-1}, 1018 cm^{-1}, and 878 cm^{-1} [26], which arose due to the vibrations of OH-st, CH-st, CH_2-b, CH_2-w, C-O-C–pyranose ring, C-O-C–st, and β-glycosidic linkage groups, respectively. In addition, in the case of the matrix, a band present at 1802 cm^{-1} (carbonyl group of ester) was missing in the spectra of the nanocomposite cotton fabrics [26]. Besides this, the band's intensity at 3334 cm^{-1} for nanocomposite cotton fabrics was lower than that of the matrix. AgNPs synthesized by banana peel extract [33], and cellulose nanofibers with AgNPs [34], a similar decrease in the intensity of the peak corresponding to OH groups was observed. Thus, these observations indicate the role of both OH and carbonyl groups in the *in situ generation* of AgNPs at elevated temperatures in the case of nanocomposite cotton fabrics [26].

The fabrics intended for medical applications must exhibit antibacterial activity. In order to examine the antibacterial activity of the nanocomposite fabrics understudy, the test was carried by disc method. It was observed that the matrix (white cotton cloth) did not form any inhibition zone indicating its inability to eradicate the bacteria. On the other hand, the nanocomposite cotton fabrics with *in situ* generated AgNPs formed inhibition (clear) zones against the standard gram-negative (*E.coli* and *Pseudomonas*) and gram-positive (*Bacillus subtilis* and *Staphylococcus aureus*) bacteria. The diameters of the clear zones in the nanocomposite cotton fabrics made using 1, 2, 3, 4, and 5 mM source solutions against *E.coli* bacteria were 7, 9, 11, and 12.5 mm, respectively. Against *Pseudomonas* bacteria, these values were 5, 6, 8, 10, and 14 mm, respectively.

Similarly, against *B.subtilis* bacteria, these values were 8, 8, 10, 12.5, and 16 mm, respectively, and against *S.aureus* bacteria, these values were found to be 6, 7, 10, 12, and 14 mm, respectively [26]. These observations indicate that, as the concentration of the source solutions increased, the antibacterial activity of the prepared nanocomposite fabrics also increased. Thus, these antibacterial nanocomposite cotton fabrics with *in situ* generated AgNPs by one-step thermal-assisted (hydrothermal) method can find applications in the medical field as antibacterial wound cleaning and dressing materials, surgical aprons, hospital bed materials, etc.

5.3.4 NANOCOMPOSITE COTTON FABRICS WITH *IN SITU* GENERATED CUNPS BY THE ONE-STEP THERMAL-ASSISTED METHOD

In order to lower the cost of the nanocomposite cotton fabrics, in the present work, CuNPs were *in situ* generated in the white cotton fabrics using 1, 5, 25, 125, and 250 mM aq.$CuSO_4 \cdot 5H_2O$ source solutions [27]. It was observed that the color of the nanocomposite cotton fabrics with *in situ* generated CuNPs was light blue, and the intensity of the color increased with source solution concentration. The change in color of the nanocomposite cotton fabrics over the matrix indicates the generation of CuNPs. For confirmation, the SEM analysis was carried out. For example, the SEM image and EDX spectrum of the nanocomposite cotton fabric with in situ generated CuNPs using a 250 mM source solution are presented in Figure 5.11.

From Figure 5.11, it can be seen that the nanocomposite cotton fabric had roughly spherical nanoparticles. The average size of the nanoparticles was found to be 85 nm [27]. In the nanocomposite cotton fabrics made using the source solutions of other concentrations, the average size of the nanoparticles varied between 87 and 92 nm. The EDX spectrum (Figure 5.11[b]) indicated copper compositions in the nanocomposite cotton fabric under study. Thus, the SEM analysis confirmed the *in situ generation* of CuNPs in the nanocomposite cotton fabrics [27]. The FTIR analysis indicated the presence of similar chemical groups in the matrix and the nanocomposite fabrics. Furthermore, the color of the nanocomposite cotton fabrics did not change even after repeated detergent washings. Thus the generated CuNPs were held in the nanocomposite cotton fabrics by electrostatic forces between the CuNPs and the matrix.

The X-ray analysis of the matrix and the nanocomposite cotton fabrics indicated the presence of familiar diffraction peaks at $2\theta = 15°$, $16.6°$, and $22°$, which arose due to the reflections from (1–10), (110), and (200) planes indicating the cellulose-II structure [27]. Furthermore, in nanocomposite cotton fabrics, additional low-intensity peaks were observed at $2\theta = 32°$ and $37°$, corresponding to Cu_2O. The other peaks observed at $2\theta = 42°$, $43.6°$, $49.8°$, and $74°$ belonged to copper [32, 35]. Thus,

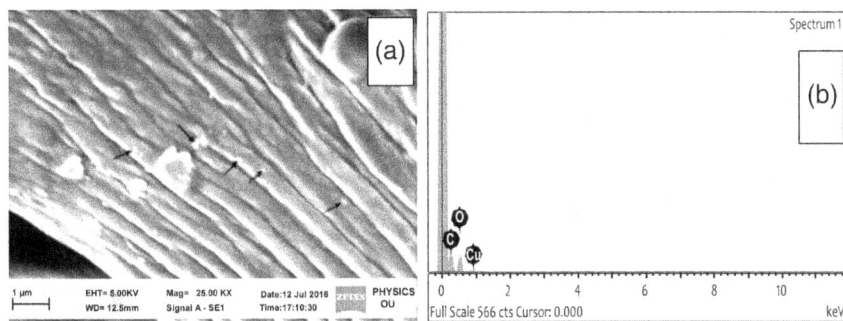

FIGURE 5.11 The SEM image (a) and the EDX spectrum (b) of the nanocomposite cellulose fabrics with *in situ* generated CuNPs using 250 mM source solution. Some of the generated nanoparticles are indicated by arrows.

the nanocomposite cotton fabrics understudy had *in situ* generated CuNPs and Cu_2O nanoparticles.

As the MNPs exhibit excellent antibacterial activity, it is expected that the nanocomposite with MNPs also exhibits antibacterial activity [36]. To examine whether the materials under study exhibit antibacterial activity, the test by disc method was carried. It was observed that though the matrix (white cotton fabric) did not show any antibacterial activity, the nanocomposite cotton fabrics formed inhibition (clear) zones indicating their good antibacterial activity against *E.coli* bacteria. The diameters of the clear zones formed by the nanocomposite cotton fabrics with *in situ* generated CuNPs using 1, 5, 25, 125, and 250 mM source solutions were reported to be 0.5, 5, 6, 10, and 12 mm, respectively. Thus, the antibacterial activity of the nanocomposite cotton fabrics increased with the increasing concentration of the source solutions. Hence, these low-cost antibacterial nanocomposite cotton fabrics with *in situ* generated CuNPs by the one-step hydrothermal method can be used as antibacterial surgical aprons, wound cleaning and dressing materials, hospital bed materials, etc., in medical field.

5.4 CONCLUSIONS

In the present chapter, the preparation and characterization of the nanocomposite cellulose films with *in situ* generated silver nanoparticles (AgNPs) and copper nanoparticles (CuNPs) using the leaf extract of the *O. sanctum*'s medicinal plant reducing agent were presented. In the same chapter, the preparation and characterization of the nanocomposite cotton fabrics with *in situ* generated AgNPs and CuNPs were also given. All the nanocomposite materials with *in situ* developed AgNPs and CuNPs were characterized by scanning electron microscopy (SEM), Fourier-transform infrared (FTIR) spectroscopy, X-ray diffraction (XRD), and antibacterial activity tests. SEM and XRD analyses confirmed the presence of the spherical metal nanoparticles (MNPs) in all these cases. The FTIR analysis indicated the role of the inherently present biochemicals of leaf extract in reducing the metal salt solutions to *in situ* generate MNPs in the nanocomposite cellulose films by the bioreduction method. The FTIR analysis also indicated the role of the OH groups of the cotton fabrics in developing the MNPs by the one-step hydrothermal method. Basing on the excellent antibacterial activity exhibited, all the systems discussed in this chapter can be used in packaging and medical fields.

REFERENCES

1. Silvera Batista, C. A., R. G. Larson, and N. A. Kotov. 2015. "Nonadditivity of nanoparticle interactions". *Science* 350(6257): 1242477–1242477. doi:10.1126/science.1242477.
2. Valenti, G., R. Rampazzo, S. Bonacchi, L. Petrizza, M. Marcaccio, M. Montalti, L. Prodi, and F. Paolucci. 2016. "Variable doping induces mechanism swapping in electrogenerated chemiluminescence of Ru(bpy)$_3$$^{2+}$core shell silica nanoparticles". *Journal of American Chemical Society.* 138(49): 15935–15942. doi:10.1021/jacs.6b08239.
3. Hajipou, M. J., K. M. Fromm, A. A. Ashkarran, D. Jimenez de Aberasturi, I. R. de Larramendi, T. Rojo, V. Serpooshan, W. J. Parak, and M. Mahmoudi. 2012. "Antibacterial properties of nanoparticles". *Trends in Biotechnology.* 30(10): 499–511. doi:10.1016/j.tibtech.2012.06.004.

4. Smekalova, M., V. Aragon, A. Panacek, R. Prucek, R. Zboril, and L. Kvitek. 2016. "Enhanced antibacterial effect of antibiotics in combination with silver nanoparticles against animal pathogens". *Veterinary Journal (London, England: 1997).* 209: 174–179. doi:10.1016/j.tvjl.2015.10.032.
5. Sathyavathi, R., M. Balamurali Krishna, S. Venugopal Rao, R. Saritha, and V. Narayana Rao. 2010. "Biosynthesis of silver nanoparticles using *Coriandrum Sativum* leaf extract and their application in nonlinear optics". *Advanced Science Letters.* 3:138–143. doi:10.1166/asl.2010.1099.
6. Banerjee, P., M. Satapathy, A. Mukhopadhayay, and P. Das. 2014. "Leaf extract mediated green synthesis of silver nanoparticles from widely available Indian plants: Synthesis, characterization, antimicrobial property and toxicity analysis". *Bioresources and Bioprocessing.* 1(3): 1–10. doi:10.1186/s40643-014-0003-y.
7. Kaviya, S., J. Santhanalakshmi, B. Viswanathan, J. Muthumary, and K. Srinivasan. 2011. "Biosynthesis of silver nanoparticles using *Citrus sinensis* peel extract and its antibacterial activity". *Spectrochimica Acta, Part A: Molecular and Biomolecular.* 79: 594–598. doi:10.1016/j.saa.2011.03.040.
8. Bindhani, B. K., and A. K. Panigrahi. 2015. "Biosynthesis and characterization of silver nanoparticles (SNPs) by using leaf extracts of *Ocimum sanctum* L (Tulsi) and study of its antibacterial activities". *Journal of Nanomedicine and Nanotechnology.* S6. doi:10.4172/2157-7439.S6-008.
9. Sutradhar, P., M. Saha, and D. Maiti. 2014. "Microwave synthesis of copper oxide nanoparticles using tea leaf and coffee powder extracts and its antibacterial activity". *Journal of Nanostructure Chemistry.* 4: 86. doi:10.1007/s40097-014-0086-1.
10. Brumbaugh, A. D., K. A. Cohen, and S. K. St. Angelo. 2014. "Ultrasmall copper nanoparticles synthesized with plant tea reducing agent". *ACS Sustainable Chemical & Engineering.* 2: 1933–1939. doi:10.1021/sc500393t.
11. Gebremedhn, K., M. H. Kahsay, and M. Aklilu. 2019. "Green synthesis of CuO nanoparticles using leaf extract of *Catha edulis* and its antibacterial activity". *Journal of Pharmacy and Pharmacology.* 7(6): 327–342. doi:10.17265/2328-2150/2019.06.007
12. Kulkarni, V., S. Suryawanshi, and P. Kulkarni, 2015. "Biosynthesis of copper nanoparticles using aqueous extract of *Eucalyptu s*sp.plant leaves". *Current Science.*109: 255–257.
13. Ananda Murthy, H. C., T. Desalegn, M. Kassa, B. Abebe, and T. Assefa. 2020. "Synthesis of green copper nanoparticles using medicinal plant *Hageniaabyssinica (Brace) JF. Gmel.* leaf extract: Antimicrobial properties". *Journal of Nanomaterials.* Article ID 3924081, 12. doi:10.1155/2020/3924081.
14. Sadanand, V., N. Rajini, B. Satyanarayana, and A. Varada Rajulu. 2016. "Preparation and properties of cellulose/silver nanoparticle composites with in situ generated silver nanoparticles using *Ocimum sanctum* leaf extract". *International Journal of Polymer Analysis and Characterization.* doi:10.1080/1023666X.2016.1161100.
15. Sadanand, V., N. Rajini, B. Satyanarayana, and A. Varada Rajulu. 2016. "Preparation of cellulose composites with in situ generated copper nanoparticles using leaf extract and their properties". *Carbohydrate Polymers.* 150: 32–39. doi:10.1016/j.carbpol.2016.04.121.
16. Sivaranjana, P., E. R. Nagarajan, N. Rajini, M. Jawaid, and A. V. Rajulu. 2017. "Cellulose nanocomposite films with in situ generated silver nanoparticles using *Cassia alata* leaf extract as a reducing agent". *International Journal of Biological Macromolecules.* 99: 223–232. doi:10.1016/j.ijbiomac.2017.02.070.
17. Sivaranjana, P., E. R. Nagarajan, N. Rajini, M. Jawaid, and A. V. Rajulu. 2017. "Formulation and characterization of in situ generated copper nanoparticles reinforced cellulose composite films for potential antimicrobial applications". *Journal of Macromolecular Science Part A.* 55: 1–8. doi:10.1080/10601325.2017.1387488.

18. Muthulakshmi, L., N. Rajini, H. Nellaiah, T. Kathiresan, M. Jawaid, and A. Varada Rajulu. 2017. "Experimental investigation of cellulose/silver nanocomposites using in situ generation method". *Journal of Polymers and the Environment*. 25: 1021–1032. doi:10.1007/s10924-016-0871-7.

19. Muthulakshmi, L., N. Rajini, H. Nellaiah, T. Kathiresan, M. Jawaid, and A. Varada Rajulu. 2017. "Preparation and properties of cellulose nanocomposite films with *in situ* generated copper nanoparticles using *Terminalia catappa* leaf extract". *International Journal of Biological Macromolecules*. 95: 1064–1071. doi:10.1016/j. ijbiomac.2016.09.114.

20. Venkateswara Rao, A., B. Ashok, M. Umamahesh, V. Chandrasekhar, G. V. Subba Reddy, and A. Veranda Rajulu. 2018. "Preparation and properties of silver nanocomposite fabrics with in situ-generated silver nano particles using red sanders powder extract as reducing agent." *International Journal of Polymer Analysis and Characterization*. 23(6): 493–501. doi:10.1080/1023666X.2018.1485200.

21. Venkateswara Rao, A., B. Ashok, M. Umamahesh, V. Chandrasekhar, G. V. Subba Reddy, and A. Veranda Rajulu. 2019. "Preparation and properties of cotton nanocomposite fabrics with *in situ* generated copper nanoparticles using Red sanders powder extract as a reducing agent". *Inorganic and Nano-Metal Chemistry*. 49(10): 343–348. doi:10.1080/24701556.2019.1661437.

22. Pusphalatha, R., B. Ashok, N. Hariram, and A. Veranda Rajulu. 2019. "Nanocomposite polyester fabrics with *in situ* generated silver nanoparticles using tamarind leaf extract reducing agent". *International Journal of Polymer Analysis and Characterization*. 24(6): 524–532. doi:10.1080/1023666X.2019.1614265.

23. Pusphalatha, R., B. Ashok, N. Hariram, and A. Veranda Rajulu. 2020. "Antibacterial polyester fabrics with *in situ* generated copper and cuprous oxide nanoparticles by biodirection method". *Inorganic and Nano-Metal Chemistry*. doi:10.1080/24701556.2020. 1791181.

24. Jaswanth, S., M. Uma Mahesh, A. Prasad, M. Arundathi, G. Venkata Ramanamurthy, N. Hariram, and A. Veranda Rajulu. 2020. "Biosynthesis and study of bimetallic copper and silver nanoparticles on cellulose cotton fabrics using *Moringa oliefiera* leaf extraction as reductant". *Inorganic and Nano-Metal Chemistry*. 50(9):828–835. doi:10.1080/2 4701556.2020.1725571.

25. Venkata Ramanamurthy, G., M. Uma Mahesh, S. Jaswanth, A, Prasad, A. Venkateswara Rao, N. Hariram, and A. Veranda Rajulu. 2020. "In situ generation of silver and silver oxide nanoparticles on cotton fabrics using *Tinospora cordifolia* as bio reductant." *SN Applied Sciences*. 2(3): 1–10. doi:10.1080/24701556.2020.1725571.

26. Sadanand, V., T. H. Feng, A. Veranda Rajulu, and B. Satyanarayana. 2017. "Antibacterial cotton fabric with *in situ* generated silver nanoparticles by one-step hydrothermal method". *International Journal of Polymer Analysis and Characterization*. 22(3): 275–279. doi:10.1080/1023666X.2017.1287828.

27. Sadanand, V., T. H. Feng, A. Veranda Rajulu, and B. Satyanarayana. 2017. "Preparation and properties of low-cost cotton nanocomposite fabrics with *in situ*-generated copper nanoparticles by simple hydrothermal method". *International Journal of Polymer Analysis and Characterization*. 22(7): 587–594. doi:10.1080/1023666X.2017.1344916.

28. Cai, J., and L. Zhang. 2005. "Rapid dissolution of cellulose in LiOH/urea and NaOH/ urea aqueous solutions". *Macromolecular Bioscience*. 5: 539–548. doi:10.1002/ mabi.200400222.

29. Raghavendra, G. M., T. Jayaramudu, K. Varaprasad, and K. Mohana Raju. 2013. "Microbial resistant nanocurcumin-gelatin-cellulose fibers for advanced medical applications". *Royal Society of Chemistry Advances*. 4: 3494–3501. doi:10.1039/ C3RA46429F.

30. Liang, S., J. Wu, H. Tian, L. Zhang, and J. Xu, 2008. "High-strength cellulose/poly(ethylene glycol) gels". *ChemSusChem*.1: 558–563. doi:10.1002/cssc.200800003.
31. Wu, J., Y. Zheng, W. Song, J. Luan, X. Wen, Z. Wu, X. Chen, Q. Wang, and S. Guo. 2014. "*In situ* synthesis of silver-nanoparticles/bacterial cellulose composites for slowreleased antimicrobial wound dressing". *Carbohydrate Polymers*. 102: 762–771. doi:10.1016/j.carbpol.2013.10.093.
32. Alekseeva, O., S. Chulovskaya, N. Bagrovskaya, and V. Parfenyuk. 2011. "Coppernanoparticle composites based on cellulose derivatives". *Chemistry and Chemical Technology*. 5: 447–450. doi:10.23939/chcht05.04.447.
33. Ibrahim, H. M. M. 2015. "Green synthesis and characterization of silver nanoparticles using banana peel extract and their antimicrobial activity against representative microorganisms". *Journal of Radiation Research and Applied Sciences*.8: 265–275. doi:10.1016/j.jrras.2015.01.007.
34. Li, R., M. He, T. Li, and L. Zhang. 2015. "Preparation and properties of cellulose/silver nanocomposite fibers". *Carbohydrate Polymers*. 115: 259–275. doi:10.1016/j.carbpol.2014.08.046.
35. Sedighi, A., M. Montazer, and N. Hemmatinejad. 2014. "Copper nanoparticles on bleached cotton fabric: In situ synthesis and characterization". *Cellulose*. 21(3): 2119–2132. doi:10.1007/s10570-014-0215-5.
36. Palza, H. 2015. "Antimicrobial polymers with metal nanoparticles". *International Journal of Molecular Sciences*. 16(1): 2099–2116. doi:10.3390/ijms16012099.

6 Antibacterial Ceramics
The Past, Present, and Future

Hideyuki Kanematsu, Dana M. Barry,
Risa Kawai, Takeshi Kogo, Akiko Ogawa,
Paul McGrath, and Toshihiro Tanaka

CONTENTS

6.1   INTRODUCTION

The antibacterial effect is defined as a characteristic of materials' surfaces that protects them from harmful environments. Materials are generally classified into three categories in terms of bonding forces: metals, ceramics (inorganic materials excluding metals), and organic ones. The first type is built by metallic bonding. The second one is ionic bonding and/or covalent bonding. The third group involves covalent bonding and/or interatomic forces. The differences among bonding forces are reflected by the interaction between bacteria and materials' surfaces and by the differences of antibacterial mechanisms.

Metallic materials exist with metallic bonding. As shown in Figure 6.1, metals produce metallic ions on surfaces (to a greater or lesser extent). The metallic ions interact with polymeric substances derived from bacterial cells. When the interaction occurs on cells' outer surfaces, bacteria do not survive. Based on our many years of experience [1–18], this metallic ion mechanism seems to be the main one for the antibacterial effect of metallic materials. However, the mechanism by radical oxygen has also been supported. Some researchers have indicated that the interaction between silver ions and bacterial cells leads to the production of hydroxy radicals [19–21]. The following reaction is well known as the Fenton reaction [22–32].

DOI: 10.1201/9781003143093-6

85

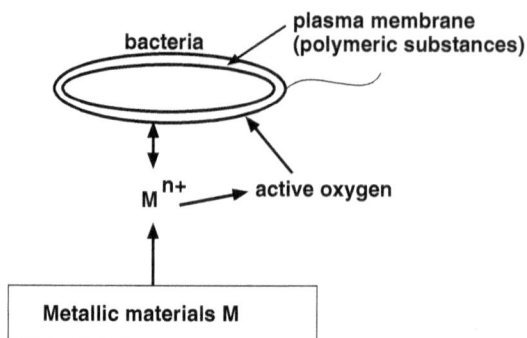

FIGURE 6.1 Antibacterial interaction between metallic materials and bacteria.

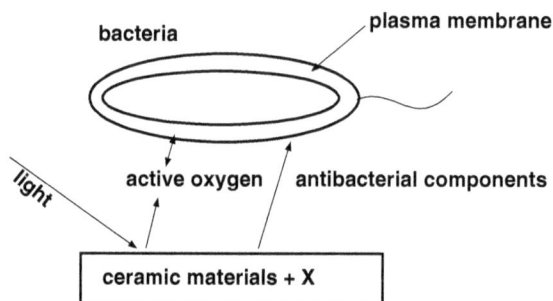

FIGURE 6.2 Antibacterial interaction between ceramics and bacteria.

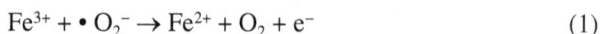

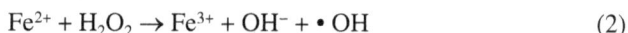

$$Fe^{3+} + \bullet O_2^- \rightarrow Fe^{2+} + O_2 + e^- \tag{1}$$

$$Fe^{2+} + H_2O_2 \rightarrow Fe^{3+} + OH^- + \bullet OH \tag{2}$$

$\bullet O_2^-$: super oxide, $\bullet OH$: hydroxy radical

And the following reaction is well known as the Haber–Weiss reaction.

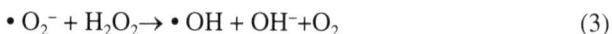

$$\bullet O_2^- + H_2O_2 \rightarrow \bullet OH + OH^- + O_2 \tag{3}$$

As for copper, the metallic ions break the plasma membranes of bacteria. On the other hand, the Fenton reaction occurs to produce hydroxy radicals in this case [33–40].

Antibacterial ceramics also break the outer part of bacterial cells, as shown in Figure 6.2 schematically. However, they are classified into several types, in terms of the mechanisms. The details will be explained in the next section.

Antibacterial organic compounds also break the outer part of bacterial cells [41–45]. The interaction between the organic compounds and the organic components of bacterial cells damages the outer part of bacteria (Figure 6.3).

In this chapter, we focus on ceramic materials. Mechanisms for the antibacterial effect by ceramics are discussed and some concrete examples of antibacterial ceramics are mentioned.

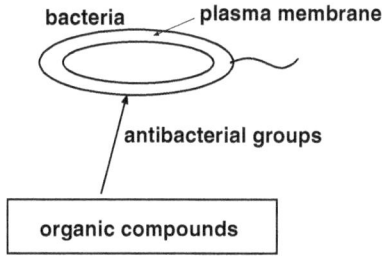

FIGURE 6.3 Antibacterial interaction between organic compounds and bacteria.

6.2 CLASSIFICATION OF ANTIBACTERIAL CERAMICS

The term ceramics was originally the name of tools our ancestors devised at the cradle of civilization, such as earthenware, porcelain, and bricks. However, ceramics nowadays encompasses a very wide area involving metallic and non-metallic elements. Oxides, carbides, nitrides, silicides, borides, and the compounds between metallic elements and non-metallic elements are representative industrial ceramics. In the past, such a crystalline inorganic material was considered as ceramic, but recently, the definition has been extended. Now it includes amorphous glasses, carbon materials, and other inorganic materials (except for metallic ones) [46]. When thinking about antibacterial ceramics, we must consider two main categories. The first category is composed of ceramics that show the antibacterial effect. Most conventional ceramics such as oxides, nitrides, and carbides have relatively stable surfaces. This means that any force fields, e.g., van der Waals force field, are not developed outside of the materials' surfaces. In this case, photocatalytic ceramics could show the antibacterial effect. Some ceramics such as titanium oxide could produce active oxygen through photocatalytic reactions to kill bacteria. Usually, the phenomenon is caused by ultraviolet light. The second category is the transition-metal-doped ceramics. When some transition metallic elements were doped into photocatalytic ceramics, the band gap between the conduction band and the valency one is decreased. Therefore, active oxygens are easily produced in this case. They are produced more than in the case of pure photocatalytic titanium oxide. As a result, such metal-doped ceramics could show the antibacterial effect by lower energy visible light. The third group is the antibacterial metal supported ceramics. This category contains antibacterial glasses, which originally do not show the antibacterial effect. The fourth category is advanced carbon materials. Particularly, graphene and carbon nanotubes can be mentioned. They often show strong antibacterial effects. Figure 6.4 shows the classification schematically.

The antibacterial ceramics (mentioned already) interact with bacterial cells in their own way. Figure 6.5 shows various interactions of antibacterial components with bacterial cells schematically. As described already, the "first contact" with antibacterial components for bacteria must be the outer part, as mentioned in the introduction [47–50]. The outer part of bacterial cells makes the first contact with materials' surfaces. Therefore, the mechanism seems to be a critical one. However,

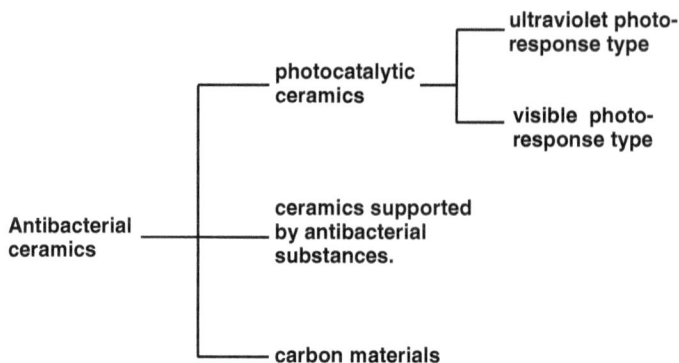

FIGURE 6.4 Classification of antibacterial ceramics.

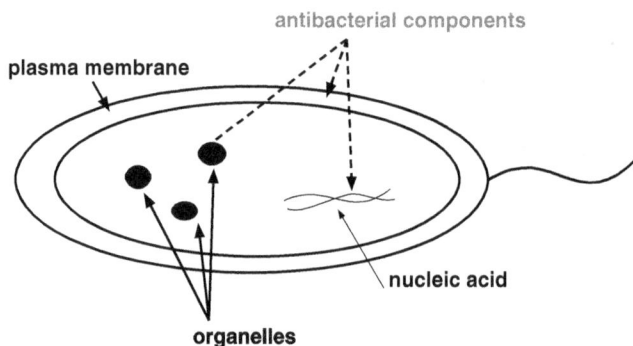

FIGURE 6.5 Overall correlations between antibacterial components in ceramics and bacterial cells.

some of the materials' components could penetrate plasma membranes to interact with organelles within the bacterial cells [51–55]. In such a case, the bacterial cells would deteriorate. As a concrete example, we can mention the antibacterial organic compounds incorporating antibiotics as components. Besides these examples, the antibacterial components could interact with nucleic acids (DNA or RNA) within bacterial cells. We can mention chitosan as an example [56–60].

6.3 PHOTOCATALYTIC CERAMICS

To apply the mechanisms described earlier to ceramic materials, they can be classified into two types as bulk materials: photocatalytic ceramics and ceramics composed of antibacterial metallic elements. Both types damage the outer part of bacterial cells. On the other hand, appropriate antibacterial substances can be inserted and supported by ceramics. In such a case, antimicrobial components could interact with organelles or nucleic acids inside the bacterial cells. In this section, photocatalytic ceramics is explained.

Photocatalytic ceramics can be classified into two more types, according to the wavelength inducing photocatalysis: ultraviolet photoresponse [61–65] and visible photoresponse [66–70]. The former one exhibits photocatalysis by ultraviolet light, while the latter one is by the visible light.

Titanium oxides have been well known as representative ultraviolet photoresponse type ceramics. Since titanium oxide has the bandgap of 3.2 eV, the ultraviolet wavelength at 380 nm and more can excite electrons in the valency band to the conduction band. Then, two kinds of reactions could occur. One of them is a photoinduced hydrophobic reaction, while the other is a photoinduced decomposition reaction.

Photoinduced hydrophobic reactions affect the surface of ceramics. In general, hydrophobic surfaces repel water and are water fearing, while hydrophilic surfaces are water loving. Ultraviolet rays decompose the organic compounds existing on materials' surfaces. However, the mechanism is not enough to explain all involved phenomena [71–73]. Hashimoto et al. attributed the cause to the change of ceramics' surface energy. At any rate, the effect would promote the photoinduced decomposition reaction.

Photoinduced decomposition reactions are defined as the reactions where positive holes and electrons produced by photocatalysis react with molecules on materials' surfaces. Basically, the reaction is reduction and oxidation (Redox reactions).

Oxidation reactions can be described as follows:

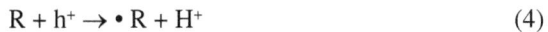

$$R + h^+ \rightarrow \bullet R + H^+ \tag{4}$$

R: organic compound, h^+: positive hole, $\bullet$ R: oxidized compound, H+: proton.

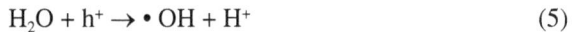

$$H_2O + h^+ \rightarrow \bullet OH + H^+ \tag{5}$$

$\bullet$ OH: Hydroxyl radical

The hydroxyl radical produced by reaction (2) also contributes to decomposition of organic compounds.

On the other hand, the reduction reaction can be described as follows:

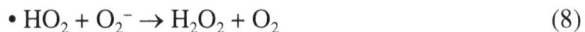

$$O_2 + e^- \rightarrow O_2^- \tag{6}$$

$$O_2^- + H^+ \rightarrow \bullet HO_2 \tag{7}$$

$$\bullet HO_2 + O_2^- \rightarrow H_2O_2 + O_2 \tag{8}$$

The reduction reaction also promotes the decomposition of organic compounds.

The main reaction for the antibacterial effect by ceramics should be the photoinduced decomposition reaction. The mechanism is illustrated in Figure 6.6 schematically. When ultraviolet light is irradiated on titanium oxide, the electrons in the valency band are excited and move to the energy level of the conduction band beyond the energy gap (3.2 eV in the case of titanium oxides). Then, the excited electrons can move freely to react with oxygen molecules on materials' surfaces and protons. They are reduced by the electrons to produce active oxygen such as "superoxide."

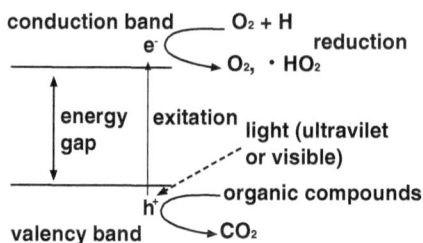

FIGURE 6.6 Photocatalytic reactions of ceramics and produced active oxygen.

On the other hand, produced holes in valency bands react with organic compounds and oxidize them to produce active oxygen and organic molecules. These products contribute to oxidize bacterial cells and show the antibacterial effect. Being compared with antibacterial metallic materials (such as silver and copper), the decrease of the antibacterial effect is caused by the formation of compounds and environmental factors (e.g., silver can easily form sulfides, and copper tends to form oxides). The ceramic products have higher resistance in relatively high temperature conditions and the minimum concentration for the antibacterial effect is relatively low (MIC: several ppm and lesser).

Many investigations have been carried out and the data have been accumulated in academic fields. Gram-negative bacteria *Escherichia coli* has been picked up as target bacteria very often [74–77]. O-157 is a type of *E. coli* and a strong pathogen. TiO_2 works well for O-157 [78–81]. *Pseudomonas aeruginosa* are also pathogenic gram-negative bacteria that cause cystic fibrosis and other opportunistic diseases. The bacteria are motile and easily form biofilms. Therefore, a lot of research results exist for them. TiO_2 also controls *P. aeruginosa* [82–85]. Many pathogenic gram-positive bacteria such as *Staphylococcus aureus* [86–88] and MRSA [89–93] have been investigated with results confirming their antibacterial effects. For many applications, TiO_2 was prepared as bulk materials, thin films, paints, even nanotubes, etc. Most of the antibacterial effects were present with light. However, in some cases, TiO_2 could show the antibacterial effect in the dark [94]. In most of those cases, the ceramics were doped or loaded with other antibacterial components, such as Co [95], Ag [96], and composites of copper and chitosan [97]. Therefore, we are afraid that those ceramics will not always be purely photocatalytic ones. We presume that other antibacterial components might contribute to the antibacterial effect in the dark by another mechanism.

When some transition metal elements are doped into titanium oxides, it is well known that the bandgap decreases from the original value of 3.23 eV, as shown in Table 6.1 [98]. The doped TiO_2 is sensitive to photocatalytic reactions in the dark to some extent.

Such doped or supported antibacterial elements in TiO_2 make the photocatalytic reactions possible in the visible light range. Particularly, Cu (II)/TiO_2 and Fe (III)/TiO_2 are well known. When we take Cu (II)/TiO_2 as an example, irradiated visible light excites and moves electrons in the valency band of TiO_2 to the nanocluster of copper [106].

TABLE 6.1
The Maximum Decrease of TiO$_2$ Doped with Transition Metal Elements

Dopant metal	The maximum decrease of bang gap (eV)	References
Vanadium	0.67	[99]
Iron	0.51	[100–101]
Cobalt	Unknown	[95]
Nickel	0.87	[102]
Copper	0.73	[103–104]
Tin	0.95	[105]

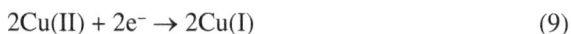

$$2Cu(II) + 2e^- \rightarrow 2Cu(I) \tag{9}$$

The copper nanocluster reduces oxygen to produce hydrogen peroxide solution.

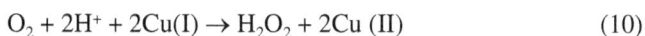

$$O_2 + 2H^+ + 2Cu(I) \rightarrow H_2O_2 + 2Cu\ (II) \tag{10}$$

On the other hand, the produced positive hole (h$^+$) by the irradiation of visible light oxidizes organic compounds on materials' surfaces. As a result, materials' surfaces are cleaned. Both effects are synchronized, so the antibacterial effect becomes effective.

The antibacterial doped or supported TiO$_2$ could also control the growth of many bacteria, such as *E. coli* [107], *S. aureus* [108–111], and MRSA [112–115].

6.4 CERAMICS COMPOSED OF ANTIBACTERIAL METALS

As described before, many ceramics do not show any antibacterial effects except for some photocatalytic ceramics. However, there are some examples without photocatalytic reactions. Cupric oxide (Cu$_2$O, monovalent copper oxide) is one of those representative antibacterial ceramics. Even though the antibacterial mechanism has not been fixed yet, it is evident that monovalent copper ion shows a very strong antibacterial effect [116]. One of the possible mechanisms is the strong affinity of monovalent copper ion to proteins derived from bacteria [117]. On the other hand, some researchers attribute the mechanism of antibacterial monovalent copper ion to the production of the OH radical (Fenton reaction) [118].

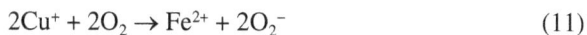

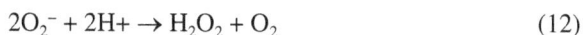

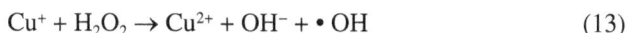

$$2Cu^+ + 2O_2 \rightarrow Fe^{2+} + 2O_2^- \tag{11}$$

$$2O_2^- + 2H+ \rightarrow H_2O_2 + O_2 \tag{12}$$

$$Cu^+ + H_2O_2 \rightarrow Cu^{2+} + OH^- + \bullet OH \tag{13}$$

In this case, antibacterial components would be the bulk materials that do not have any original antibacterial effects. Such a non-antibacterial material could show an antibacterial effect, by supporting antibacterial components. However, there are some antibacterial ceramics with bulk components.

Conventional industrial ceramics such as silica and alumina can be mentioned as examples. The antibacterial metallic materials such as silver, zinc, and copper are mixed into those ceramics.

A representative ceramic in this category is zeolite [119–121]. Zeolite is basically a complex oxide composed of alumina and silica containing water molecules. It contains regular tube-shaped channels and cavities. Metallic ions can be inserted into those channels and cavities to show antibacterial effects. Among those antibacterial metal supporting zeolites is Ag-Zeolite that is well known [122–124]. Usually, they are white micropowders (diameter: 10^{-6} m) that are in commercial use [125–127]. The second method is the mixing into paints which would be used for coatings.

The principle of Ag-Zeolite can be applied to other ceramics. To name a few, silica gels [128], zirconium phosphate [129], calcium phosphate [130], silicic acid compounds [131], etc. can be mentioned. Antibacterial glasses are also produced in similar ways. In these cases, the key points are how antibacterial components should be incorporated into the bulk ceramics. The antibacterial metallic ions should be produced in minimum amounts (over a specific period of time), since they often lose their antibacterial effects by the production of compounds with environmental factors such as oxygen, chloride ions, sulfide ions, and organic compounds. When those compounds form, the ionization in aqueous environments would stop with the antibacterial effects in many cases. Therefore, the knowledge and know-how in the materials science and engineering fields must play important roles to produce antibacterial ceramics. Such a concept of composite antibacterial ceramics is recently being applied in practical fields. We are talking about the design, investigation, and development of antibacterial metals, organic compounds such as antibiotics, and other biocides.

6.5   CONCLUSIONS AND FUTURE PERSPECTIVE

In this chapter, we described antibacterial ceramics and their mechanisms by classifying them into three categories. Antibacterial effects differ for each one. Photocatalytic ceramics express the antibacterial effect by producing radical oxygen. Ceramics doped with antibacterial metals produce antibacterial ions as well as the active oxygen. On the other hand, ceramics supporting antibacterial metals show the metal ions' antibacterial effects. Similar principles can be applied to other antibacterial components such as organic compounds.

Antibacterial effects are important characteristics needed to control bacteria. However, they are not enough in the light of practicality. Generally, bacteria do not live individually, but live in groups. The bacterial state where individual bacteria are floating in environments is called "planktonic." However, such a situation is not favorable for bacteria to survive. In most cases, the state is oligotrophic. Therefore, bacteria usually exist in biofilms. This state is more common for bacteria. Actually, more than 90% of natural bacteria exist in biofilms. From the viewpoint, the antibiofilm properties of ceramics should be investigated much more. Both topics are closely related, but do not usually overlap completely. The time dependencies are sometimes lacking or weak for the concept of the antibacterial effect, while they are more important for biofilms because biofilms are formed through multi-step processes with time. One more big difference is the contribution of killed and broken bacteria. In the case of the antibacterial effect, only the viable bacteria should be considered. On the other hand, dead and collapsed bacteria are also important components of biofilms, since they are still organic compounds and polymeric substances including nucleic acids in biofilms. Therefore, the antibiofilm properties should be investigated more in the future.

Antiviral effects and characteristics should also be investigated more. Humans are now suffering from COVID-19. Therefore, we are concentrating on the antiviral properties of materials. From that viewpoint, antiviral properties of ceramics should be investigated further. Most antibacterial ceramics also show antiviral properties at this point. However, we should also focus on their differences. A new door to control infections through ceramics will be open in the future.

ACKNOWLEDGMENTS

A part of this work was supported by the GEAR 5.0 Project of the National Institute of Technology (KOSEN) in Japan as well as JSPS KAKENHI (Grants-in-Aid for Scientific Research from the Japan Society for the Promotion of Science), Grant Number 20K05185 and 21K12739. We also appreciate SIAA (The Society of International Sustaining Growth for Antimicrobial Articles) for their useful advice. And we also appreciate Prof. Peerawatt Nunthavarawong for his well-timed advice, kind consideration, encouragement, and patience.

REFERENCES

1. Ikigai, H., H. Kanematsu, K. Kuroda, and Y. Kikuchi. "Antibacterial effect of the plating metals to some bacteria." *CAMP-ISIJ* 17 (2004): 1125–1126.
2. Ikigai, H., H. Kanematsu, K. Kuroda, and A. Ohmori. "Antibacterial activity by alloying of tin & copper plating." *SFIC Sur/Fin* (2005): 497–503.
3. Kanematsu, H., H. Ezaki, H. Ikegai, T., and T. Oki. *Sn-Cu Alloy Thin Film Having Antibacterial Property, Sn-Cu Alloy Thin film-Formed Article Having Antibacterial Property, and Method for Producing Sn-Cu Alloy Thin Film-Formed Article Having Antibacterial Property*, 2005. https://www.zhangqiaokeyan.com/patent-detail/06130436025553.html.
4. Kanematsu, H., H. Ikigai, and M. Yoshitake. "Antibacterial eco-plating based on HACCP system." *Bulletin of Tokai Kagaku Kougyoukai (The Society of Chemical Industry in Midland of Japan)* 252 (2006): 9–14.
5. Kanematsu, H., H. Ikigai, and M. Yoshitake. "Alloying of tin plating film with silver by combination of multistage plating and heat treatment for antibacterial property." *Sur/Fin* (2007): 13–15.
6. Kanematsu, H., H. Ikigai, D. Kuroda, M. Yoshitake, and S. Yagyu. "Tin-cobalt alloy film formation through heat treatment and its antibacterial property." *The 17th IFHTSE Congress* (2008): 210.
7. Kanematsu, H., H. Ikigai, and M. Yoshitake. "Antibacterial eco-plating based on HACCP and biofilm." *Bulletin of the Iron and Steel Institute of Japan* 13 (2008): 27–34.
8. Kanematsu, H., H. Ikigai, and M. Yoshitake. "Antibacterial tin-silver plating by the combination of multistage plating and heat treatment." *The Journal of Applied Surface Finishing* 2008 (2008): 114–118.

9.   Kanematsu, H., H. Ikigai, D. Kuroda, M. Yoshitake, and S. Yagyu. "Tin-cobalt alloy film formation through heat treatment and its antibacterial property." *Proceedings of the 17th IFHTSE Congress* 49 (2009): 284–287.
10. Kanematsu, H., H. Ikigai, D. Kuroda, M. Yoshitake, S. Yagyu, and A. Ogawa. "Tin-palladium alloy formation by heat treatment-alloy plating process and antibacterial effect of its film." *The Journal of Japan Society for Heat Treatment* 49 (2009): 274–278.
11. Kuroda, D., H. Ikigai, H. Kanematsu, and A. Ogawa. "Difference between antibacterial effect and inhibition capability against biofilm formation by surface coatings." *Processing and Fabrication of Advanced Materials-XVIII* 3 (2009): 1149–1158.
12. Kanematsu, H. *Antibacterial Materials for Safety, Security and Reliability.* Yoneda Shuppan Co., 2010, p. 154.
13. Ikegai, H., and H. Kanematsu. "Mechanism for antibacterial effects by metallic elements and their inhibition of bacterial infections." *Journal of Japanese Society for Biomaterials* 29 (2011): 232–239.
14. Kanematsu, H., H. Ikegai, and M. Yoshitake. "Patents for antibacterial metallic coating and its future trend in Japan." *Research Inventy: International Journal of Engineering and Science* 3 (2013): 47–55.
15. Kanematsu, H., and D.M. Barry. "Antibacterial effect of materials and biofilm." *Biofilm and Materials Science* (2015): 169–174. doi:10.1007/978-3-319-14565-5_21.
16. Kanematsu, H., and M. Yoshitake. *Nanocomposite Coating for Antibacterial Purposes.* A.S.H. Makhlouf and D. Sharnweber, Eds. Elsevier, 2015, pp. 498–513.
17. Kanematsu, H. "A new international standard for testing antibacterial effects." *Advanced Materials & Processing* 175 (2017): 26–29.
18. Kanematsu, H., R. Kawai, and R. Satoh. "Antibacterial, antiviral and antibiofilm coatings." *The Journal of Japan Thermal Spray Society (JTSS)* 57 (2020): 183–190.
19. Barras, Frédéric, Laurent Aussel, and Benjamin Ezraty. "Silver and antibiotic, new facts to an old story." *Antibiotics* 7, no. 3 (2018): 79.
20. Morones-Ramirez, Jose Ruben, Jonathan A. Winkler, Catherine S. Spina, and James J. Collins. "Silver enhances antibiotic activity against gram-negative bacteria." *Science Translational Medicine* 5, no. 190 (2013): 190ra81.
21. Park, Hee-Jin, Jee Yeon Kim, Jaeeun Kim, Joon-Hee Lee, Ji-Sook Hahn, Man Bock Gu, and Jeyong Yoon. "Silver-ion-mediated reactive oxygen species generation affecting bactericidal activity." *Water Research* 43, no. 4 (2009): 1027–1032.
22. Winterbourn, Christine C. "Toxicity of iron and hydrogen peroxide: The Fenton reaction." *Toxicology Letters* 82 (1995): 969–974.
23. Gutteridge, John M.C. "Iron promoters of the Fenton reaction and lipid peroxidation can be released from haemoglobin by peroxides." *FEBS Letters* 201, no. 2 (1986): 291–295.
24. Salgado, Pablo, Victoria Melin, David Contreras, Yanko Moreno, and Hector D. Mansilla. "Fenton reaction driven by iron ligands." *Journal of the Chilean Chemical Society* 58, no. 4 (2013): 2096–2101.
25. Toyokuni, Shinya. "Iron and carcinogenesis: From Fenton reaction to target genes." *Redox Report* 7, no. 4 (2002): 189–197.
26. Hug, Stephan J., and Olivier Leupin. "Iron-catalyzed oxidation of arsenic (III) by oxygen and by hydrogen peroxide: pH-dependent formation of oxidants in the Fenton reaction." *Environmental Science & Technology* 37, no. 12 (2003): 2734–2742.
27. Zhang, Chen, Wenbo Bu, Dalong Ni, Shenjian Zhang, Qing Li, Zhenwei Yao, Jiawen Zhang, Heliang Yao, Zheng Wang, and Jianlin Shi. "Synthesis of iron nanometallic glasses and their application in cancer therapy by a localized Fenton reaction." *Angewandte Chemie* 128, no. 6 (2016): 2141–2146.
28. Cohen, Gerald. "The Fenton reaction." *Handbook of Methods for Oxygen Radical Research* (1985): 55–64.

29. Wang, Chuan, Hong Liu, and Zhimin Sun. "Heterogeneous photo-Fenton reaction catalyzed by nanosized iron oxides for water treatment." *International Journal of Photoenergy* 2012 (2012).
30. Engelmann, Mark D., Robert T. Bobier, Terrance Hiatt, and I. Francis Cheng. "Variability of the Fenton reaction characteristics of the EDTA, DTPA, and citrate complexes of iron." *Biometals* 16, no. 4 (2003): 519–527.
31. Engelmann, Mark D., Robert T. Bobier, Terrance Hiatt, and I. Francis Cheng. "Variability of the Fenton reaction characteristics of the EDTA, DTPA, and citrate complexes of iron." *Biometals* 16, no. 4 (2003): 519–527.
32. Burkitt, M.J., and B.C. Gilbert. "Model studies of the iron-catalysed Haber-Weiss cycle and the ascorbate-driven Fenton reaction." *Free Radical Research Communications* 10, no. 4–5 (1990): 265–280.
33. Sutton, Harry C., and Christine C. Winterbourn. "On the participation of higher oxidation states of iron and copper in Fenton reactions." *Free Radical Biology and Medicine* 6, no. 1 (1989): 53–60.
34. Lloyd, Daniel R., and David H. Phillips. "Oxidative DNA damage mediated by copper (II), iron (II) and nickel (II) Fenton reactions: Evidence for site-specific mechanisms in the formation of double-strand breaks, 8-hydroxydeoxyguanosine and putative intra-strand cross-links." *Mutation Research/Fundamental and Molecular Mechanisms of Mutagenesis* 424, no. 1–2 (1999): 23–36.
35. Gutteridge, John M.C. "Inhibition of the Fenton reaction by the protein caeruloplasmin and other copper complexes: Assessment of ferroxidase and radical scavenging activities." *Chemico-Biological Interactions* 56, no. 1 (1985): 113–120.
36. Pham, A. Ninh, Guowei Xing, Christopher J. Miller, and T. David Waite. "Fenton-like copper redox chemistry revisited: Hydrogen peroxide and superoxide mediation of copper-catalyzed oxidant production." *Journal of Catalysis* 301 (2013): 54–64.
37. Li, Xia, Sijia Hao, Ailing Han, Yayu Yang, Guozhen Fang, Jifeng Liu, and Shuo Wang. "Intracellular Fenton reaction based on mitochondria-targeted copper (ii) – peptide complex for induced apoptosis." *Journal of Materials Chemistry B* 7, no. 25 (2019): 4008–4016.
38. Yao, Tongjie, Yi Qi, Yuqing Mei, Yang Yang, Rashed Aleisa, Xin Tong, and Jie Wu. "One-step preparation of reduced graphene oxide aerogel loaded with mesoporous copper ferrite nanocubes: A highly efficient catalyst in microwave-assisted Fenton reaction." *Journal of Hazardous Materials* 378 (2019): 120712.
39. Gutteridge, John M.C., and Joe V. Bannister. "Copper+ zinc and manganese superoxide dismutases inhibit deoxyribose degradation by the superoxide-driven Fenton reaction at two different stages: Implications for the redox states of copper and manganese." *Biochemical Journal* 234, no. 1 (1986): 225–228.
40. Valenzuela, Roberto, David Contreras, Claudia Oviedo, Juanita Freer, and Jaime Rodríguez. "Copper catechol-driven Fenton reactions and their potential role in wood degradation." *International Biodeterioration & Biodegradation* 61, no. 4 (2008): 345–350.
41. Buffet-Bataillon, Sylvie, Pierre Tattevin, Martine Bonnaure-Mallet, and Anne Jolivet-Gougeon. "Emergence of resistance to antibacterial agents: The role of quaternary ammonium compounds – a critical review." *International Journal of Antimicrobial Agents* 39, no. 5 (2012): 381–389.
42. Makvandi, Pooyan, Rezvan Jamaledin, Mostafa Jabbari, Nasser Nikfarjam, and Assunta Borzacchiello. "Antibacterial quaternary ammonium compounds in dental materials: A systematic review." *Dental Materials* 34, no. 6 (2018): 851–867.
43. Eley, B.M. "Antibacterial agents in the control of supragingival plaque – a review." *British Dental Journal* 186, no. 6 (1999): 286–296.

44. Yongjun, Chen, Li Bengao, and Wang Xieqing. "Advances in organic antibacterial agents [J]." *Petroleum Processing and Petrochemicals* 1 (1997).
45. Chapman, John S. "Biocide resistance mechanisms." *International Biodeterioration & Biodegradation* 51, no. 2 (2003): 133–138.
46. Callister, William D., and David G. Rethwisch. *Callister's Materials Science and Engineering.* John Wiley & Sons, 2020.
47. Trombetta, Domenico, Francesco Castelli, Maria Grazia Sarpietro, Vincenza Venuti, Mariateresa Cristani, Claudia Daniele, Antonella Saija, Gabriela Mazzanti, and Giuseppe Bisignano. "Mechanisms of antibacterial action of three monoterpenes." *Antimicrobial Agents and Chemotherapy* 49, no. 6 (2005): 2474–2478.
48. Bondarenko, Olesja M., Mariliis Sihtmäe, Julia Kuzmičiova, Lina Ragelienė, Anne Kahru, and Rimantas Daugelavičius. "Plasma membrane is the target of rapid antibacterial action of silver nanoparticles in *Escherichia coli* and *Pseudomonas aeruginosa*." *International Journal of Nanomedicine* 13 (2018): 6779.
49. Corre, J., J.J. Lucchini, G.M. Mercier, and A. Cremieux. "Antibacterial activity of phenethyl alcohol and resulting membrane alterations." *Research in Microbiology* 141, no. 4 (1990): 483–497.
50. Corre, J., J.J. Lucchini, G.M. Mercier, and A. Cremieux. "Antibacterial activity of phenethyl alcohol and resulting membrane alterations." *Research in Microbiology* 141, no. 4 (1990): 483–497.
51. Thatiparti, Thimma R., Andrew J. Shoffstall, and Horst A. Von Recum. "Cyclodextrin-based device coatings for affinity-based release of antibiotics." *Biomaterials* 31, no. 8 (2010): 2335–2347.
52. Stigter, M., J. Bezemer, K. De Groot, and P. Layrolle. "Incorporation of different antibiotics into carbonated hydroxyapatite coatings on titanium implants, release and antibiotic efficacy." *Journal of Controlled Release* 99, no. 1 (2004): 127–137.
53. Brohede, Ulrika, Johan Forsgren, Stefan Roos, Albert Mihranyan, Håkan Engqvist, and Maria Strømme. "Multifunctional implant coatings providing possibilities for fast antibiotics loading with subsequent slow release." *Journal of Materials Science: Materials in Medicine* 20, no. 9 (2009): 1859–1867.
54. Song, Jiankang, Qiang Chen, Yang Zhang, Mani Diba, Eva Kolwijck, Jinlong Shao, John A. Jansen, Fang Yang, Aldo R. Boccaccini, and Sander CG Leeuwenburgh. "Electrophoretic deposition of chitosan coatings modified with gelatin nanospheres to tune the release of antibiotics." *ACS Applied Materials & Interfaces* 8, no. 22 (2016): 13785–13792.
55. Pan, Chenhao, Zubin Zhou, and Xiaowei Yu. "Coatings as the useful drug delivery system for the prevention of implant-related infections." *Journal of Orthopaedic Surgery and Research* 13, no. 1 (2018): 1–11.
56. Sudarshan, N.R., D.G. Hoover, and D. Knorr. "Antibacterial action of chitosan." *Food Biotechnology* 6, no. 3 (1992): 257–272.
57. Fei Liu, Xiao, Yun Lin Guan, Dong Zhi Yang, Zhi Li, and Kang De Yao. "Antibacterial action of chitosan and carboxymethylated chitosan." *Journal of Applied Polymer Science* 79, no. 7 (2001): 1324–1335.
58. Qi, Lifeng, Zirong Xu, Xia Jiang, Caihong Hu, and Xiangfei Zou. "Preparation and antibacterial activity of chitosan nanoparticles." *Carbohydrate Research* 339, no. 16 (2004): 2693–2700.
59. Raafat, Dina, Kristine Von Bargen, Albert Haas, and Hans-Georg Sahl. "Insights into the mode of action of chitosan as an antibacterial compound." *Applied and Environmental Microbiology* 74, no. 12 (2008): 3764–3773.
60. Chung, Ying-Chien, and Chih-Yu Chen. "Antibacterial characteristics and activity of acid-soluble chitosan." *Bioresource Technology* 99, no. 8 (2008): 2806–2814.

61. Liu, Chien-Min, Chih Chen, and Hsyi-En Cheng. "Ultraviolet photoresponse of TiO_2 nanotube arrays fabricated by atomic layer deposition." *Electrochemical and Solid State Letters* 14, no. 6 (2011): K33.

62. Mondal, Sulakshana, and Durga Basak. "Very high photoresponse towards low-powered UV light under low-biased condition by nanocrystal assembled TiO_2 film." *Applied Surface Science* 427 (2018): 814–822.

63. Yu, Hongtao, Shuo Chen, Xie Quan, Huimin Zhao, and Yaobin Zhang. "Silicon nanowire/TiO_2 heterojunction arrays for effective photoelectrocatalysis under simulated solar light irradiation." *Applied Catalysis B: Environmental* 90, no. 1–2 (2009): 242–248.

64. Li, Shasha, Tao Deng, Yang Zhang, Yuning Li, Weijie Yin, Qi Chen, and Zewen Liu. "Solar-blind ultraviolet detection based on TiO_2 nanoparticles decorated graphene field-effect transistors." *Nanophotonics* 8, no. 5 (2019): 899–908.

65. Zheng, Xin, Yihui Sun, Haiying Qin, Zhenguo Ji, and Hongzhong Chi. "Interface engineering on ZnO/Au based Schottky junction for enhanced photoresponse of UV detector with TiO_2 inserting layer." *Journal of Alloys and Compounds* 816 (2020): 152537.

66. Land, C.E., and P.S. Peercy. "A review of the effects of ion implantation on the photoferroelectric properties of PLZT ceramics." *Ferroelectrics* 45, no. 1 (1982): 25–43.

67. Lv, Jianguo, Jinhua Xu, Min Zhao, Pengpeng Yan, Sicong Mao, Fengjiao Shang, Gang He, Miao Zhang, and Zhaoqi Sun. "Effect of seed layer on optical properties and visible photoresponse of ZnO/Cu2O composite thin films." *Ceramics International* 41, no. 10 (2015): 13983–13987.

68. He, Xiang, Chen Chen, Chunbo Li, Huarong Zeng, and Zhiguo Yi. "Ferroelectric, photoelectric, and photovoltaic performance of silver niobate ceramics." *Advanced Functional Materials* 29, no. 28 (2019): 1900918.

69. Wang, Wenhao, Shun Wang, Jianguo Lv, Min Zhao, Miao Zhang, Gang He, Chenxu Fang, Lele Li, and Zhaoqi Sun. "Enhanced photoresponse and photocatalytic activities of graphene quantum dots sensitized Ag/TiO_2 thin film." *Journal of the American Ceramic Society* 101, no. 12 (2018): 5469–5476.

70. Zhong, Haoyin, Hongyuan Xiao, Nan Jiao, and Yiping Guo. "Boosting piezoelectric response of KNN-based ceramics with strong visible-light absorption." *Journal of the American Ceramic Society* 102, no. 11 (2019): 6422–6426.

71. Miyauchi, Masahiro, Akira Nakajima, Akira Fujishima, Kazuhito Hashimoto, and Toshiya Watanabe. "Photoinduced surface reactions on TiO_2 and $SrTiO_3$ films: Photocatalytic oxidation and photoinduced hydrophilicity." *Chemistry of Materials* 12, no. 1 (2000): 3–5.

72. Watanabe, T., A. Nakajima, R. Wang, M. Minabe, S. Koizumi, A. Fujishima, and K. Hashimoto. "Photocatalytic activity and photoinduced hydrophilicity of titanium dioxide coated glass." *Thin Solid Films* 351, no. 1–2 (1999): 260–263.

73. Sun, Ren-De, Akira Nakajima, Akira Fujishima, Toshiya Watanabe, and Kazuhito Hashimoto. "Photoinduced surface wettability conversion of ZnO and TiO_2 thin films." *The Journal of Physical Chemistry B* 105, no. 10 (2001): 1984–1990.

74. Ireland, John C., Petra Klostermann, Eugene W. Rice, and Robert M. Clark. "Inactivation of *Escherichia coli* by titanium dioxide photocatalytic oxidation." *Applied and Environmental Microbiology* 59, no. 5 (1993): 1668–1670.

75. Christensen, P.A., T.P. Curtis, T.A. Egerton, S.A.M. Kosa, and J.R. Tinlin. "Photoelectrocatalytic and photocatalytic disinfection of *E. coli* suspensions by titanium dioxide." *Applied Catalysis B: Environmental* 41, no. 4 (2003): 371–386.

76. Mantravadi, Hima Bindu. "Effectivity of titanium oxide based nano particles on *E. coli* from clinical samples." *Journal of Clinical and Diagnostic Research: JCDR* 11, no. 7 (2017): DC37.

77. Bekbölet, M. "Photocatalytic bactericidal activity of TiO$_2$ in aqueous suspensions of *E. coli*." *Water Science and Technology* 35, no. 11–12 (1997): 95–100.

78. Sani, Mahmood Alizadeh, Ali Ehsani, and Mohammad Hashemi. "Whey protein isolate/cellulose nanofibre/TiO$_2$ nanoparticle/rosemary essential oil nanocomposite film: Its effect on microbial and sensory quality of lamb meat and growth of common foodborne pathogenic bacteria during refrigeration." *International Journal of Food Microbiology* 251 (2017): 8–14.

79. Azizi-Lalabadi, Maryam, Ali Ehsani, Babak Ghanbarzadeh, and Bahark Divband. "Polyvinyl alcohol/gelatin nanocomposite containing ZnO, TiO$_2$ or ZnO/TiO$_2$ nanoparticles doped on 4A zeolite: Microbial and sensory qualities of packaged white shrimp during refrigeration." *International Journal of Food Microbiology* 312 (2020): 108375.

80. Fujishima, A.K.I.R.A., Tata N. Rao, and Donald A. Tryk. "TiO$_2$ photocatalysts and diamond electrodes." *Electrochimica Acta* 45, no. 28 (2000): 4683–4690.

81. Alizadeh-Sani, Mahmood, Arezou Khezerlou, and Ali Ehsani. "Fabrication and characterization of the bionanocomposite film based on whey protein biopolymer loaded with TiO$_2$ nanoparticles, cellulose nanofibers and rosemary essential oil." *Industrial Crops and Products* 124 (2018): 300–315.

82. Mohammed Sadiq, I., N. Chandrasekaran, and A.J.C.N. Mukherjee. "Studies on effect of TiO$_2$ nanoparticles on growth and membrane permeability of *Escherichia coli*, *Pseudomonas aeruginosa*, and *Bacillus subtilis*." *Current Nanoscience* 6, no. 4 (2010): 381–387.

83. Arora, Bindu, Madhura Murar, and Vinayak Dhumale. "Antimicrobial potential of TiO$_2$ nanoparticles against MDR *Pseudomonas aeruginosa*." *Journal of Experimental Nanoscience* 10, no. 11 (2015): 819–827.

84. Amezaga-Madrid, P., G.V. Nevarez-Moorillon, E. Orrantia-Borunda, and M. Miki-Yoshida. "Photoinduced bactericidal activity against *Pseudomonas aeruginosa* by TiO$_2$ based thin films." *FEMS Microbiology Letters* 211, no. 2 (2002): 183–188.

85. Horst, Allison M., Andrea C. Neal, Randall E. Mielke, Patrick R. Sislian, Won Hyuk Suh, Lutz Mädler, Galen D. Stucky, and Patricia A. Holden. "Dispersion of TiO$_2$ nanoparticle agglomerates by *Pseudomonas aeruginosa*." *Applied and Environmental Microbiology* 76, no. 21 (2010): 7292–7298.

86. Jalvo, Blanca, Marisol Faraldos, Ana Bahamonde, and Roberto Rosal. "Antimicrobial and antibiofilm efficacy of self-cleaning surfaces functionalized by TiO$_2$ photocatalytic nanoparticles against *Staphylococcus aureus* and *Pseudomonas putida*." *Journal of Hazardous Materials* 340 (2017): 160–170.

87. Shiraishi, Koutaro, Hironobu Koseki, Toshiyuki Tsurumoto, Koumei Baba, Mariko Naito, Koji Nakayama, and Hiroyuki Shindo. "Antibacterial metal implant with a TiO$_2$-conferred photocatalytic bactericidal effect against *Staphylococcus aureus*." *Surface and Interface Analysis: An International Journal Devoted to the Development and Application of Techniques for the Analysis of Surfaces, Interfaces and Thin Films* 41, no. 1 (2009): 17–22.

88. Pérez-Jorge, Concepción, Ana Conde, Maria A. Arenas, Ramón Pérez-Tanoira, Endhze Matykina, Juan J. de Damborenea, Enrique Gómez-Barrena, and Jaime Esteban. "In vitro assessment of *Staphylococcus epidermidis* and *Staphylococcus aureus* adhesion on TiO$_2$ nanotubes on Ti – 6Al – 4V alloy." *Journal of Biomedical Materials Research Part A* 100, no. 7 (2012): 1696–1705.

89. Ullah, Kaleem, Shujaat A. Khan, Abdul Mannan, Romana Khan, Ghulam Murtaza, and Muhammad A. Yameen. "Enhancing the antibacterial activity of erythromycin with titanium dioxide nanoparticles against MRSA." *Current Pharmaceutical Biotechnology* 21, no. 10 (2020): 948–954.

90. Tsai, Ting-Mi, Hsin-Hou Chang, Kia-Chih Chang, Yu-Lin Liu, and Chun-Chieh Tseng. "A comparative study of the bactericidal effect of photocatalytic oxidation by

TiO$_2$ on antibiotic-resistant and antibiotic-sensitive bacteria." *Journal of Chemical Technology & Biotechnology* 85, no. 12 (2010): 1642–1653.

91. Chow, Wai Leng, Aung Soe Tin, Woan Wui Lim, Jeremy Lim, Asok Kurup, Moi Lin Ling, Ai Ling Tan, and Biauw Chi Ong. "Efficacy of titanium dioxide compounds in preventing environmental contamination by methicillin resistant *Staphylococcus aureus* (MRSA)." *International Journal of Infection Control* 9, no. 3 (2013).

92. Ansari, Mohammad Azam, Hani Manssor Albetran, Muidh Hamed Alheshibri, Abdelmajid Timoumi, Norah Abdullah Algarou, Sultan Akhtar, Yassine Slimani et al. "Synthesis of electrospun TiO$_2$ nanofibers and characterization of their antibacterial and antibiofilm potential against gram-positive and gram-negative bacteria." *Antibiotics* 9, no. 9 (2020): 572.

93. Subbiah, Geetha, Mariappan Premanathan, Sang Jae Kim, Karthikeyan Krishnamoorthy, and Kadarkaraithangam Jeyasubramanian. "Preparation of TiO$_2$ nanopaint using ball milling process and investigation on its antibacterial properties." *Materials Express* 4, no. 5 (2014): 393–399.

94. Kangwansupamonkon, W., V. Lauruengtana, S. Surassmo, and U. Ruktanonchai. "Antibacterial activity of apatite-coated titanium dioxide." *Nanomedicine: Nanotechnology, Biology and Medicine* 5(2009): 240.

95. Amna, Touseef, M. Shamshi Hassan, Muthuraman Pandurangan, Myung-Seob Khil, Hak-Kyo Lee, and I. H. Hwang. "Characterization and potent bactericidal effect of cobalt doped titanium dioxide nanofibers." *Ceramics International* 39, no. 3 (2013): 3189–3193.

96. Zhang, Qijun, Chenghua Sun, Yong Zhao, Shuyun Zhou, Xiujie Hu, and Ping Chen. "Low Ag-doped titanium dioxide nanosheet films with outstanding antimicrobial property." *Environmental Science & Technology* 44, no. 21 (2010): 8270–8275.

97. Chen, Shiguo, Yujuan Guo, Shaojun Chen, Huimin Yu, Zaochuan Ge, Xuan Zhang, Peixin Zhang, and Jiaoning Tang. "Facile preparation and synergistic antibacterial effect of three-component Cu/TiO$_2$/CS nanoparticles." *Journal of Materials Chemistry* 22, no. 18 (2012): 9092–9099.

98. Yadav, Hemraj Mahipati, Jung-Sik Kim, and Shivaji Hariba Pawar. "Developments in photocatalytic antibacterial activity of nano TiO$_2$: A review." *Korean Journal of Chemical Engineering* 33, no. 7 (2016): 1989–1998.

99. Fu, Guifen, Patricia S. Vary, and Chhiu-Tsu Lin. "Anatase TiO$_2$ nanocomposites for antimicrobial coatings." *The Journal of Physical Chemistry B* 109, no. 18 (2005): 8889–8898.

100. Yadav, Hemraj M., Tanaji V. Kolekar, Shivaji H. Pawar, and Jung-Sik Kim. "Enhanced photocatalytic inactivation of bacteria on Fe-containing TiO$_2$ nanoparticles under fluorescent light." *Journal of Materials Science: Materials in Medicine* 27, no. 3 (2016): 57.

101. Trapalis, Christos C., P. Keivanidis, George Kordas, Maria Zaharescu, Maria Crisan, Alexandra Szatvanyi, and M. Gartner. "TiO$_2$ (Fe^{3+}) nanostructured thin films with antibacterial properties." *Thin Solid Films* 433, no. 1–2 (2003): 186–190.

102. Yadav, Hemraj M., Sachin V. Otari, Raghvendra A. Bohara, Sawanta S. Mali, Shivaji H. Pawar, and Sagar D. Delekar. "Synthesis and visible light photocatalytic antibacterial activity of nickel-doped TiO2 nanoparticles against gram-positive and gram-negative bacteria." *Journal of Photochemistry and Photobiology A: Chemistry* 294 (2014): 130–136.

103. Karunakaran, C., G. Abiramasundari, P. Gomathisankar, G. Manikandan, and V. Anandi. "Cu-doped TiO$_2$ nanoparticles for photocatalytic disinfection of bacteria under visible light." *Journal of Colloid and Interface Science* 352, no. 1 (2010): 68–74.

104. Wang, Mei, Qianfei Zhao, He Yang, Dai Shi, and Juncen Qian. "Photocatalytic antibacterial properties of copper doped TiO2 prepared by high-energy ball milling." *Ceramics International* 46, no. 10 (2020): 16716–16724.

105. Sayılkan, Funda, Meltem Asiltürk, Nadir Kiraz, Esin Burunkaya, Ertuğrul Arpaç, and Hikmet Sayılkan. "Photocatalytic antibacterial performance of Sn4+-doped TiO_2 thin films on glass substrate." *Journal of Hazardous Materials* 162, no. 2–3 (2009): 1309–1316.

106. Irie, Hiroshi, Kazuhide Kamiya, Toshihiko Shibanuma, Shuhei Miura, Donald A. Tryk, Toshihiko Yokoyama, and Kazuhito Hashimoto. "Visible light-sensitive Cu (II)-grafted TiO_2 photocatalysts: Activities and X-ray absorption fine structure analyses." *The Journal of Physical Chemistry C* 113, no. 24 (2009): 10761–10766.

107. Rengifo Herrera, Julian Andres, and Cesar Pulgarin. "Photocatalytic activity of N, S co-doped and N-doped commercial anatase TiO_2 powders towards phenol oxidation and *E. coli* inactivation under simulated solar light irradiation." *Solar Energy* 84, no. 1 (2010): 37–43.

108. Necula, Bogdan S., Lidy E. Fratila-Apachitei, Sebastian A.J. Zaat, Iulian Apachitei, and Jurek Duszczyk. "In vitro antibacterial activity of porous TiO_2 – Ag composite layers against methicillin-resistant *Staphylococcus aureus*." *Acta Biomaterialia* 5, no. 9 (2009): 3573–3580.

109. Jiang, Xuhong, Bin Lv, Yuan Wang, Qianhong Shen, and Xinmin Wang. "Bactericidal mechanisms and effector targets of TiO_2 and $Ag-TiO_2$ against *Staphylococcus aureus*." *Journal of Medical Microbiology* 66, no. 4 (2017): 440.

110. Kustiningsih, Indar, Asep Ridwan, Devi Abriyani, Muhammad Syairazy, Teguh Kurniawan, and Ria Barleany Dhena. "Development of chitosan-TiO_2 nanocomposite for packaging film and its ability to inactive *Staphylococcus aureus*." *Oriental Journal of Chemistry* 35, no. 3 (2019): 1132.

111. Natarajan, Kandasamy. "Antibiofilm activity of epoxy/$Ag-TiO_2$ polymer nanocomposite coatings against *Staphylococcus aureus* and *Escherichia coli*." *Coatings* 5, no. 2 (2015): 95–114.

112. Marulasiddeshwara, Roopesh, M.S. Jyothi, Khantong Soontarapa, Rangappa S. Keri, and Rajendran Velmurugan. "Nonwoven fabric supported, chitosan membrane anchored with curcumin/TiO_2 complex: Scaffolds for MRSA infected wound skin reconstruction." *International Journal of Biological Macromolecules* 144 (2020): 85–93.

113. Chokesawatanakit, Nuttaporn, Pasakorn Jutakridsada, Sophon Boonlue, Jesper T.N. Knijnenburg, Phillip C. Wright, Mika Sillanpää, and Khanita Kamwilaisak. "Ag-doped Cobweb-like structure of TiO_2 nanotubes for antibacterial activity against Methicillin-resistant *Staphylococcus aureus* (MRSA)." *Journal of Environmental Chemical Engineering* (2021): 105843.

114. Roy, Aashis S., Ameena Parveen, Anil R. Koppalkar, and MVN Ambika Prasad. "Effect of nano-titanium dioxide with different antibiotics against methicillin-resistant *Staphylococcus aureus*." *Journal of Biomaterials and Nanobiotechnology* 1, no. 1 (2010): 37.

115. Chen, Wei-Jen, Pei-Jane Tsai, and Yu-Chie Chen. "Functional Fe_3O_4/TiO_2 core/shell magnetic nanoparticles as photokilling agents for pathogenic bacteria." *Small* 4, no. 4 (2008): 485–491.

116. Popov, S., O. Saphier, M. Popov, M. Shenker, S. Entus, Y. Shotland, M. Saphier. Factors enhancing the antibacterial effect of monovalent copper ions. *Current Microbiology* 77 (2020): 361–368. doi:10.1007/s00284-019-01794-6.

117. Festa, Richard A., and Dennis J. Thiele. "Copper: An essential metal in biology." *Current Biology* 21, no. 21 (2011): R877–R883.

118. Masarwa, Mohamed, Haim Cohen, Dan Meyerstein, David L. Hickman, Andreja Bakac, and James H. Espenson. "Reactions of low-valent transition-metal complexes with hydrogen peroxide: Are they 'Fenton-like' or not? 1. The case of Cu^+ aq and Cr^{2+} aq." *Journal of the American Chemical Society* 110, no. 13 (1988): 4293–4297.

119. Ma, Ying, Wei Tong, Hua Zhou, and Steven L. Suib. "A review of zeolite-like porous materials." *Microporous and Mesoporous Materials* 37, no. 1–2 (2000): 243–252.

120. Marambio-Jones, Catalina, and Eric M.V. Hoek. "A review of the antibacterial effects of silver nanomaterials and potential implications for human health and the environment." *Journal of Nanoparticle Research* 12, no. 5 (2010): 1531–1551.

121. Serati-Nouri, Hamed, Amir Jafari, Leila Roshangar, Mehdi Dadashpour, Younes Pilehvar-Soltanahmadi, and Nosratollah Zarghami. "Biomedical applications of zeolite-based materials: A review." *Materials Science and Engineering: C* 116 (2020): 111225.

122. Inoue, Yoshihiro, Masanobu Hoshino, Hiroo Takahashi, Tomoko Noguchi, Tomomi Murata, Yasushi Kanzaki, Hajime Hamashima, and Masanori Sasatsu. "Bactericidal activity of Ag – zeolite mediated by reactive oxygen species under aerated conditions." *Journal of Inorganic Biochemistry* 92, no. 1 (2002): 37–42.

123. Shameli, Kamyar, Mansor Bin Ahmad, Mohsen Zargar, Wan Md Zin Wan Yunus, and Nor Azowa Ibrahim. "Fabrication of silver nanoparticles doped in the zeolite framework and antibacterial activity." *International Journal of Nanomedicine* 6 (2011): 331.

124. Nakane, T., H. Gomyo, I. Sasaki, Y. Kimoto, N. Hanzawa, Y. Teshima, and T. Namba. "New antiaxillary odour deodorant made with antimicrobial Ag-zeolite (silver-exchanged zeolite)." *International Journal of Cosmetic Science* 28, no. 4 (2006): 299–309.

125. Llorens, Amparo, Elsa Lloret, Pierre A. Picouet, Raul Trbojevich, and Avelina Fernandez. "Metallic-based micro and nanocomposites in food contact materials and active food packaging." *Trends in Food Science & Technology* 24, no. 1 (2012): 19–29.

126. Hodgson, Steven C., R. John Casey, and Stephen W. Bigger. "Review of zeolites as deodorants for polyethylene resins used in food packaging applications." *Polymer-Plastics Technology and Engineering* 41, no. 5 (2002): 795–818.

127. Zhu, Hua-yu, Sheng-juan Yan, Huai-Cheng Chen, and Hong-yi Zhao. "The research progress of natural zeolite applied in the field of building materials [J]." *Bulletin of the Chinese Ceramic Society* 5 (2012).

128. Payami, Roya, Mohammad Ghorbanpour, and Aiyoub Parchehbaf Jadid. "Antibacterial silver-doped bioactive silica gel production using molten salt method." *Journal of Nanostructure in Chemistry* 6, no. 3 (2016): 215–221.

129. Tan, Shaozao, Yousheng Ouyang, Liling Zhang, Yiben Chen, and Yingliang Liu. "Study on the structure and antibacterial activity of silver-carried zirconium phosphate." *Materials Letters* 62, no. 14 (2008): 2122–2124.

130. Cheng, Lei, Michael D. Weir, Hockin H.K. Xu, Alison M. Kraigsley, Nancy J. Lin, Sheng Lin-Gibson, and Xuedong Zhou. "Antibacterial and physical properties of calcium – phosphate and calcium – fluoride nanocomposites with chlorhexidine." *Dental Materials* 28, no. 5 (2012): 573–583.

131. Weber, Florian, Alejandro Barrantes, and Hanna Tiainen. "Silicic acid-mediated formation of tannic acid nanocoatings." *Langmuir* 35, no. 9 (2019): 3327–3336.

7 Materials Characterization Using Advanced Synchrotron Radiation Techniques for Antimicrobial Materials

*Chatree Saiyasombat, Prae Chirawatkul,
Suittipong Wannapaiboon, Catleya
Rojviriya, Siriwat Soontaranon, Nuntaporn
Kamonsutthipaijit, Sirinart Chio-Srichan, Chanan
Euaruksakul, and Nichada Jearanaikoon*

CONTENTS

DOI: 10.1201/9781003143093-7

7.1 INTRODUCTION

A tremendous increase in the demand for novel antimicrobial materials emerges from global pandemic diseases and the antibiotic resistance capability in pathogenic microorganisms. Research works in antimicrobial materials have been built upon multidisciplinary knowledge both in synthesis and characterization. The development of antimicrobial materials involves a deeper scientific insight of the materials and detailed information from characterization techniques. The scientific and technological research for antimicrobial materials is based on three main strategies: (1) the antiadhesive, (2) contact-killing, and (3) release-killing mechanism. For material development in each strategy, different perspectives of materials are investigated, ranging from the atomic scale, nanoscale up to microscale. The requirement of higher advanced characterization tools exceeding the capability of benchtop tools is eminent. Synchrotron-based techniques have better resolution and faster acquisition time compared to their conventional laboratory counterparts. Due to substantially higher photon flux, tunable energy capability, together with highly monochromatic, and collimated beams from the synchrotron, many *operando* and *in situ* experiments deemed too complicated are achievable.

In this chapter, different characterization techniques are separated into four main perspectives: (1) atomic scale, (2) nanoscale and molecular scale, (3) microscale, and (4) surface and interface. Various synchrotron-based techniques could be applied to study antimicrobial materials, namely, X-ray absorption spectroscopy and X-ray powder diffraction, small-angle X-ray scattering, Fourier-transform infrared spectroscopy and microscopy, X-ray microtomography, X-ray fluorescence spectroscopy, and microscopy, grazing-incidence X-ray diffraction, X-ray reflectivity, and X-ray photoelectron spectroscopy are presented. The essential background of each technique and its applications are discussed. Current limitations and future perspectives of synchrotron-based techniques are also noted.

7.2 ATOMIC SCALE

7.2.1 X-Ray Absorption Spectroscopy

X-ray absorption spectroscopy (XAS) is a synchrotron-based technique for structural characterization [1–2]. The method has proven powerful as structural information obtained from crystalline or non-crystalline materials and measurements are relatively simple. Samples could be measured in solid or liquid forms, and the measurement configuration is straightforward. Absorption is determined from the absorption coefficient, μ. Following the Beer–Lambert law,

$$I = I_0 e^{-\mu x} \tag{7.1}$$

where I is the intensity of transmitted X-rays, I_0 is the intensity of incoming X-rays, and x is the sample thickness. The absorption is determined from the measurement of X-ray intensity before and after samples. The schematic of a typical absorption measurement is shown in Figure 7.1(a). Also shown in Figure 7.1(b) is the illustration

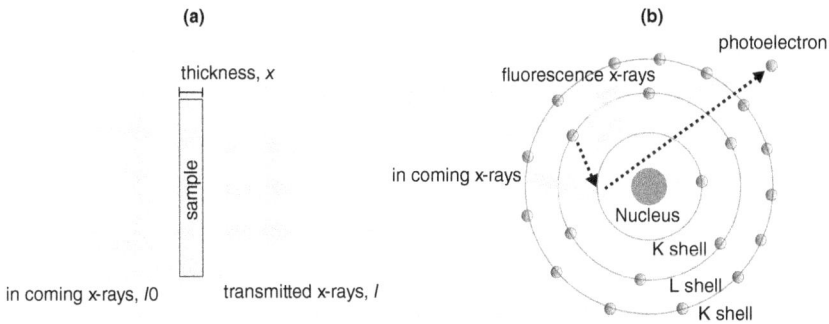

FIGURE 7.1   (a) Schematic of a typical XAS measurement showing transmission mode measurement where X-rays intensity before and after samples are collected. (b) Diagram illustrating the photoelectric effect.

of the photoelectric effect describing the phenomena where an atom is exposed to X-rays with energy higher than but in the proximity of the energy level of the core electrons. Because of the photoelectric effect, the absorption coefficient is modulated. The modulation originates from the interference between outgoing and backscattered photoelectrons [2]. Local structures of the interested atoms are thus revealed by analyzing these features. Figure 7.2 shows an example of XAS spectra measured at the Fe K-edge. The spectrum is divided into two parts. The XANES (X-ray Absorption Near-Edge Structure) part gives information regarding oxidation states and the local symmetry of the atoms of interest. The EXAFS (Extended X-ray Absorption Fine Structure) part provides quantitative information of their atomic local coordination environments. Many XAS data analysis programs are available, both free and commercial, including the widely used Demeter package [3]. And as XAS spectra are unique to each local environment, they can be compared to measurements of reference compounds, and fingerprinting could be used for speciation in XANES or EXAFS.

For most antimicrobial materials, the concentration of exciting elements is low and not appropriate for direct measurements. Instead, they are often measured indirectly using fluorescence (FL) yield mode. Following the photoelectric effect, as X-rays are absorbed, and the core electron leaves its energy level, the electron in the higher energy level will replace the recently evacuated level and gives out the excess energy in the form of fluorescence X-rays. In this way, the intensity of fluorescence X-rays could indirectly represent absorption. By measuring the spectrum in an FL mode, the lower limit concentration of interesting elements could be reduced to around 10–100 ppm.

The XAS technique has been applied to various materials, including semiconductors, catalytic materials, transition metal complex systems, and biological and environmental science [4–7]. Structural information such as oxidation states, local symmetry, local coordination environment, not directly obtained via other techniques, has also been applied fruitfully to characterize antimicrobial materials. The XANES spectra measured at the C K-edge were used to identify the C=C and C–F bonds of the antimicrobial quaternary ammonium compounds (QACs) used against

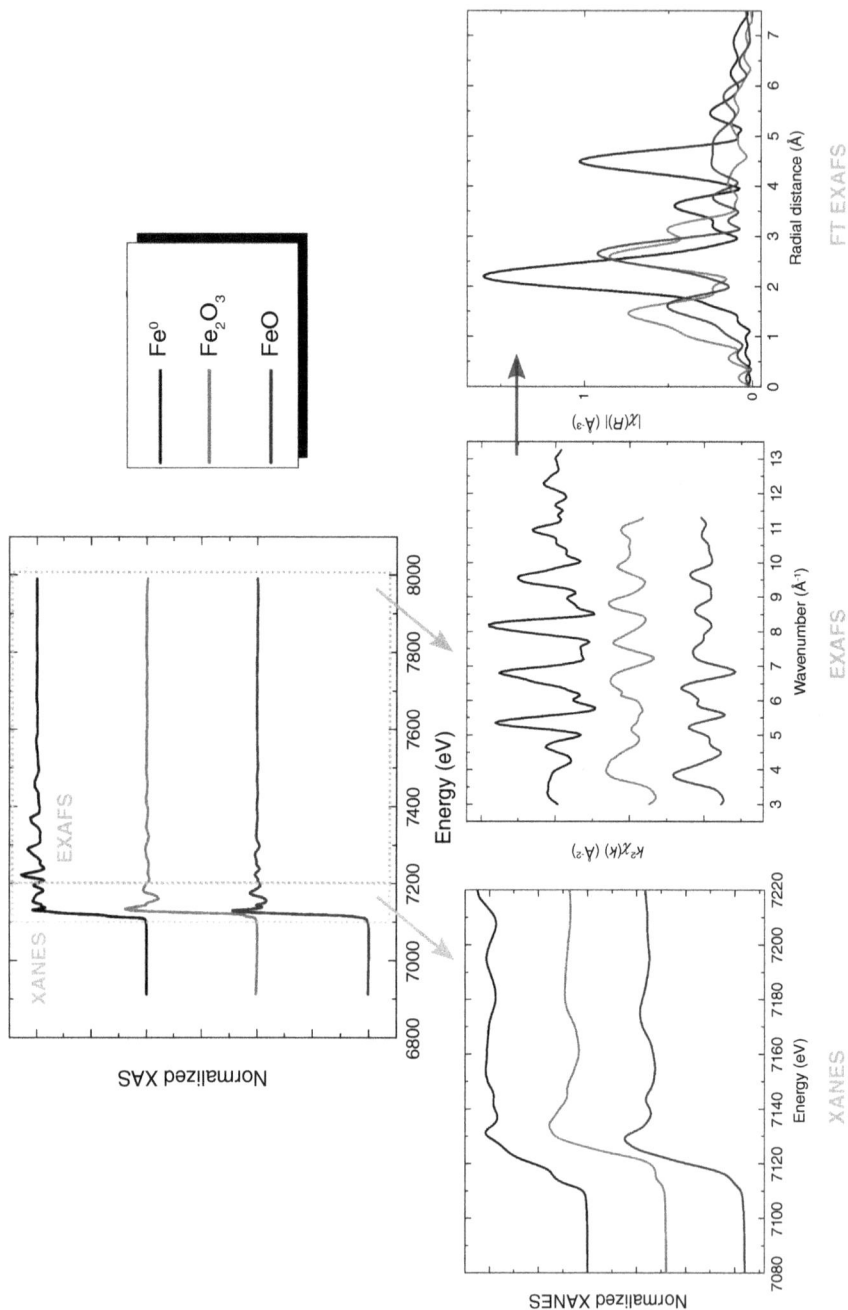

FIGURE 7.2 XAS spectra of Fe^0, Fe$_2$O$_3$, and FeO showing the XANES part plotted as a function of energy, the EXAFS part which are extractions of the high-energy oscillations plotted as a function of a wavevector k and the Fourier transform of the k space EXAFS. The spectra are unique for different environments of Fe atoms. They were measured at the BL1.1W beamline, Synchrotron Light Research Institute (SLRI), Thailand.

airborne and marine microorganisms semifluorinated-quaternized triblock copoly-mers (SQTC-F8H6Br-H6Br) [8]. The surface reconstruction upon introducing the hydrophobic hexyl groups to the SQTC-F8H6Br was shown to reduce the C–F bonds. The Zn K-edge XANES and EXAFS were used to confirm the formation of chitosan-ZnO-based complex [9] as the XANES spectra of the prepared complex were signifi-cantly different from those of the pure ZnO nanoparticle. The structure was furthered confirmed by refining a theoretical model to the measured EXAFS spectrum.

Speciation of metal antimicrobial agents by XAS has been used to elucidate their toxicity mechanism and delivery means. Oxidation of Fe was determined from the XANES spectra measured at the Fe K-edge of zero-valent iron nanoparticles (ZVI NPs) used against gram-positive *Bacillus subtilis* and *Bacillus thuringiensis* [10]. The XAS result showed that ZVI NPs enter the cells before oxidized to Fe_2O_3. The increased concentration of intracellular ROS (reactive oxygen species) disrupted cell membrane integrity and, subsequently, cell viability. The factors affecting the release of Ga^{3+} from the gallium-doped bioresorbable and biocompatible phosphate-based glasses were studied using XAS [11]. The XANES spectra measured at the Ga K-edge showed that Ga^{3+} occupied octahedral sites, which helped stabilize the glass network affecting the dissolution of the glass network and, consequently, the release of Ga^{3+}. XAS has also been applied to determine local structures of Ag in Ag-containing materials. The XANES spectra measured at the Ag K-edge were employed to iden-tify the preference-bonding site of Ag^+ to *Staphylococcus aureus*, *Listeria monocy-togenes*, and *Escherichia coli* [12]. The local structure of Ag was used to explain the increased photocatalytic and antimicrobial activities of Ag-doped dip-coated TiO_2 anatase film [13]. The XAS results showed that Ag was not incorporated into TiO_2 lattice as a solid solution, but the film was composed of TiO_2 and Ag_2O composite and that Ag_2O acted as an electron source and charge separators.

Attentions have also been given to the chemical transformation of antimicrobial materials in the environment. The XAS result showed that most Ag^0 in Ag-treated fabric remained in their metallic form, although some underwent sulfidation to form AgS when the fabric was incubated in soil [14]. The linear combination of the Ag K-edge XANES spectra was used to monitor the rate of sulfidation. The effect of washing for a different type of Ag-treated fabric was studied. The XAS result sug-gested that the chemical transformation to AgCl or AgS was both textile and deter-gent type-dependent [15]. It has also been found that oxidation reaction is crucial for the transform to AgCl [16]. Biotransformation of nanoparticle (NPs) ZnO to nitrate forms was identified using XAS in the investigation of the effect of NPs ZnO on the seedling of alfalfa (*Medicago sativa*), cucumber (*Cucumis sativus*), and tomato (*Solanum lycopersicum*) [17].

In situ or *in vitro* study of antimicrobial materials is in high demand [18]. Although XAS has already been employed to study many antimicrobial materials, *in situ* or *in vitro* studies are still scarce. With high flux X-rays from the synchrotron, one XAS spectrum could be measured in minutes down to milliseconds appropriated for *in situ* measurements. Speciation could be used to monitor structural change dur-ing material synthesis [19], and time-dependent chemical transformation could be studied. In addition, many synchrotron beamlines are equipped with various sample environments such as furnaces, cryocoolers, and flow cells; the sample environment could be adjusted to resemble realistic operational conditions, and its effect on chemical transformation could be studied.

7.2.2 POWDER X-RAY DIFFRACTION

Understanding geometrical structures of materials potentially provides the design and control of their characteristic features, which can be further used for desired applications. Practically, most of the candidate materials are synthesized as bulk powders, of which properties and performances are thoroughly characterized prior to applying for practical uses. For decades, powder X-ray diffraction (PXRD) is well recognized as one of the crucial techniques for revealing the long-range periodic ordering of atoms and/or molecules in crystalline materials. Crystal structure, crystalline phase compositions, and purity of materials can be qualitatively and quantitatively examined by employing the PXRD technique. Moreover, specific structural data responsible for their characteristic features of materials, i.e., lattice parameters, atomic positions, site occupancy, domain size, texture, microstrain, and macrostrain, can be obtained and refined from PXRD patterns. In addition, PXRD provides structural information concerning microstructure, dislocations, defects, and structural disordering, which are often crucial evidence for an explanation of emerging properties of materials [20–22].

PXRD of crystalline materials can be explained as a coherent elastic scattering of X-ray by electrons bounded to atoms in various sets of lattice planes, which are periodically separated by regions of much lower electron density. The constructive interference is observed only when the conditions of the Bragg equation (as shown in the following) are fulfilled, which consequently illustrates PXRD peak at a specific diffracted angle (θ) corresponding to each spacing between lattice plane (d) in the material and the incident and diffracted X-ray wavelength (λ).

$$2d\sin\theta = n\lambda \tag{7.2}$$

Polycrystalline powder sample consists of thousands of randomly orientated tiny single crystals. For every set of planes, a statistically relevant number of crystallites are adequately oriented to diffract the incident X-ray. In PXRD, a set of planes possessing similar d-spacing shows the diffracted spots with the same distance but in a random direction, consequently forming continuous "Debye diffraction cones." Linear (or one-dimensional) diffraction pattern is measured as the detector scans along an arc that intersects each Debye cone at a single point. The PXRD pattern can identify crystalline phases and compositions in materials [20–22].

Synchrotron-based PXRD has been carried out to overcome the limitations and enhance the detection performance of laboratory PXRD instruments. For example, synchrotron PXRD eliminates a significant source of low-angle peak broadening found in conventional laboratory PXRD. Due to continuous spectra of synchrotron radiation, synchrotron PXRD provides a possibility to select well-defined X-ray wavelength to avoid the unwanted fluorescence background of some elements in the probed materials. Moreover, synchrotron X-ray offers a highly intense and highly collimated nature of radiation, leading to superior statistics, better spatial precision, and a high measurement speed. Hence, the *in situ* experiments can be straightforwardly carried out at synchrotron facilities to monitor the structural change of materials upon external stimuli and controlled sample environment such as temperature dependence, pressure dependence, and guest-induced incorporation. There are two primary setup geometries of synchrotron-based PXRD, as shown in Figure 7.3. The Debye–Scherrer geometry measures diffracted X-ray that is transmitted from powder samples packed in a capillary. The grazing incidence geometry (GIXRD) measures diffracted X-rays reflected from the very small (grazing) incident angle of the X-ray on surfaces of materials. Note that GIXRD is suitable to identify crystalline phases of thin films, coatings, and surface compositions.

Considering the development of novel materials for disinfection technology, the materials should possess high efficacy to reduce the emerging pathogens, good environmental safety, low toxicity, and should be able to expand for large-scale production with cost-effectiveness [23–24]. Regarding these aspects, inorganic antimicrobial materials attract significant attention. PXRD is a primary and crucial technique to identify the formation of desired materials and investigate their structural characteristics and stability upon antimicrobial reaction conditions. Specifically, PXRD is carried out to identify phase compositions, physical and chemical stability of the antimicrobial materials themselves (such as metal, metal oxides, and metal sulfides nanoparticles), and the microporous/mesoporous matrix used impregnating the reactive antimicrobial substances [13, 23–27].

For example, the successful impregnations of silver (Ag), zinc oxide (ZnO), and composited Ag/ZnO nanoparticles on highly porous activated carbon (AC) have been revealed by the coexisting of characteristics PXRD patterns assigned to each component in the obtained nanohybrid materials. Noteworthy, the Ag/ZnO impregnated AC hybrid material exhibited the highest antimicrobial activity and killing kinetics against both gram-negative and gram-positive bacteria by employing the disc diffusion method [23]. In addition, PXRD was used to examine the degree of aggregation of gold nanoparticles, which were incorporated into different types of zeolite supports (namely clinoptilolite, mordenite, and faujasite). The XRD peaks indexed to metallic gold were clearly observed in containing gold nanoparticles into mordenite,

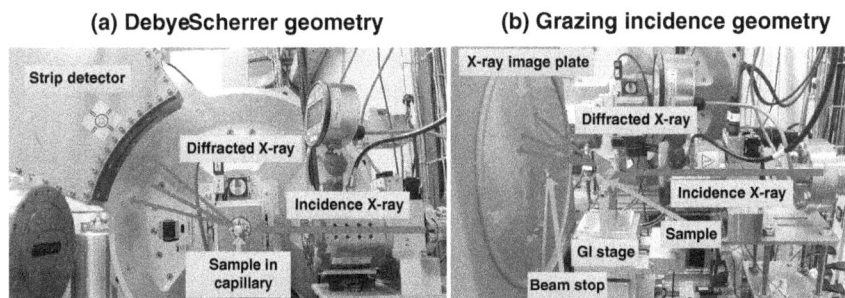

(a) DebyeScherrer geometry   **(b) Grazing incidence geometry**

FIGURE 7.3 Synchrotron-based PXRD geometries: (a) Debye–Scherrer geometry for powder samples packed in capillary and (b) grazing incidence geometry (GIXRD) for thin-films, coatings, and surface compositions.

which indicated the high degree of aggregation and poor dispersion of biocide materials on the support surface. The corresponding data obtained from solid-state ^{29}Si nuclear magnetic resonance (NMR) and transmission electron microscopy (TEM) were combined with PXRD for better understanding. Note that the gold nanoparticles incorporated in zeolites exhibited high performance for eliminating *E. coli* and *Salmonella typhi* bacteria, which are two common microorganisms contaminated in water and can develop a resistance toward the commonly used bactericides [25]. Moreover, GIXRD was used to characterize antimicrobial materials in the form of films and coating. For example, GIXRD revealed the crystalline phase compositions of anatase (TiO$_2$) and silver-doped anatase films deposited on glass substrates by employing a sol-gel dip-coating method, which interestingly exhibited the photocatalytic-enhanced antimicrobial activity [13].

Additionally, synchrotron-based PXRD and GIXRD have been used for phase identification and crystalline compositional analysis of antimicrobial materials, especially in the cases that require high-resolution PXRD patterns for better clarification of phase compositions [11, 28–29]. As a demonstrating example, crystalline phase compositions of the complex so-called ruthenium (II) chloro-phenanthroline-trithiacyclononane powdered materials have been thoroughly identified by high-resolution synchrotron PXRD beamlines at the European Synchrotron Radiation Facility (ESRF), Grenoble, France. Excellent line resolution of synchrotron 1D-PXRD pattern unambiguously confirmed the presence of mixed crystalline phases, of which their space group and the corresponding unit cell parameters were assigned and refined ideally. Note that the presence of mixed crystalline phases, in this case, could not be clearly distinguished by the laboratory PXRD instrument due to the convolution of PXRD reflection lines [29].

As a highlight, time-resolved synchrotron-based PXRD facilities provide a straightforward way to monitor the structural transformation of the obtained antimicrobial materials upon altering temperature, the crystallization process, and the chemical reaction [20, 30–31]. For example, the temperature-dependent supramolecular structures of antimicrobial amphiphilic ionic complexes between hyaluronic acid and alkyl-trimethyl phosphonium soaps with different alkyl chains have been investigated by synchrotron PXRD using heating and cooling interval between 10 and 120 °C. Both small-angle X-ray scattering (SAXS) and wide-angle X-ray scattering (WAXS) regions have been probed simultaneously to study the influences of temperature on the nanoscale (1–10 nm) and sub-nanoscale (0.1–0.6 nm) structural ordering of the targeted complexes, respectively. Interestingly, these complexes could be a promising candidate for further biocompatible/biodegradable antimicrobial films [30]. Moreover, time-resolved synchrotron PXRD in simultaneous SAXS/WAXS study provides the information of dynamic crystallization evolution of bio-nanocomposites and the effect of cellulose nanocrystal (CNC) loadings on the crystallite nucleation control of poly(3-hydroxybutyrate-co-3-hydroxy valerate) (PHBV) composites. The obtained PHBV/CNC bio-nanocomposites were used as a host substrate to incorporate zinc oxides and silver nanoparticles, which exhibited such suitable antimicrobial inhibition activities and biocompatibility [31].

In addition, synchrotron-based PXRD was used for real-time monitoring of the structural transformation upon the ongoing chemical reaction to investigate the chemical mechanism and the kinetic transformation process. Since silver nanoparticles

(AgNPs) are well known and widely used as the reactive antimicrobial agent, the understanding of AgNPs transformation in practical uses to elucidate their toxicity once discharged into the environment and interact with natural organic matter is of interest. *In situ* synchrotron PXRD revealed the real-time alteration of crystalline phases of the AgNPs to silver sulfide (Ag_2S) concerning the prolongation of the sulfidation reaction (as shown in Figure 7.4). The obtained results also indicate

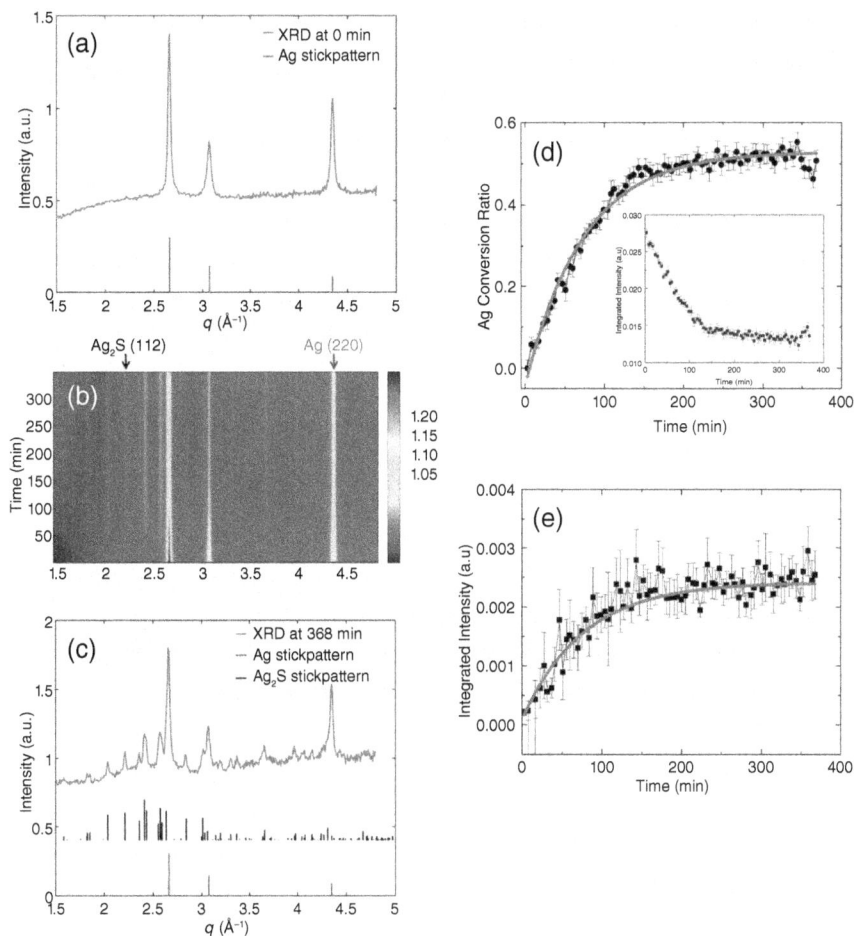

FIGURE 7.4   (a) XRD pattern recorded from pristine AgNP suspension. (b) Two-dimensional contour plot of the in situ XRD patterns showing the time-dependent evolution of crystalline phases present during sulfidation. (c) XRD pattern recorded from AgNP suspension at 368 min after the sulfidation process was initiated. The reference stick patterns were simulated using the space groups and lattice parameters shown in the TEM section. (d) The conversion ratio of Ag to Ag_2S, based on the integrated intensity of Ag (220) peak shown in its inset. (e) Time-dependent evolution of the integrated intensity of Ag_2S (112) peak. In (d) and (e), the solid lines represent least-squares fits of the kinetics data using an exponential decay function.

Source: Reproduced from Ref. [20] with permission from the Royal Society of Chemistry.

the first-order kinetics of response and the dependency of the AgNPs sulfidation on the crystallographic orientation of the crystal facets. Interestingly, the normalized integration of peak intensity of AgNPs and Ag_2S from the starting point and during the sulfidation reaction is preserved. This observation suggested that there was no leaching of Ag^+ to the environment during the sulfidation transformation from Ag to Ag_2S, indicating the less environmental toxicity of AgNPs [20].

In summary, the *in situ* monitoring of structural change by employing synchrotron-based PXRD complimented with other practical characterization techniques such as solid-state NMR, *in situ* Raman spectroscopy, scanning electron microscopy (SEM), and transmission electron microscopy (TEM), and XAS could provide the crucial information to understand the materials and to be able to apply for realistic applications.

7.3 NANOSCALE AND MOLECULAR SCALE

7.3.1 SMALL-ANGLE X-RAY SCATTERING

Small-angle X-ray scattering (SAXS) is a non-destructive tool for the structural characterization of materials with electron density fluctuation on the length scale of approximately 1–100 nm. In the SAXS experiment, a monochromatic X-ray beam is employed to illuminate the sample. In contrast, the scattered X-ray is recorded by a 2D area detector placed at a distance behind the sample, as schematically shown in Figure 7.5. In general, the scattering intensity I(q) at the detector can be mathematically expressed by

$$I(q) = \phi \, \Delta\rho^2 V \, P(q) S(q) \tag{7.3}$$

where φ is the number density of scattering particles, $\Delta\rho$ is the electron density contrast between the scattering particles and the medium, and V is the scattering particles volume. $P(q)$ is the form factor corresponding to the scattering from a single particle, while the structure factor $S(q)$ is accounted for the interparticle interference effects. Here, the magnitude of scattering vector q is defined by

$$q = \frac{4\pi\sin\theta}{\lambda} \tag{7.4}$$

where λ is the wavelength of the X-ray and 2θ is the scattering angle.

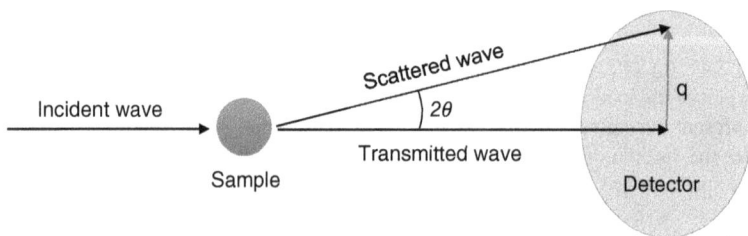

FIGURE 7.5 Schematic representation of a typical SAXS experiment.

SAXS experiment can be done using either a conventional X-ray source or X-rays from synchrotron radiation. The extremely bright and low divergence synchrotron light results in the SAXS pattern with a higher signal-to-noise ratio and a more negligible smearing effect. Time-resolved study as a function of applied external parameters such as temperature or tension is also possible with the synchrotron SAXS experiment. Because of these advantages, demand for using SAXS beamline is increasing, as can be seen from the increasing number of SAXS beamlines at the synchrotron facilities worldwide. Figure 7.6 illustrates the SAXS experimental station of the BL1.3W: SAXS/WAXS at the Synchrotron Light Research Institute (SLRI), Thailand.

SAXS measurements are sensitive to electron density contrast in materials. The measured SAXS patterns give quantitative information regarding the sizes and shapes of nanometer-sized structures. A general small-angle scattering pattern of a monodisperse and homogeneous system comprises two regions along the q scale. The low q region is where the curve follows Guinier's laws, providing the structures' radius of gyration (R_g). The curve at the middle q region gives information regarding the shapes of scattering particles. For polydisperse systems, the Porod law describes the behavior of the scattering intensity in the high-q region.

Antimicrobial peptides (AMPs) were developed in various nanostructure materials, including nanosheets, fibrils, vesicles, and nanotubes, with a range of potential applications. SAXS profiles of antimicrobial peptides (RA6R) with different concentrations

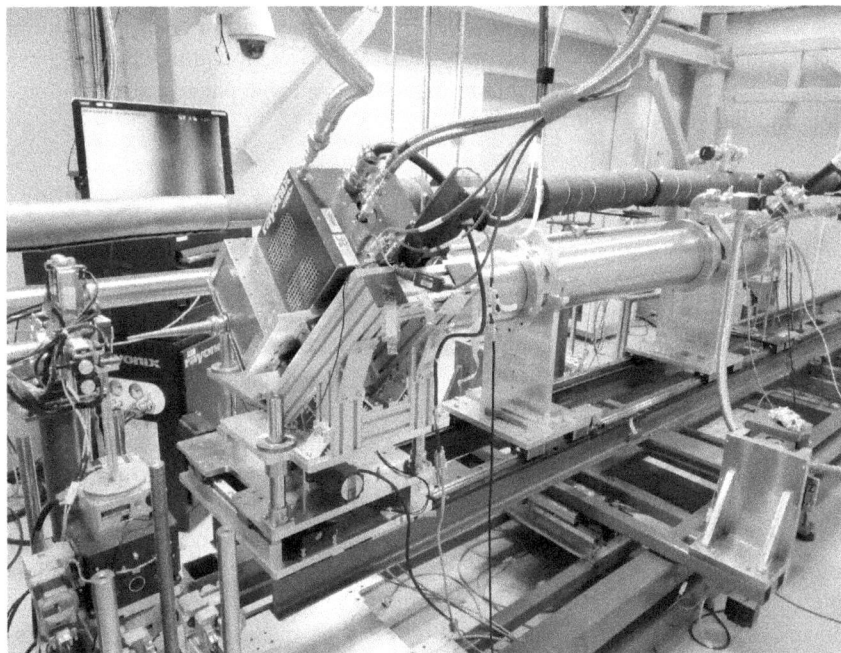

FIGURE 7.6   BL1.3W: SAXS/WAXS experimental station at SLRI, Thailand.

were constructed assuming a scattering entity of known shape, Gaussian coil model in this case [32]. Each scattering intensity curve is related to a set of peptides with different radii of gyration (R_g), with R_g = 7.0, 7.16, and 6.94 Å for 1, 5, and 15 wt.% RA6R, respectively. The SAXS result agreed with the Cryo-TEM images for the formation of occasional clusters of monomers.

Another example is antimicrobial peptides (RA9R) with a long cylindrical shell [32]. SAXS can provide the details of the core radius, the shell thickness, and the scattering length density of the core, shell, and solvent. The structural information obtained from SAXS and those from the Cryo-TEM confirmed the presence of the cylindrical shells with an average diameter of 7.6 nm.

Apart from structural characterization, to understand the antimicrobial activity of antimicrobial peptides, SAXS was also used to probe the interaction between the peptide residues and lipid membranes [32–36]. The SAXS profiles of the mixture between the model bacterial and lipid membrane, represented by DPPG and anti-microbial peptides (RA6R and RA9R), were investigated [32]. The pure lipids were found to be unilamellar vesicles displayed by a broad peak positioned at approximately q = 0.15 Å^{-1}. Upon adding RA9R, the SAXS data indicated that some correlation between the bilayers was introduced, as shown by the presence of two small Bragg peaks with d-spacing values of 83.1 and 44.8 Å ($d = 2\pi/q_0$; q_0 denotes the peak maxima), and the structure became multilamellar.

Likewise, G. C. L. Wong and co-workers have extensively studied the topological changes upon the addition of AMPs in their synthetic mimics against lipid membranes by SAXS [35–36]. Their study showed that the cationic phenylene ethynyl-ene antimicrobial oligomers (AMOs) induced the transition from small unilamellar vesicles to an inverted hexagonal phase [35]. On the other hand, polydisperse cationic methacrylate-based random copolymers (SMAMPs) were found to induce the topological transition of the lipid membranes into inverse cubic phase, corresponding to $Pn3m$ and $Im3m$ lattices [36].

7.3.2 FOURIER-TRANSFORM INFRARED SPECTROSCOPY

The infrared (IR) region of the electromagnetic spectrum is divided into three areas, known in increasing wavelength coverage, as the near-, mid-, and far-IR; these cover the wavelength ranges of about 780 nm (0.8 μm) to 2500 nm (2.5 μm), 2.5 μm to 25 μm and 25 μm to about 1000 μm. The energies of infrared radiation range from 1.5 eV at 0.8 μm to 0.001 eV at 1000 μm which are insufficient to cause electron translations but molecular vibration. The wavelengths and energies that have generally been used in research areas of biophysics and biochemistry are shown in Table 7.1.

The basic principle of Fourier-transform infrared spectroscopy (FTIR) spectros-copy is the measurement of infrared radiation emitted or absorbed by a sample. The absorption of specific wavelengths upon interacting with specific molecular bond-ing happens when the frequency of the IR radiation matches the molecular resonant frequency. The absorbed wavelength ranges can be measured and represented in identifiable peaks. Thus, it is possible to determine the significant chemical bonding present in the sample [37].

TABLE 7.1
The Infrared Regions and Energy Ranges

	Wavenumber (cm⁻¹)	Wavelength (μm)	Energy (eV)
NIR	12500–4000	0.8–2.5	1.5–0.5
MIR	4000–400	2.5–25	0.5–0.05
FIR (THz)	400–10	25–1000	0.05–0.001

FTIR spectroscopy is a fast and non-destructive analytical method complementary to chemometrics, and it becomes a powerful tool for the pharmaceutical industry. The potential of FTIR spectroscopy in pharmaceutical drugs analysis was reviewed in detail by Bunaciu et al., 2010 [38]. The antimicrobial material characterization and identification using FTIR spectroscopy have become routinely used in the pharmaceutical industry. FTIR has been applied in drug delivery development. It has been used to characterize molecular interaction between vehicles and drugs. The interaction between tobramycin and lipid components of solid lip nanoparticles was evaluated using FTIR spectroscopy [39]. Moreover, FTIR analysis has been used to follow the presence of encapsulated compounds in nanoparticles by analyzing the functional groups of doxycycline presented in encapsulated drugs [40].

In recent years, the search for new antimicrobial and antiviral agents has accelerated. With this speed, faster means to identify mechanisms of action of the new potential candidates are needed. With the advantage of a high-throughput method for screening whole cells, FTIR spectroscopy was used to study the biochemical effect of a new drug on bacterial cells [41]. The antimicrobial activity of gallic acid conjugated with gold nanoparticles on foodborne pathogens was analyzed using FTIR spectroscopy. The analysis revealed that the conjugated AuNP-GA caused alterations to lipids, proteins, and nucleic acids in the bacterial cell membrane [42].

The application of modern mid-IR FTIR spectrometers utilized higher sensitivity to analyze tiny samples or localized areas of larger samples. The development includes systems in which an FTIR spectrometer is interfaced to an optical microscope or is equipped with a liquid nitrogen-cooled high sensitivity detector. Additionally, synchrotron radiation has been coupled with FTIR spectrometer and IR microscope in IR beamlines worldwide to gain the advantages of the bright and high collimated synchrotron radiation. This leads to the application of FTIR microspectroscopy in the cellular and sub-cellular level study. The study of the interaction of the drug and the bacteria at single-cell is challenging. Recently, Meneghel et al. developed a custom-built attenuated total reflection inverted microscope coupling to a synchrotron-based FTIR spectrometer and achieved a projected spot size of 1×1 micron^2 allowed spectral acquisition at the single-cell level in the 1800–1300 cm⁻¹ region (Amide I and II of proteins) [43]. This achievement leads to future study mechanisms of antibacterial agents against bacterial at the single-cell level.

The advantages of synchrotron FTIR microspectroscopy, including higher signal-to-noise ratio, high-energy throughput, and high accuracy and stability, gain this technique more interest in advanced material characterization. However, the application of this technique is suitable to solid-phase samples while working with samples in the liquid phase is feasible but remains challenging. Furthermore, multiple background scans and post-processing analysis are undeniable limitations of this technique.

7.4 MICROSCALE

7.4.1 X-Ray Tomography

X-ray tomography (XTM) has emerged as an X-ray imaging approach that provides three-dimensional information not long after discovering X-rays by Wilhelm Conrad Röntgen (1845–1923) [44]. Nowadays, X-ray microtomography is applied in medical imaging and is widely used as a non-invasive assessment tool in materials science research. The tomographic images are allowed for three-dimensional (3D) visualization to analyze the microstructures, including porosity and defects such as fatigue cracks of most types of materials with sub-micron resolution [45]. Recently, third-generation synchrotron X-ray radiation sources have established themselves as invaluable experimental facilities for X-ray microtomography. The 3D information of the internal structure of materials can be obtained with excellent spatial and temporal resolution [46–49]. The principal difference between synchrotron X-rays and the X-rays used in hospitals is the brilliance. Synchrotron radiation (SR) is emitted from electrons traveling at almost the speed of light in a tangential direction to its circular orbit as a magnetic field bends the electron's path in a storage ring. SR is characterized by high directionality, variable polarization, and brightness more than 10^6-times brighter than radiation from laboratory or medical X-ray sources. This brightness is attributable to the fine collimation of the X-ray beam. Utilizing insertion devices of the storage ring such as superconducting multipole wiggler or superconducting undulator, higher photon flux, higher energy, and coherence X-ray beam can be produced to serve a broader range of specimens; from poorly X-ray absorbed systems such as soft tissue to highly X-ray immersed systems such as metal alloys. Given the high intensity of the synchrotron radiation, tomographic scanning can be achieved in a few minutes. This has made it possible to visualize the microstructure of materials in realistic synthesis environments and operating conditions, at high or low temperatures or under tensile strength—the structural change in real time or investigations in non-equilibrium states [50]. Moreover, tuning the X-ray energy of SR source by crystals or multilayers offers the single-wavelength monochromatic beam that allows for the qualitative analysis of selected elements and eliminates the beam hardening artifacts due to the energy dependence of X-ray absorption. One more advantage of synchrotron light source to X-ray imaging system is the flexible experiment station that can be adjusted to accommodate large specimens or equipped with the custom-made apparatus for *in situ* experiments.

SR microtomography beamline in most synchrotron facilities usually consists of a specimen rotator, single-crystal scintillator (X-ray phosphor), optical lens, and an area detector such as a CCD. Depicted in Figure 7.7, the polychromatic X-rays generated from a bending magnet or an insertion device (an undulator or a multipole wiggler) are converted to a monochromatic beam by a double-crystal monochromator

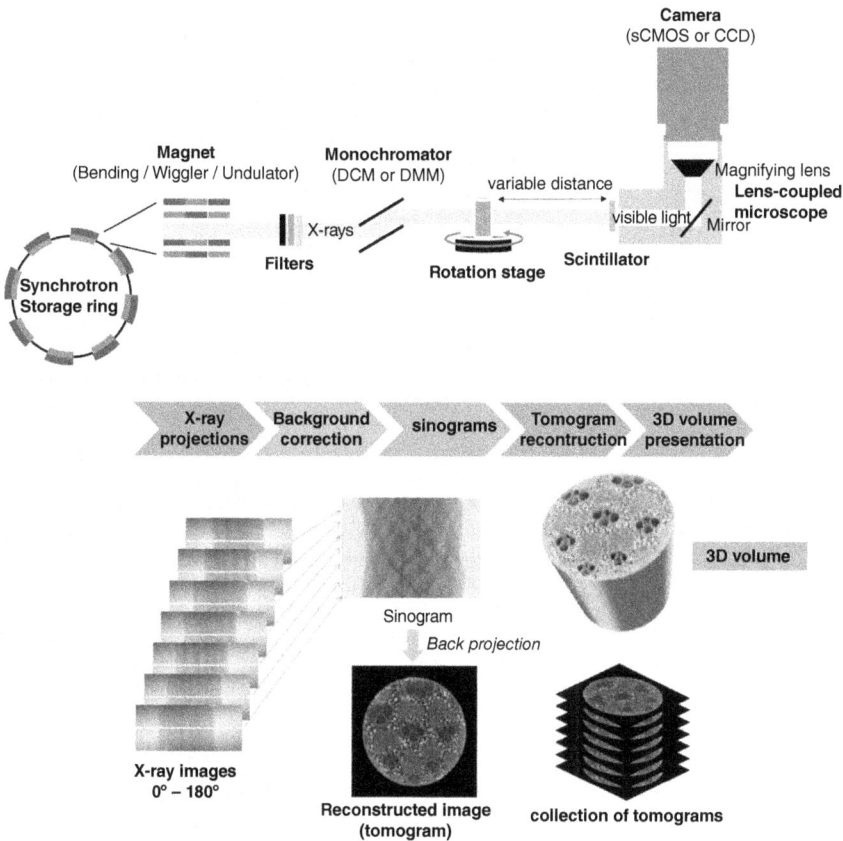

FIGURE 7.7 SR microtomography beamline layout (upper) and the standard X-ray microtomography procedure (lower).

(DCM) or a double-multilayer monochromator (DMM). When the monochromatic X-ray beam passes through a specimen mounted on the rotation stage, the X-rays are attenuated due to interactions with the electrons in the specimen. A detection system records the attenuated X-ray beam. It is converted into visible light by a scintillator, then collected and magnified by an objective lens, and forms a real-space image on the area detector.

In tomography, a collection of X-ray images is acquired when the specimen is rotated. Given the parallel beam geometry of the synchrotron source, a typical tomography scan requires X-ray projections from 180 degrees around the specimen to reconstruct a complete 3D image representing the local mass distribution in the specimen. Illustrated in Figure 7.8 is the tomographic reconstruction procedure based on the backprojection algorithm [51–52]. The backprojection reconstruction algorithm takes each projection to build a sinogram and mathematically projects it back along the angle θ at which it is recorded. So, the mass represented by each line profile is distributed uniformly along the ray path at each angle. This virtual

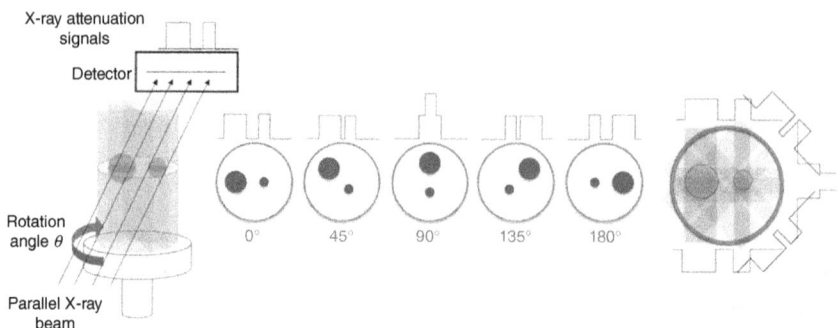

FIGURE 7.8 Backprojection of tomographic image and their X-ray attenuation signals from different rotation angles.

mass is constructed at positions where the intensities from different projections intersect. Therefore, to reconstruct an original cross-section image of the specimen, an increasing number of X-ray projections is required. A standard X-ray microtomography procedure is illustrated in Figure 7.8.

In materials science research, SR microtomography is increasingly being used as an additional characterizing technique to SEM/TEM that mostly limits surface characterization to provide the information in 3D, such as microstructural features and porosity in porous materials [52]. The absorption contrast between matter and air allows for the segmentation of pores or voids via binary image. A recent study led by Synchrotron Light Research Institute, Thailand, has applied SR microtomography to functional designs of fine-silk fabric face masks for particles 2.5 microns (PM2.5) and COVID-19 protection. The microstructures of various natural and synthetic fibers were studied along with the weaving thread and patterns used, which contribute to their filtration efficiency. The 3D information of the porosity was involved in designing and engineering the thread and the weaving pattern for high filtration efficiency as well as good ventilation to the wearers. SR microtomography revealed the microstructural sieves tightly formed in a cross-sectional view of the designed Thai-fine silk fabric accounted for 32% porosity (Figure 7.9). The designed face mask displayed more than 80% filtration efficiency to prevent PM2.5 particles and more than 70% to particles 0.3 microns (unpublished data).

Many advanced materials nowadays rely mostly on silver nanoparticles (AgNPs) to deliver the antibacterial property. The distribution of AgNPs in the material, therefore, can be a factor affecting antibacterial activity. SR microtomography can offer a visualization to trace the AgNPs [53]. Since the amount of X-rays absorbed as they pass through the specimen depends on the density and composition of the material being imaged, AgNPs are speculated to attenuate X-rays more than their surrounded materials and thus visible in tomographic images. Using SR monochromatic X-ray beam with this system can also minimize the scattering artifacts contributed by AgNPs and allow for quantitative analysis. However, the quality of tomographic images can be disturbed if the material surrounding AgNPs has similar X-ray attenuation to AgNPs. Illustrated in Figure 7.10 is an example of the 3D tomographic

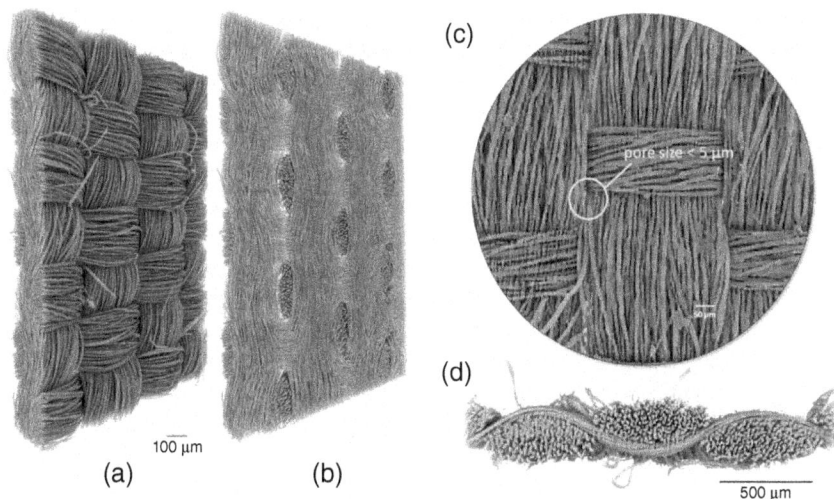

FIGURE 7.9   3D visualization of microstructure of Thai silk fabric face mask. (a) 3D tomographic volume presentation of Thai silk fabric, (b) cross-sectional view of the tomographic volume of Thai silk fabric, (c) magnified view of Thai silk fabric and the pore distributed across the fabric of less than 5 microns in size, (d) cross-sectional view of Thai silk fabric along z-axis.

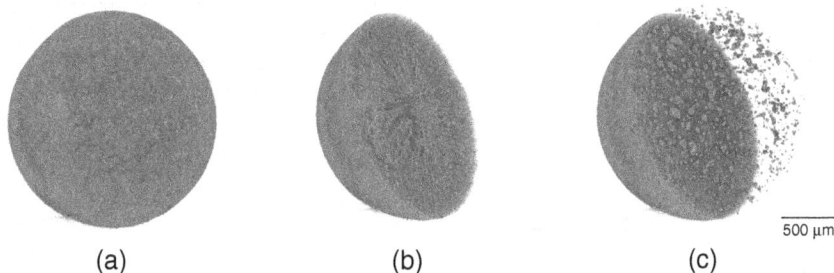

FIGURE 7.10   Tomographic images of silver nanoparticle augmented PVDF microcapsules. (a) 3D tomographic volume of the PVDF microcapsule (blue color), (b) cross-sectional view of the PVDF microcapsule reveals the pores inside, (c) cross-sectional view of the PVDF microcapsule with the other half renders the agglomerated AgNPs (red color).

volume of polyvinylidene difluoride (PVDF) microcapsule augmented with AgNPs. The microstructure and the pores inside the microcapsule are revealed. The agglomerated AgNPs can be segmented on the absorption contrast between PVDF and AgNPs, as shown in Figure 7.10.

7.4.2   X-Ray Fluorescence Spectroscopy

X-ray fluorescence spectroscopy (XRF) is one of the well-established characterization techniques. It is a non-destructive probe and has been used in a wide range of applications for elemental analysis. The basic principle of XRF is based on recording characteristic X-rays, so-called fluorescent X-rays, generated from the interaction between the inner shell electrons and X-rays as the materials are exposed to X-rays. Suppose the energy of incoming X-rays are higher than the binding energy of the inner shell electrons. In that case, the interaction will result in the electrons in that shell being ejected from the atom, become photoelectrons and leave holes in that energy level. The holes are then filled by cascading of electrons from higher energy levels to fill the inner shell vacancies and emitting characteristic fluorescent X-rays (Figure 7.1[b]). By measuring the energy of the emitted characteristic X-rays, all elements in the material are qualitatively and quantitatively identified.

The same basic principle of the XRF technique aforementioned is applied for synchrotron-based-X-ray fluorescence (SR-XRF) but with the advantage of small size X-ray spots and high brilliance X-ray source. For SR-XRF, an X-ray beam is focused (by focusing optics, e.g., KB-mirror, compound refractive lens, zone plates) onto the specimen with the size ranging from microns to nanometers, whereas the conventional XRF uses millimeter-sized X-ray beam. In most XRF measurements, samples are subjected to raster scans to obtain 2D elemental mapping therefore, the SR-XRF provides much better spatial resolution than conventional XRF. Moreover, high brilliance synchrotron X-rays allow better detection ability for low elemental concentration down to a few ppm [54]. Table 7.2 lists some examples of SR-XRF beamlines and end stations at different synchrotron facilities with the available energy ranges and spatial resolutions.

Many studies on novel antimicrobial materials have been conducted. The characterization methods used for antimicrobial metals and metal oxides are usually based on FTIR microspectroscopy, X-ray diffraction, X-ray photoelectron spectroscopy, energy dispersive scanning X-ray microscopy, and X-ray fluorescence spectroscopy

TABLE 7.2
List of Some SR-XRF Beamlines at Synchrotron Facilities [94–99]

Beamline/SR facility	Flux at the sample	Energy range	Spatial resolution
XFM beamline/Australian Synchrotron, Australia	2×10^{10} ph/s at 10 keV	4–27 keV	Down to 2×2 μm^2 (H × V)
Microprobe XRF beamline/ Indus-2, India	10^7–10^8 ph/s at 10 keV	4–20 keV	7.5×4.3 μm^2 (H × V)
Microfocus spectroscopy beamline (I18)/Diamond, UK	2×10^{12} ph/s at 10 keV	2–20 keV	2.1×2.5 μm^2 (H × V)
TES beamline/NSLS-II, USA	Up to 10^{11} ph/s	2–8 keV	2 to 25 μm spot size
ID16BX-ray nanoprobe/ ESRF, France	N/A	5–70 keV	~50 nm spot size
BL37XU/Spring-8, Japan	10^{10}–10^{11} ph/s	6–17 keV	1.35×0.83 μm^2 (H × V)
BL5.1WB/SLRI, Thailand (under construction)	~10^8 ph/s (calculated)	4–30 keV	20–40 μm spot size

techniques [55–57]. For the XRF technique, most characterization works have been conducted to verify the incorporation of antimicrobial metals into composite materials [58–59] or to prove the homogeneity of antimicrobial metals in the matrix or on the surface of products [60]. Metals, metal oxides, or metal salt-based materials (e.g., silver [Ag], zinc oxide [ZnO], titanium oxide [TiO_2], and iron oxide [Fe_3O_4]) have been known for their bactericidal activities and widely used as antimicrobial materials [61]. As the very high spatial distribution of such antimicrobial agents in sub-micron resolution is unnecessary, the laboratory XRF is usually adequate for material characterization without the need for SR-XRF spectroscopy. The use of SR-XRF in antimicrobial material characterization is limited to experiments not achievable using laboratory XRF. Those cases include the elemental localization at the cellular or sub-cellular level. For example, the effect of silver nanoparticles in the wound dressing to the healing mechanism of the skin wounds has been studied using SR-XRF. This study showed the information of spatial distribution and speciation (studied by SR-XAS spectroscopy) of the silver nanoparticle that were released to the wound surface [62]. Takeuchi et al. [14] used synchrotron micro-XRF and micro-XANES to investigate the Ag in sock fabric buried in the soil. Distribution of Ag and Ag speciation in the soil section revealed that silver in the sock fabric is relatively stable and has a negligible effect on soil enzymes. The work done by Smulders et al. [63] investigated the effect of inhalation of silver nanoparticles on the mice's lung tissues. The XRF mapping revealed the co-location of Fe and Cu in the Ag-rich spots, which suggested a formation of metallothioneins (MTs). SR-XRF spectroscopy can be used in complementary with other synchrotron-based techniques such as XAS, synchrotron-FTIR microspectroscopy, and SR-XTM to elucidate the antimicrobial mechanism of nanoparticle in the antimicrobial product after being contacted to living cells or to study the effect of these nanoparticles released into the natural resources such as aquatic environments, terrestrial environments, or even in the atmosphere.

7.5   SURFACE AND INTERFACE

7.5.1   GRAZING INCIDENCE X-RAY DIFFRACTION

Grazing incidence X-ray diffraction (GIXRD) is a surface-sensitive technique providing phase compositions, crystalline-phase purity, crystallographic information, structural ordering, and crystallite orientation of chemicals in the forms of thin films, coatings, and membranes. In GIXRD setup, the incident monochromatic X-ray beam is parallelly exposed to the surface (or interface) of a sample at the very-small (grazing) incidence angle (α_i), which consequently interacts with the material only at a low depth profile but with a wide footprint (i.e., surface probing). The diffracted (also called Bragg scattered) X-ray is detected by a position-sensitive detector (PSD), mainly using area detectors such as X-ray image plate and CCD detector.

Two-dimensional (2D) GIXRD pattern is used to identify preferred crystallite orientation within a thin-film sample, which correspondingly exhibits a discrete diffracted pattern on an area detector. In detail, each Bragg scattered peak illustrates a high intensity at a specific position on an area detector corresponding to the crystallite orientation on a substrate surface. Performing the vertical line cut profile of the

2D-GIXRD pattern, so-called the out-of-plane component, gives structural information on the crystallite planes aligned parallelly to the substrate surface (stacking crystallite planes on the film growth direction). The horizontal line cut profile of the 2D-GIXRD pattern, so-called the in-plane component, provides periodic orientation of crystallite planes aligned in the normal direction to the substrate surface.

Comparing to laboratory GIXRD, synchrotron GIXRD offers various advantages such as the possibility to select X-ray wavelength, well-defined parallel beam nature, high intensity, and high resolution. Moreover, sample stages and sample environmental-controlled units can be straightforwardly modified to suit each specific experiment. Hence, synchrotron facilities have attracted significant attention for GIXRD measurements required *in situ* monitoring and high-resolution data. Generally, synchrotron GIXRD has been carried out to study phase compositions, physical and chemical stability of antimicrobial substances distributed in various fabricated materials such as polymer composite films, porous membranes, woven textiles, and coatings.

Interestingly, synchrotron GIXRD has been effectively used to study phospholipid membranes' structural orientation, including the highly oriented multilamellar samples, the formation of phospholipid monolayers on the air/liquid interface, and the phospholipid bilayers [64–67]. In addition, synchrotron GIXRD has been carried out to monitor the interaction between antimicrobial peptides and phospholipid membranes to understand the mechanistic activity of antimicrobial peptides at a molecular level. The obtained information can be further used to design and develop novel peptide-based antibiotics to overcome the dramatically increased number of multidrug-resistant bacteria strains.

As an example, synchrotron GIXRD was used to characterize the structural ordering of a neutral multilamellar membrane, so-called 1,2-dimyristoyl-*sn*-glycerol-3-phosphatidylcholine (DMPC) deposited on cleaned silicon wafers or glass substrates. Regarding the out-of-plane GIXRD pattern, the well-defined Bragg peaks with periodic intervals were observed, suggesting the highly oriented multilamellar structure of DMPC with a well-defined lamellar periodicity of 4.96 nm. Addition of antimicrobial peptide, namely "magainin 2" to DMPC under biologically relevant liquid Lα phase led to a substantial decay of GIXRD Bragg peak intensity assigned to the periodic lamellar structure of DMPC. This result indicated that the intercalation of the "magainin 2" peptide affected the structural ordering of DMPC in both the lamellar stacking and the local molecular ordering of the hydrophobic tails in the multilamellar membrane. The interference of lamellar ordering of phospholipid multilamellar membrane utilizing the antimicrobial peptide subsequently increased membrane permeability and finally led to cell lysis. This work proposed the perspective of *in situ* investigations of antimicrobial activity of peptides by employing GIXRD and the possibility of further developing the novel peptide-based antibiotics [64].

In addition, synchrotron GIXRD was applied to investigate the selective interaction of antimicrobial peptides with various kinds of phospholipid monolayers at the air/liquid interphase. The antimicrobial frog skin isolated so-called peptide peptidyl-glycyl-leucine-carboxamide (PGLa) was used to study the selective interference toward the ordered phospholipid monolayers assembled at the air/liquid interphase: namely (a) the negatively charged phosphatidylglycerol monolayers (PG, a representative component of bacterial membranes) and (b) the zwitterionic phos-phatidylcholine monolayers (PC, a representative component of mammalian cyto-plasmic membranes). According to GIXRD patterns, the Bragg peak of pristine PG monolayers vanished after the addition of PGLa peptide, which indicated the pen-etration of PGLa into the lipid chain region and consequently the induction of a strong tilt or disordering of the aliphatic chains within the PG lipid monolayers. On the contrary, the Bragg peak of pristine PC monolayers remained observable after adding the PGLa peptide. Even though, slightly lower peak intensity was observed due to the dilution effect. This result indicated that the antimicrobial PGLa peptide did not alter the 2D periodic structure of PC monolayers. In other words, the anti-microbial PGLa peptide preferentially interacted with liposomes of PG monolayers, which induced lipid segregation and phase separation in the PG-based membranes. It suggested a high selectivity of the antimicrobial peptide to the bacterial phospholipid membranes than the mammalian ones based on the molecular mechanism of phos-pholipid-peptide interactions. Moreover, it clearly exhibited the high performance of synchrotron GIXRD as a sensitive technique to investigate the ordering of assembled molecules at the surfaces and interfaces on an atomic length scale [65].

7.5.2   X-Ray Reflectivity

X-ray reflectivity (XRR) is a non-destructive method for investigating properties of single or multilayered thin films. XRR is used to determine the thickness, density, and surface or interface roughness of exciting layers. This technique is based on measuring total reflection intensity as a function of incident angles concerning the thin film surface. Single-crystalline, polycrystalline, or amorphous materials can be non-destructively analyzed.

A reflectivity profile exhibits oscillations caused by interference between X-ray reflected from the surface of the coated layer and the interface between the coated layer and the substrate. This oscillation is known as Kiessing fringes [68]. The period of the oscillation depends on the film thickness; the thicker film, the shorter the period of the oscillation. When X-rays are applied to a sample flat surface at grazing angles of incidence, a total reflection will occur at or below a critical angle (θ_c). The density difference between the film and the substrate affects the amplitude of the oscillation and the critical angle; the more significant the density, the higher the amplitude of the oscillation and the higher the critical angle. The value of the critical angle of a film is determined from,

$$\theta_c = \sqrt{2\delta} \qquad (7.5)$$

where δ is a real part of the refractive index which is proportionated to wavelength and density following the relation,

$$\delta \propto \lambda^2 \rho \qquad (7.6)$$

The decay rate of the reflectivity profile is modified by surface roughness; the larger the roughness of the film, the faster the decay rate of reflectivity. The interface roughness comprises both the physically uneven interface and the transitional boundary where the density continuously changes. These two origins of interface roughness can be identified as a continuous variation of electron density along the thickness direction; the larger the interface roughness, the lower the oscillation amplitude. Thin-film information can be extracted from the XRR profile, as shown in Figure 7.11. The optimal solution from refining experimental to theoretical curve, based on layer structure model, provides thickness, density, and roughness of the film. From the non-linear least squares fitting, the optimal parameter values are based on Parratt formalism [69], coupled with the Nevot and Croce theory to include roughness [70].

The detailed surface properties of the active layer of antimicrobial materials coated on substrates are extensively studied in hard and soft materials. The thickness of atomic layer deposition (ALD) ZnO and Al_2O_3 on polymer films was indirectly determined [71]. The actual polymer thin films had poor thermal stability, film flatness, and surface roughness. Therefore, the silicon wafers were used as substrates. The polymer layers were deposited using similar conditions to those used to fabricate the polymer films, and the properties of the surrogate systems were analyzed. XRR can provide the surface properties of a hard active layer on a substrate, but it can also be used to study the thin lipid layer. As X-rays produce relatively small incoherent background scattering than neutrons, the involved momentum transfers are more vital. Therefore, XRR has an advantage over neutron reflectivity (NR) in resolving broad interference fringes [72–73]. In fact, Martynowycz et al. [74] explored the interaction between lipopolysaccharides (LPS) from *Salmonella enterica* and the human antimicrobial peptides (AMPs) LL-37. There was evidence of a significant increase of the electron density based on XRR measurement when LL-37 interacted with AMPs. The increased electron density was less pronounced in the case of modified lipopolysaccharides (LPS). A liquid cell has been developed to study soft matter nanofilms at the mica–water interface [75].

The disadvantages and limitations of XRR mostly come from the sample rather than the limit of the instrument in synchrotron facilities. XRR has suffered from a sub-nanometer film, non-reflecting layers, laterally inhomogeneous layers, and

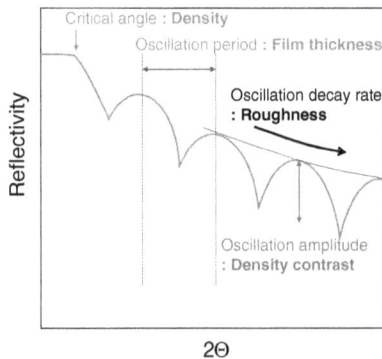

FIGURE 7.11 Features that can be obtained from XRR profile of thin films.

multi-elemental composite thin film systems [76]. X-rays are also ionizing and can lead to sample damage in soft matter systems [77]. The benefits and limitations of using *in situ* XRR for the study of protein adsorption were reviewed in detail by Richter and Kuzmenko [78].

New approaches to reflectivity data analysis and detectors have been developed. A combination of molecular dynamics (MD) simulations and XRR has been used to study soft biomolecular interfaces [77, 79–80]. The unphysical model in the fitting is limited with MD, and MD's structure can be corrected with real-world data. Fujii developed the new, improved formalism to correct the surface and interface roughness effect. This new XRR formalism depends on the size of coherent X-rays probing area, derived the roughness correlation function and the lateral correlation length [81]. A New 2D detector with low noise and fast readout allows a much quicker measurement time suitable for *in situ* experiments [82–84]. The background in the 2D detector can be obtained simultaneously from regions of interest (ROI) using offset area by a few pixels away from ROI of reflectivity.

7.5.3 X-Ray Photoelectron Spectroscopy

X-ray photoelectron spectroscopy (XPS) is one of the most widely used techniques to investigate chemical compositions of materials non-destructively. It works by using excitation by a monochromatic X-ray to the electrons inside materials. If the X-ray has energy higher than the binding energy of certain shells, the excited electrons from those shells can be removed from the atoms by the energy transfer. These emitted electrons are called *photoelectrons*. Their kinetic energy is equal to the difference between the X-ray energy and the *electron shell's binding energy*. As electrons in each shell have characteristic binding energy specific to the atomic species, the kinetic energy and the number of the photoelectrons represent atomic species and the amount of the particular atoms inside the samples. A survey scan in XPS that produces a spectrum covering a wide range of photoelectron kinetic energy (typically up to more than 1000 eV) can give detailed information about how many species of atoms and how much for each of them are in the sample. XPS users can rely on a binding energy table in X-ray Data Booklet (*https://xdb.lbl.gov/Section1/Sec_1-1.html*), one of the most widely used references for elemental identifications in XPS. Schematic diagrams related to the XPS principle and an example of XPS measurement are shown in Figure 7.12.

One of the unique features of XPS is the very high surface sensitivity of the measurements. This is due to the very shallow escape depth of the photoelectrons (from around 0.5 to 10 nm depending on the kinetic energy), so the XPS signal only comes from the topmost part of the samples. This makes XPS very useful to acquire chemical information specifically from fragile layers of materials that otherwise may give weak signals had it been measured by other bulk characterization techniques. With a suitable selection of X-ray energy, sub-monoatomic layers of materials on the surface can be well characterized by XPS (usually done using tunable energy of synchrotron sources). The high surface sensitivity can sometimes be a challenge if the chemical information inside the bulk is needed. This can be overcome by using an in-vacuum etching technique such as Ar^+ sputtering to remove the material until the desired

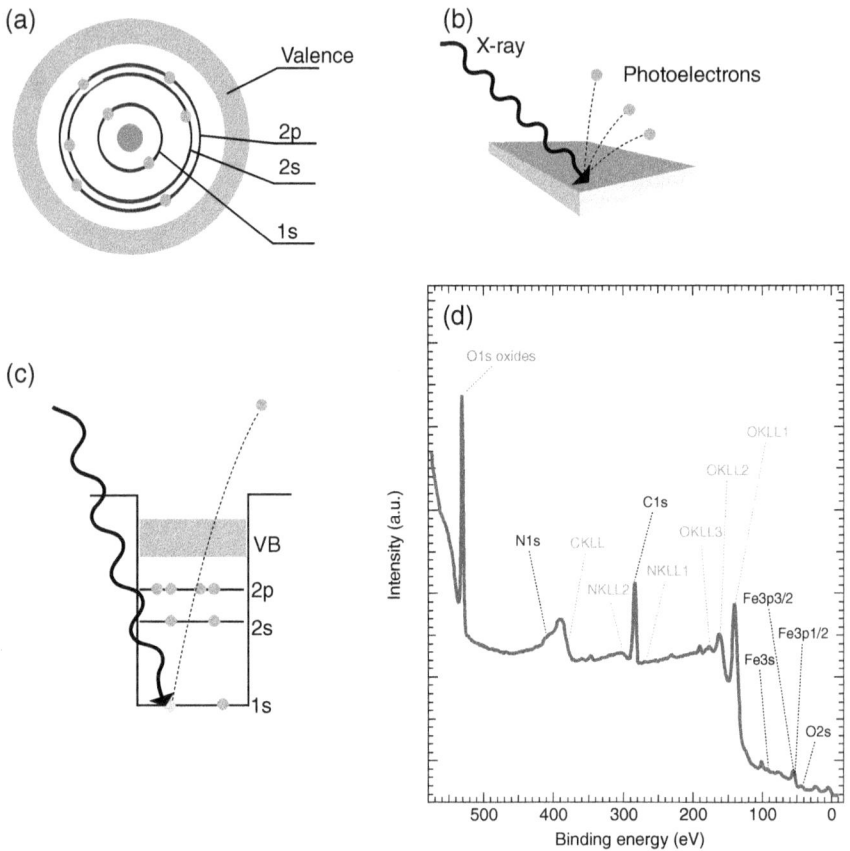

FIGURE 7.12 XPS principle: (a) electrons in atoms, (b) photoelectric effect, (c) energy band diagram and excitation, and (d) XPS spectrum of Fe surface taken by photoemission electron microscopy with synchrotron X-ray (Beamline 3.2U, Synchrotron Light Research Institute, Nakhon Ratchasima).

depth is reached (this turns XPS into a destructive measurement). With a well-controlled sputtering rate, depth profiling by XPS is also possible.

XPS tells the amounts of atomic species in the sample. It also describes the chemical states of the atoms by a slight shift of the binding energy due to the change of electrostatic screening from the valence electrons surrounding the atoms. To explain this, we need to consider that the binding energy measured by XPS is a *final state* which means that the energy required to move an electron from the core level in an atom to the continuum is measured. First, the inward electrostatic force by the positive charge in the nucleus is considered to find the binding energy. In addition to that, the electrostatic screening by the negative valence electrons (electrons in the outermost electron shell that form chemical bonds with other atoms in molecules or solids) reduces the total energy required for the electron removal (as shown in

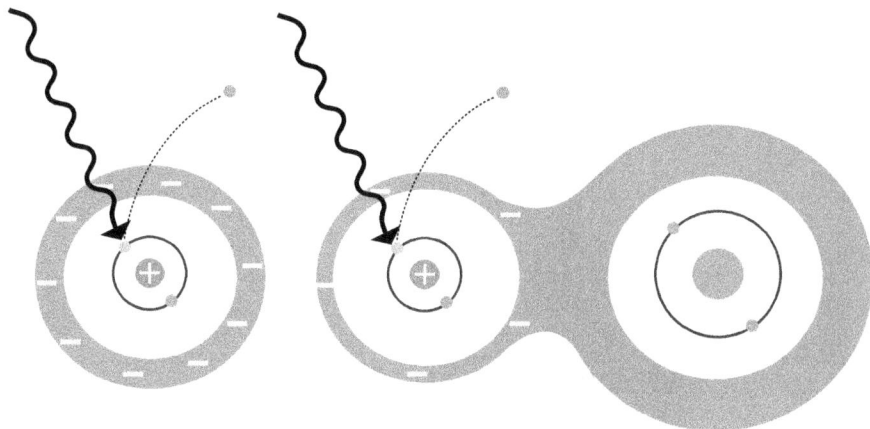

FIGURE 7.13 A diagram explaining the chemical shifts in XPS due to a change in the screening effect from a neighbor atom which has higher electronegativity.

Figure 7.13). Since the valence electrons are affected by the chemical bonds that form with surrounding neighbor atoms, e.g., when the measured atom forms a covalent bond with another atom with higher electronegativity, the valence electrons are pulled away screening effect smaller. In XPS, we see this as a slight but measurable shift to the higher binding energy. For example, in C atoms, the 1s core level in XPS shifts to higher binding energy if the C atoms bond with N, O, or F (the shift gets larger by the same order). For transition metals, the chemical shift is also larger with a higher oxidation number. For materials with multiple covalent bonding to different atoms or with many oxidation states, XPS analysis can quantitatively determine the amount of each chemical state typically by deconvolution of XP spectra into multiple Gaussian–Lorentzian peaks. The area under each peak represents the quantitative amount. Details of the deconvolution/peak fitting procedures can be found in many sources elsewhere [85].

Most XPS systems consist of double metal hemispheres and channeltrons/MCP detectors to measure photoelectrons' energy dispersion and counts. It works by applying different bias voltages to the inner and outer hemispheres, resulting in an electric field in the gap between them that makes the incoming electrons travel in an arc. For an electron with specific kinetic energy, the radius of the arc is proportional to the kinetic energy. Therefore, for a fixed analyzer geometry, only electrons which have the right kinetic energy within a small energy window will reach the detectors (Figure 7.14). The electrons that exit the double hemisphere can either be counted by a set of channeltrons (a device that amplifies electron counts using high voltage) or a position-sensitive detector such as a microchannel plate or a delay-line detector.

Because electrons cannot travel far under atmospheric pressure, XPS must be performed inside a vacuum chamber. Conventionally XPS operates under the pressure of 10^{-8} mbar or below (this is in the *ultrahigh vacuum* regime). Because of this environment, samples that are suitable for XPS should be in a solid form. Volatile materials with high vapor pressure may degas inside the vacuum system and make

(a)   (b)

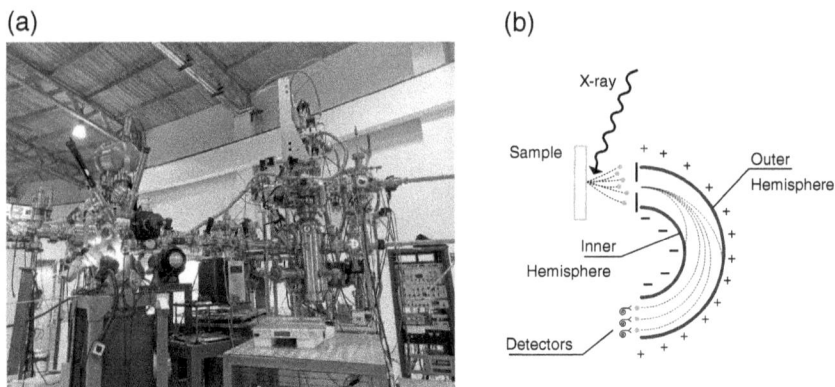

FIGURE 7.14   (a) XPS system at Beamline 3.2U of the Synchrotron Light Research Institute, Nakhon Ratchasima, Thailand. (b) A schematic diagram of photoelectrons' kinetic energy measurement by a double-hemisphere electron energy analyzer.

XPS measurements difficult. Also, because the generation of photoelectrons makes the sample surface positively charged, if the sample is not electrically conductive, the charge compensation (generally with a small electrical current from the earth ground) is small, and there can be a significant shift of binding energy for the entire XP spectrum. It can sometimes be compensated using an electron flood gun that shoots an electron beam toward the sample surface to neutralize the accumulated charges.

The X-ray source in XPS can be a small X-ray gun that produces X-ray by applying a high-energy electron beam to an anode material made from Mg or Al, resulting in Kα radiation with the fixed energy of 1254 eV and 1487 eV, respectively. Higher-intensity X-ray can be made at synchrotron facilities with a soft X-ray monochromator that consists of an X-ray grating and slits to produce highly brilliant monochromatic X-rays. For the latter, XPS users can select photon energy by adjusting the grating angle relative to the slit position to change the probing depth and also to scan the X-ray energy to perform complementary techniques such as near-edge X-ray absorption fine structure (NEXAFS) to gain more information about the chemical states of the surface (examples can be found in Krishnan et al. [86]).

Many metals and metal oxide nanoparticles have bactericidal effects so that they can be used as antimicrobial agents. Certain metals with the appropriate chemical states kill bacteria or prevent bacterial growths and biofilm formations [87]. XPS is one of the main tools to confirm that the synthesized metals and metal nanoparticles have the correct oxidation states from chemical shifts of the metal peaks in XP spectra. As XPS is widely used to identify oxidation states for metals in other applications, several useful databases are freely accessible (e.g., NIST's XPS database: *https://srdata.nist.gov/xps/main_search_menu.aspx* and Thermo Scientific's XPS database: *https://xpssimplified.com/periodictable.php*). Table 7.3 summarizes the binding energy values of metals at different oxidation states used in antimicrobial applications.

TABLE 7.3

Binding Energy Table for Metal with Different Oxidation States Related to the Antimicrobial Applications (All Data Are from $2p_{3/2}$ Core Levels Except Ag Which Uses $3d_{5/2}$ Level)

Element/ compounds	Binding energy (eV)	Element/ compounds	Binding energy (eV)	Element/ compounds	Binding energy (eV)
Cu	933.0	Ni	852.6	Zn	1021.7
CuO	933.5	NiO	853.7	ZnO	1022.0
Ag	368.2	Mg	49.8	Ti	454.1
		MgF_2	51.0	TiO_2	458.5

Source: Data from https://xpssimplified.com

XPS also works effectively to characterize hydrocarbon molecules, so the technique is suitable for studying polymers. Usually, to add the antimicrobial properties, regular polymers (or block copolymers) must be modified by grafting active functional groups into the polymer chains. Similar to the characterization of metal nanoparticles, XPS can measure the number of functional groups by either detecting chemical shifts in C and O or detecting key elements such as N (e.g., in quaternary ammonium compounds) and F (e.g., in hydrophobic fluorinated functional groups) to confirm the successful synthesis of the polymers that are active for bacteria. As XPS is surface sensitive, it can also detect accumulations of active functional groups on the surface in direct contact with bacteria in some applications. One example can be seen from the modification of poly(vinylidene fluoride) (PVDF) with poly(hexamethylene) guanidine hydrochloride (PHMG) to make PVDF-g-AGE-PHMG for antibiofouling membrane in water treatment applications [88]. XPS detects an increase in N from the successful grafting of PHMG into PVDF and the antimicrobial performance of the polymers. XPS also explains that the high performance of 10.0 wt.% of PVDF-g-AGE-PHMG in the PVDF membrane is due to the surface enrichment of the active PHMG. Table 7.4 summarizes the ranges of binding energies for C, N, and O in different chemical states. It is crucial to note that there is still an ongoing issue related to the consistency of binding energy values reported in the literature to date. This is primarily due to different energy calibrations for XPS systems in other laboratories or from different manufacturers [89–91]. It is thus essential for XPS users to apply the basic principle of the chemical shifts in their peak assignments (e.g., by comparing influence from neighboring atoms with higher and lower electronegativities).

XPS is also used to characterize other antimicrobial materials such as graphene oxide (GO) [92]. The C/O ratio from XPS is an indicator for the successful oxidation of graphene. XPS can also detect chemical contamination (S and N) in the GO structure. While XPS with laboratory X-ray sources is adequate for checking the successful synthesis of antimicrobial materials, understanding how the surface chemical states affect the bacteria-fighting mechanism may require more detailed chemical analysis. This can be helped by the higher X-ray flux, which results in a much higher energy resolution in XPS. The X-ray can also be tuned to minimize the escape depth

TABLE 7.4

Binding Energy Table (1s Levels) for C, N, and O in Different Functional Groups Which Indicate the Chemical States of Different Polymers

Element/ functional groups	Binding energy (eV)	Element/ functional groups	Binding energy (eV)	Element/ functional groups	Binding energy (eV)
C–C	285.0[a]	C–N	285.0–286.0[c]	CF	288.0–289.0[d]
C–O	286.3–286.7[a]	N-pyridine	399.0[b]	CF_2	291.0–292.0[b,d]
C=O	287.8–288.3[a]	N-pyridine (quaternized)	402.0[b]	CF_3	293.0–294.0[b,d]
COO	289.0–289.5[a]	C=O	532.3[a]	C–O–C	532.9–533.5[a]

[a][100], [b][86], [c][101], and [d][102]

of the photoelectrons to make the measurement even more sensitive to the surface molecules. Ambient-pressure XPS currently available at many synchrotron facilities is another promising candidate to study the antimicrobial surface in action. The technique bridges the gap between conventional analysis under ultrahigh vacuum and the more realistic near ambient pressure environment. The chemical reaction between the surface and the microorganism may be studied *in situ*. Using XPS in this way is still under development. Users still need to be careful about beam damage to both the bacteria and the material in a study using intense synchrotron X-rays. A summary of how XPS can be used to study bacteria (including how materials affect parts of bacteria such as cell walls) can be found from [93].

7.6   CONCLUSIONS

Synchrotron-based techniques have proved especially powerful and practical tools in material characterization. Each technique offers different information of the materials, in bulk or surface. Much research on antimicrobial materials requires detailed information on the material characteristics from atomic scale, nanoscale, and microscale. Understanding each technique's basic knowledge, advantages, and limitations can help one choose the right tool for the research. This book chapter covers each technique's brief fundamental background, including its benefits, limitations, and case studies. The case studies reviewed in this chapter show that synchrotron-based techniques with their high brightness, tunable energy, and highly polarized radiation source are invaluable tools for frontier research in the antimicrobial field. In order to better control and optimize the materials, it is crucial to understand both their static and dynamic properties. For dynamic studies, *operando* and *in situ* capabilities of beamline end-stations surpass those of benchtop tools. Complicated experiments can be achieved with better resolution and faster acquisition. The synchrotron end-stations can face challenges of complex or non-ambient setups due to their flexible nature. Finally, combining multiple techniques with *operando* and *in situ* experiments, which is the trend of the end-station development in most beam-lines, will help support antimicrobial material research like never before.

REFERENCES

1. Calvin, S., *XAFS for Everyone*. CRC Press, 2013.
2. Bunker, G., *Introduction to XAFS: A Practical Guide to X-Ray Absorption Fine Structure Spectroscopy*. Cambridge University Press, 2010.
3. Ravel, B., and M. Newville, ATHENA, ARTEMIS, HEPHAESTUS: Data analysis for x-ray absorption spectroscopy using IFEFFIT. *Journal of Synchrotron Radiation*, 2005. **12**(4): pp. 537–541.
4. Schnohr, C.S., and M.C. Ridgway, *X-ray absorption spectroscopy of semiconductors*. Springer, 2015.
5. Li, Q., et al., Quantitative probe of the transition metal redox in battery electrodes through soft x-ray absorption spectroscopy. *Journal of Physics D: Applied Physics*, 2016. **49**(41): p. 413003.
6. Solomon, E.I., et al., Ligand K-edge x-ray absorption spectroscopy: Covalency of ligand – metal bonds. *Coordination Chemistry Reviews*, 2005. **249**(1–2): pp. 97–129.
7. Parsons, J., M. Aldrich, and J. Gardea-Torresdey, Environmental and biological applications of extended x-ray absorption fine structure (EXAFS) and x-ray absorption near edge structure (XANES) spectroscopies. *Applied Spectroscopy Reviews*, 2002. **37**(2): pp. 187–222.
8. Park, D., et al., Antimicrobial behavior of semifluorinated-quaternized triblock co-polymers against airborne and marine microorganisms. *ACS Applied Materials & Interfaces*, 2010. **2**(3): pp. 703–711.
9. Perelshtein, I., et al., Chitosan and chitosan – ZnO-based complex nanoparticles: Formation, characterization, and antibacterial activity. *Journal of Materials Chemistry B*, 2013. **1**(14): pp. 1968–1976.
10. Hsueh, Y.-H., et al., Antimicrobial effects of zero-valent iron nanoparticles on gram-positive Bacillus strains and gram-negative *Escherichia coli* strains. *Journal of Nanobiotechnology*, 2017. **15**(1): pp. 1–12.
11. Pickup, D.M., et al., Structural characterization by x-ray methods of novel antimicro-bial gallium-doped phosphate-based glasses. *The Journal of Chemical Physics*, 2009. **130**(6): p. 064708.
12. Bovenkamp, G.L., et al., X-ray absorption near-edge structure (XANES) spectroscopy study of the interaction of silver ions with *Staphylococcus aureus, Listeria monocyto-genes*, and *Escherichia coli*. *Applied and Environmental Microbiology*, 2013. **79**(20): pp. 6385–6390.
13. Page, K., et al., Titania and silver – titania composite films on glass – potent antimicro-bial coatings. *Journal of Materials Chemistry*, 2007. **17**(1): pp. 95–104.
14. Takeuchi, S., et al., Chemical speciation and enzymatic impact of silver in antimicrobial fabric buried in soil. *Journal of Hazardous Materials*, 2016. **317**: pp. 602–607.
15. Lombi, E., et al., Silver speciation and release in commercial antimicrobial textiles as influenced by washing. *Chemosphere*, 2014. **111**: pp. 352–358.
16. Impellitteri, C.A., T.M. Tolaymat, and K.G. Scheckel, The speciation of silver nanopar-ticles in antimicrobial fabric before and after exposure to a hypochlorite/detergent solu-tion. *Journal of Environmental Quality*, 2009. **38**(4): pp. 1528–1530.
17. de la Rosa, G., et al., Effects of ZnO nanoparticles in alfalfa, tomato, and cucumber at the germination stage: Root development and x-ray absorption spectroscopy studies. *Pure and Applied Chemistry*, 2013. **85**(12): pp. 2161–2174.

18. Oei, J.D., et al., Antimicrobial acrylic materials with in situ generated silver nanopar-
     ticles. *Journal of Biomedical Materials Research Part B: Applied Biomaterials*, 2012.
     100(2): pp. 409–415.
19. Pickup, D.M., et al., In situ high temperature x-ray diffraction measurements on a (TiO_2)
     0.18 (SiO_2) 0.82 xerogel using a curved image-plate. *Journal of Physics: Condensed
     Matter*, 2000. **12**(15): p. 3521.
20. Zhang, F., et al., Transformation of engineered nanomaterials through the prism of sil-
     ver sulfidation. *Nanoscale Advances*, 2019. **1**(1): pp. 241–253.
21. Dinnebier, R.E., and S.J. Billinge, Principles of powder diffraction. *Powder Diffraction:
     Theory and Practice*, 2008: pp. 1–19.
22. Waseda, Y., E. Matsubara, and K. Shinoda, *X-Ray Diffraction Crystallography:
     Introduction, Examples and Solved Problems*. Springer Science & Business Media,
     2011.
23. Kumar, T.P., et al., Highly efficient performance of activated carbon impregnated with
     Ag, ZnO and Ag/ZnO nanoparticles as antimicrobial materials. *RSC Advances*, 2015.
     5(130): pp. 108034–108043.
24. Sambhy, V., et al., Silver bromide nanoparticle/polymer composites: Dual action tun-
     able antimicrobial materials. *Journal of the American Chemical Society*, 2006. **128**(30):
     pp. 9798–9808.
25. Lima, E., et al., Gold nanoparticles as efficient antimicrobial agents for *Escherichia coli*
     and *Salmonella typhi*. *Chemistry Central Journal*, 2013. **7**(1): pp. 1–7.
26. Stanić, V., et al., Synthesis, characterization and antimicrobial activity of copper and
     zinc-doped hydroxyapatite nanopowders. *Applied Surface Science*, 2010. **256**(20):
     pp. 6083–6089.
27. Cano, A.P., et al., Copper sulfate-embedded and copper oxide-embedded filter paper
     and their antimicrobial properties. *Materials Chemistry and Physics*, 2018. **207**:
     pp. 147–153.
28. Veranitisagul, C., et al., Antimicrobial, conductive, and mechanical properties of
     AgCB/PBS composite system. *Journal of Chemistry*, 2019. **2019**.
29. Marques, J., et al., Cyclodextrins improve the antimicrobial activity of the chloride salt
     of Ruthenium (II) chloro-phenanthroline-trithiacyclononane. *Biometals*, 2009. **22**(3):
     pp. 541–556.
30. Gamarra, A., et al., Amphiphilic ionic complexes of hyaluronic acid with organo-
     phosphonium compounds and their antimicrobial activity. *International Journal of
     Biological Macromolecules*, 2018. **118**: pp. 2021–2031.
31. Malmir, S., et al., Poly(3-hydroxybutyrate-co-3-hydroxyvalerate)/cellulose nanocrystal
     films: Artificial weathering, humidity absorption, water vapor transmission rate, anti-
     microbial activity and biocompatibility. *Cellulose*, 2019. **26**(4): pp. 2333–2348.
32. Edwards-Gayle, C.J., et al., Self-assembly, antimicrobial activity, and membrane inter-
     actions of arginine-capped peptide bola-amphiphiles. *ACS Applied Bio Materials*, 2019.
     2(5): pp. 2208–2218.
33. Castelletto, V., et al., Arginine-containing surfactant-like peptides: Interaction
     with lipid membranes and antimicrobial activity. *Biomacromolecules*, 2018. **19**(7):
     pp. 2782–2794.
34. Edwards-Gayle, C.J., et al., Selective antibacterial activity and lipid membrane interac-
     tions of arginine-rich amphiphilic peptides. *ACS Applied Bio Materials*, 2020. **3**(2):
     pp. 1165–1175.
35. Yang, L., et al., Synthetic antimicrobial oligomers induce a composition-dependent
     topological transition in membranes. *Journal of the American Chemical Society*, 2007.
     129(40): pp. 12141–12147.
36. Hu, K., et al., A critical evaluation of random co-polymer mimesis of homogeneous
     antimicrobial peptides. *Macromolecules*, 2013. **46**(5): pp. 1908–1915.

37. Stuart, B., *Infrared Spectroscopy*. Kirk-Othmer Encyclopedia of Chemical Technology, 2000.
38. Bunaciu, A.A., H.Y. Aboul-Enein, and S. Fleschin, Application of Fourier transform infrared spectrophotometry in pharmaceutical drugs analysis. *Applied Spectroscopy Reviews*, 2010. **45**(3): pp. 206–219.
39. Chetoni, P., et al., Solid lipid nanoparticles as promising tool for intraocular tobramycin delivery: Pharmacokinetic studies on rabbits. *European Journal of Pharmaceutics and Biopharmaceutics*, 2016. **109**: pp. 214–223.
40. Hosseini, S.M., et al., Doxycycline-encapsulated solid lipid nanoparticles as promising tool against *Brucella melitensis* enclosed in macrophage: A pharmacodynamics study on J774A. 1 cell line. *Antimicrobial Resistance & Infection Control*, 2019. **8**(1): p. 62.
41. Ribeiro da Cunha, B., L.P. Fonseca, and C.R. Calado, Metabolic fingerprinting with Fourier-transform infrared (FTIR) spectroscopy: Towards a high-throughput screening assay for antibiotic discovery and mechanism-of-action elucidation. *Metabolites*, 2020. **10**(4): p. 145.
42. Rattanata, N., et al., Gallic acid conjugated with gold nanoparticles: Antibacterial activity and mechanism of action on foodborne pathogens. *International Journal of Nanomedicine*, 2016. **11**: p. 3347.
43. Meneghel, J., et al., FTIR micro-spectroscopy using synchrotron-based and thermal source-based radiation for probing live bacteria. *Analytical and Bioanalytical Chemistry*, 2020. **412**(26): pp. 7049–7061.
44. Filler, A., The history, development and impact of computed imaging in neurological diagnosis and neurosurgery: CT, MRI, and DTI. *Nature Precedings*, 2009: p. 1.
45. Withers, P.J., X-ray nanotomography. *Materials Today*, 2007. **10**(12): pp. 26–34.
46. Stock, S.R., *Microcomputed Tomography: Methodology and Applications*. CRC Press, 2019.
47. Stock, S., Recent advances in x-ray microtomography applied to materials. *International Materials Reviews*, 2008. **53**(3): pp. 129–181.
48. Maire, E., and P.J. Withers, Quantitative x-ray tomography. *International Materials Reviews*, 2014. **59**(1): pp. 1–43.
49. Banhart, J., *Advanced Tomographic Methods in Materials Research and Engineering*. Vol. 66. Oxford University Press, 2008.
50. Marone, F., et al., Time resolved in situ x-ray tomographic microscopy unraveling dynamic processes in geologic systems. *Frontiers in Earth Science*, 2020. **7**: p. 346.
51. Zeng, G.L., Model based filtered backprojection algorithm: A tutorial. *Biomedical Engineering Letters*, 2014. **4**(1): pp. 3–18.
52. Withers, P.J., et al., X-ray computed tomography. *Nature Reviews Methods Primers*, 2021. **1**(1): pp. 1–21.
53. Molnar, I.L., et al., Method for obtaining silver nanoparticle concentrations within a porous medium via synchrotron x-ray computed microtomography. *Environmental Science & Technology*, 2014. **48**(2): pp. 1114–1122.
54. Haschke, M., *Laboratory Micro-X-Ray Fluorescence Spectroscopy*. Vol. 55. Springer, 2014.
55. Fierascu, I., et al., Analytical characterization and potential antimicrobial and photocatalytic applications of metal-substituted hydroxyapatite materials. *Analytical Letters*, 2019. **52**(15): pp. 2332–2347.
56. Hui, F., and C. Debiemme-Chouvy, Antimicrobial N-halamine polymers and coatings: A review of their synthesis, characterization, and applications. *Biomacromolecules*, 2013. **14**(3): pp. 585–601.

57.   Khattab, T.A., et al., Development of illuminant glow-in-the-dark cotton fabric coated by luminescent composite with antimicrobial activity and ultraviolet protection. *Journal of Fluorescence*, 2019. **29**(3): pp. 703–710.

58.   Karetsi, V., et al., An efficient disinfectant, composite material {SLS@[Zn$_3$(CitH)$_2$]} as ingredient for development of sterilized and non infectious contact lens. *Antibiotics*, 2019. **8**(4): p. 213.

59.   de Araújo, L.O., K. Anaya, and S.B.C. Pergher, Synthesis of antimicrobial films based on low-density polyethylene (LDPE) and zeolite A containing silver. *Coatings*, 2019. **9**(12): p. 786.

60.   Lotfiman, S., and M. Ghorbanpour, Antimicrobial activity of ZnO/silica gel nano-composites prepared by a simple and fast solid-state method. *Surface and Coatings Technology*, 2017. **310**: pp. 129–133.

61.   Beyth, N., et al., Alternative antimicrobial approach: Nano-antimicrobial materials. *Evidence-Based Complementary and Alternative Medicine*, 2015. **2015**.

62.   Roman, M., et al., Spatiotemporal distribution and speciation of silver nanoparticles in the healing wound. *Analyst*, 2020. **145**(20): pp. 6456–6469.

63.   Smulders, S., et al., Lung distribution, quantification, co-localization and speciation of silver nanoparticles after lung exposure in mice. *Toxicology Letters*, 2015. **238**(1): pp. 1–6.

64.   Münster, C., et al., Grazing incidence x-ray diffraction of highly aligned phospholipid membranes containing the antimicrobial peptide magainin 2. *European Biophysics Journal*, 2000. **28**(8): pp. 683–688.

65.   Konovalov, O., et al., Lipid discrimination in phospholipid monolayers by the antimi-crobial frog skin peptide PGLa: A synchrotron x-ray grazing incidence and reflectivity study. *European Biophysics Journal*, 2002. **31**(6): pp. 428–437.

66.   Neville, F., et al., Lipid headgroup discrimination by antimicrobial peptide LL-37: Insight into mechanism of action. *Biophysical Journal*, 2006. **90**(4): pp. 1275–1287.

67.   Majerowicz, M., et al., Interaction of the antimicrobial peptide dicynthaurin with mem-brane phospholipids at the air– liquid interface. *The Journal of Physical Chemistry B*, 2007. **111**(14): pp. 3813–3821.

68.   Kiessig, H., Interferenz von Röntgenstrahlen an dünnen Schichten. *Annalen der Physik*, 1931. **402**(7): pp. 769–788.

69.   Parratt, L.G., Surface studies of solids by total reflection of x-rays. *Physical Review*, 1954. **95**(2): p. 359.

70.   Nevot, L., and P. Croce, Caractérisation des surfaces par réflexion rasante de rayons X: Application à l'étude du polissage de quelques verres silicates. *Revue de Physique Appliquée*, 1980. **15**(3): pp. 761–779.

71.   Vähä-Nissi, M., et al., Antibacterial and barrier properties of oriented polymer films with ZnO thin films applied with atomic layer deposition at low temperatures. *Thin Solid Films*, 2014. **562**: pp. 331–337.

72.   Clifton, L.A., et al., The role of protein hydrophobicity in thionin – phospholipid inter-actions: A comparison of α1 and α2-purothionin adsorbed anionic phospholipid mono-layers. *Physical Chemistry Chemical Physics*, 2012. **14**(39): pp. 13569–13579.

73.   Tarabia, M., et al., Neutron and x-ray reflectivity studies of self-assembled hetero-structures based on conjugated polymers. *Journal of Applied Physics*, 1998. **83**(2): pp. 725–732.

74.   Martynowycz, M.W., et al., Salmonella membrane structural remodeling increases resistance to antimicrobial peptide LL-37. *ACS Infectious Diseases*, 2019. **5**(7): pp. 1214–1222.

75.   Briscoe, W.H., et al., Synchrotron XRR study of soft nanofilms at the mica – water interface. *Soft Matter*, 2012. **8**(18): pp. 5055–5068.

76. Das, G., et al., Simultaneous measurements of X-ray reflectivity and grazing incidence fluorescence at BL-16 beamline of Indus-2. *Review of Scientific Instruments*, 2015. **86**(5): p. 055102.
77. Skoda, M.W., Recent developments in the application of X-ray and neutron reflectivity to soft-matter systems. *Current Opinion in Colloid & Interface Science*, 2019. **42**: pp. 41–54.
78. Richter, A.G., and I. Kuzmenko, Using in situ x-ray reflectivity to study protein adsorption on hydrophilic and hydrophobic surfaces: Benefits and limitations. *Langmuir*, 2013. **29**(17): pp. 5167–5180.
79. Hughes, A.V., et al., On the interpretation of reflectivity data from lipid bilayers in terms of molecular-dynamics models. *Acta Crystallographica Section D: Structural Biology*, 2016. **72**(12): pp. 1227–1240.
80. Scoppola, E., and E. Schneck, Combining scattering and computer simulation for the study of biomolecular soft interfaces. *Current Opinion in Colloid & Interface Science*, 2018. **37**: pp. 88–100.
81. Fujii, Y., Recent developments in the x-ray reflectivity analysis. *American Journal of Physics and Applications*, 2016. **4**(2): p. 27.
82. Mocuta, C., et al., Fast x-ray reflectivity measurements using an x-ray pixel area detector at the DiffAbs beamline, synchrotron SOLEIL. *Journal of Synchrotron Radiation*, 2018. **25**(1): pp. 204–213.
83. Wirkert, F., et al. *Study of Time and Pressure Dependent Phenomena at the Hard X-Ray Beamline BL9 of DELTA*. Journal of Physics: Conference Series, IOP Publishing, 2013.
84. Wirkert, F.J., et al., X-ray reflectivity measurements of liquid/solid interfaces under high hydrostatic pressure conditions. *Journal of Synchrotron Radiation*, 2014. **21**(1): pp. 76–81.
85. Sherwood, P.M., The use and misuse of curve fitting in the analysis of core x-ray photoelectron spectroscopic data. *Surface and Interface Analysis*, 2019. **51**(6): pp. 589–610.
86. Krishnan, S., et al., Surfaces of fluorinated pyridinium block co-polymers with enhanced antibacterial activity. *Langmuir*, 2006. **22**(26): pp. 11255–11266.
87. Hajipour, M.J., et al., Antibacterial properties of nanoparticles. *Trends in Biotechnology*, 2012. **30**(10): pp. 499–511.
88. Chen, F., et al., Permanent antimicrobial poly(vinylidene fluoride) prepared by chemical bonding with poly(hexamethylene guanidine). *ACS Omega*, 2020. **5**(18): pp. 10481–10488.
89. Greczynski, G., and L. Hultman, C1s peak of adventitious carbon aligns to the vacuum level: dire consequences for material's bonding assignment by photoelectron spectroscopy. *ChemPhysChem*, 2017. **18**(12): p. 1507.
90. Greczynski, G., and L. Hultman, X-ray photoelectron spectroscopy: Towards reliable binding energy referencing. *Progress in Materials Science*, 2020. **107**: p. 100591.
91. Crist, B.V., XPS in industry – Problems with binding energies in journals and binding energy databases. *Journal of Electron Spectroscopy and Related Phenomena*, 2019. **231**: pp. 75–87.
92. Fallatah, H., et al., Antibacterial effect of graphene oxide (GO) nano-particles against pseudomonas putida biofilm of variable age. *Environmental Science and Pollution Research*, 2019. **26**(24): pp. 25057–25070.
93. Ramstedt, M., L. Leone, and A. Shchukarev, *Bacterial Surfaces in Geochemistry – How Can X-Ray Photoelectron Spectroscopy Help?: Analytical Geomicrobiology: A Handbook of Instrumental Techniques*. Cambridge University Press, 2019: pp. 262–287.
94. Howard, D.L., et al., The XFM beamline at the Australian synchrotron. *Journal of Synchrotron Radiation*, 2020. **27**(5): pp. 1447–1458.

95. Tiwari, M., et al., *A Microprobe-XRF Beamline on Indus-2 Synchrotron Light Source.* Journal of Physics: Conference Series, IOP Publishing, 2013.
96. Mosselmans, J.F.W., et al., I18 – the microfocus spectroscopy beamline at the diamond light source. *Journal of Synchrotron Radiation*, 2009. **16**(6): pp. 818–824.
97. Northrup, P., The TES beamline (8-BM) at NSLS-II: Tender-energy spatially resolved x-ray absorption spectroscopy and x-ray fluorescence imaging. *Journal of Synchrotron Radiation*, 2019. **26**(6).
98. Martinez-Criado, G., et al., ID16B: A hard X-ray nanoprobe beamline at the ESRF for nano-analysis. *Journal of Synchrotron Radiation*, 2016. **23**(1): pp. 344–352.
99. Terada, Y., et al., *High-Resolution X-Ray Microprobe Using a Spatial Filter and Its Application to Micro-XAFS Measurements.* AIP Conference Proceedings, American Institute of Physics, 2011.
100. Beamson, G., *High Resolution XPS of Organic Polymers.* The Scienta ESCA 300 Database, 1992.
101. Cen, L., K. Neoh, and E. Kang, Surface functionalization technique for conferring antibacterial properties to polymeric and cellulosic surfaces. *Langmuir*, 2003. **19**(24): pp. 10295–10303.
102. Ma, Y., et al., Structural and electronic properties of low dielectric constant fluorinated amorphous carbon films. *Applied Physics Letters*, 1998. **72**(25): pp. 3353–3355.

8 Emerging Antiviral Technology

Vinaya Tari, Karthik Kannan,
and Vinita Vishwakarma

CONTENTS

8.1 INTRODUCTION

Microorganisms such as viruses, bacteria, and fungi are causing infectious diseases in plants, animals, and humans. Infectious diseases have been recognized since 1000 BC that they are the primary cause of death in the world [1]. Nearly about 40% of the 14 million deaths are occurring per year [2–3]. Therefore, this is a global public health concern. Viruses are more notorious as they will be more spread, and they have the ability to evolve through genetic mutation [4–5]. Viruses are microscopic intracellular parasites with DNA or RNA as genetic material enclosed in a protein coat called capsid [1, 5]. Sometimes lipid bilayer membranes also present external to protein coat, known as 'Envelope' [5]. Several viruses such as severe acute respiratory syndrome (SARS), Middle East Respiratory Syndrome, and Novel coronavirus, i.e., Novel COVID-19 or severe acute respiratory syndrome coronavirus-2

DOI: 10.1201/9781003143093-8

137

(SARS-CoV-2), have recently emerged and caused major disease outbreaks along with a threat to health and global economy [6]. To date, antiviral drugs do not exist for all types of viruses.

Antiviral drug development is a challenging task. However, the detection of stages involved in viral duplication is essential for the same [5]. Basic steps involved in developing antiviral drugs are, viz. identification of the target, lead generation, optimization, preclinical study, clinical trials, and finally registration of the drug (Figure 8.1). Major obstacles in approval of drugs are mainly two; side effects of

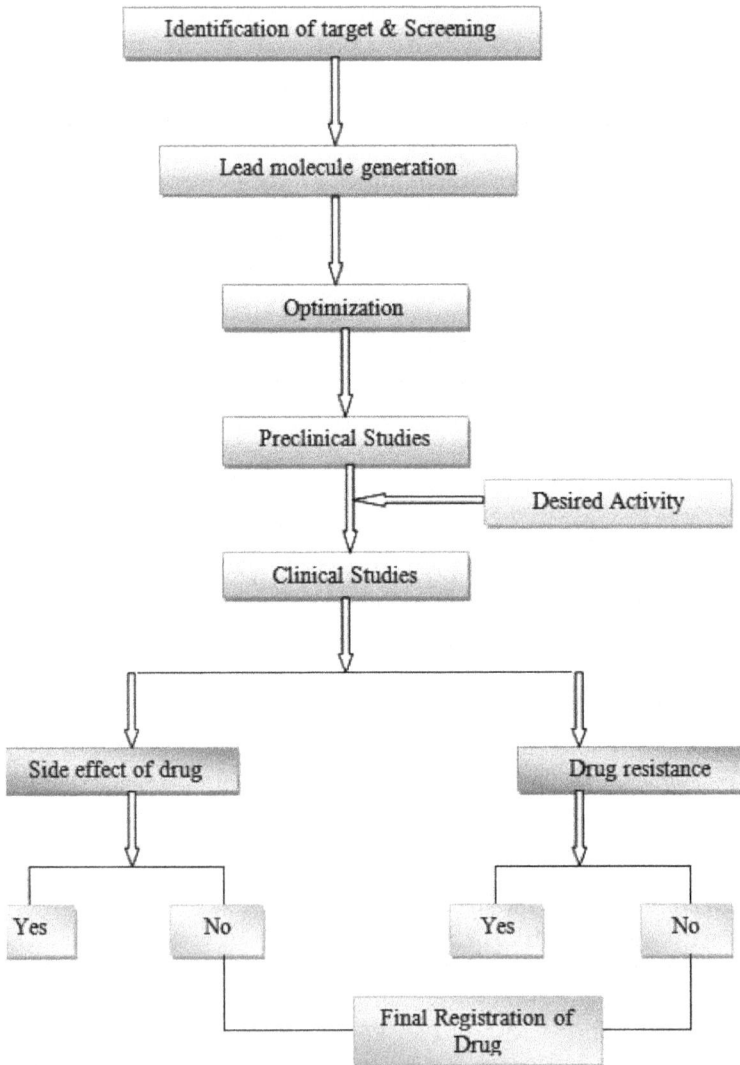

FIGURE 8.1   Drug development process.

respective drugs and development of resistance [1, 7]. Antiviral drugs are administered orally, intramuscularly, intravenously, in ointments, creams, eye drops, or can be inhaled in powder form [1]. The demand for antiviral drugs is more from very ancient times to get rid of deadly infectious diseases.

There are also many existing technologies in drug discovery to combat infectious diseases, viz. artificial neural networks (ANNs), proteomics and genomics, high throughput molecular screening, etc. [7].

8.2 APPLICATIONS OF NANOMATERIALS IN EMERGING ANTIVIRAL TECHNOLOGIES

Nanotechnology is a multidisciplinary field that mainly revolves around scales ranging between 1 and 100 nm (10^{-9}, i.e., 1 billionth of a meter). Materials that fall in that size are called 'Nanomaterials' [2]. These Nanomaterials, viz. nanoparticles, nanotubes, nanowires, nanorods, etc., are distinguished with their unique properties such as electronic, optical, mechanical, and magnetic [8]. Nanotechnology poses an essential part in growth arrest of the microorganism. Nanomaterials are proved to be clean, low cost, eco-friendly, and have a wide range of applications in various fields such as environmental, agricultural, biomedical, bio-labeling, and defense [2, 4, 8]. These nanomaterials have distinctive physical and chemical properties, viz. surface modification is possible, its large surface area to volume ratio, small size, hydrophobic and lipophilic nature, etc. [2, 5]. Due to these properties, it easily targets specific biological sites. Eventually, smooth delivery of antiviral agents to the site results in fewer side effects on non-infected cells. However, multiple antiviral entities can be integrated into a single nanoparticle, and it facilitates better bioavailability and biodistribution of therapeutics compared to molecular medicines [5]. The nanomaterials introduced intravenously can be circulated in the bloodstream and not meeting lung capillaries and mononuclear phagocytic cells [5]. Many metal and metal oxide-based nanomaterials have antimicrobial, antifungal, and antiviral properties because they disturb the respiratory enzymes leading to DNA damage of the microorganism [2, 4].

8.3 NANOPARTICLES AND THEIR APPLICATIONS

Nanomaterials are used as an alternative material for detection, treatment, and antiviral activity [4–5]. Several researchers reported that nanomaterials such as quantum dots, organic nanomaterials, silver and gold nanoparticles, polymer, dendrimers, and liposomes are effective against many viral diseases like severe acute respiratory syndrome (SARS), Middle East Respiratory Syndrome, human immunodeficiency virus, i.e., HIV, Respiratory Syncytial Virus, Hepatitis B virus, H1N1 influenza 'A' virus, Tacaribe virus, monkey poxvirus, Herpes simplex virus type 1, and Hemagglutinin type 5 and neuraminidase type 1 (H5N1) of influenza virus [6, 21–31]. Schematic presentation of various properties of nanoparticles and their application of which they fit to be used in emerging antiviral technology are shown in Table 8.1 and Figure 8.2.

TABLE 8.1
Types of Nanomaterials Used in Antiviral Therapy

Sr. no.	Types of nanomaterials used in antiviral therapeutics	Advantages	Limitations	Ref.
1	**Liposome bound**: Hydrophilic therapeutic agents with an aqueous core and lipophilic agents are incorporated in the lipid bilayer. Engulfment of liposomes by the phagocytic cells can be reduced with the help of polyethylene glycol (PEG) through chemical modification.	• Its efficiency depends on hydrophobicity and membrane fluidity. • Suitable for transdermal delivery and cellular translocation	• Poor stability *in vivo* and *in vitro* • High production cost and low efficiency of incorporation of therapeutics in the lipid bilayer and aqueous core • Biological as well as physical stability of the antiretroviral	[5, 9–10]
2	**Noisome bound (Vesicle)**: Analogous to liposome in structure. Consist of non-ionic surfactant instead of lipid bilayers	• Superior loading and slow release of drug		[5]
3	**Micelles**: The core of the micelle is made up of hydrophobic fragments, and its outer layer form of hydrophilic fragments, i.e., polar or hydrophilic head & hydrophobic tail	• Carrier for antiviral therapeutic in aqueous media • A slow rate of dissociation • Retention of the drug for a longer time • Heavy accumulation of therapeutic at the target site	• Polymeric micelle shows more excellent stability in vivo. • Irritation in the mucus membrane	[5, 9]
4	**Microspheres**: Prepared from the biodegradable poly-D,L-lactide and poly(D,L-lactide-co-glycolide) captured with antiviral drug	• Carriers for drug delivery, prolonged release of the drug, carrier for vaccine delivery	• Biodegradable	[5]
5	**Dendrimer bound**: Branched polymeric nanostructure which can bind different ligands	• Delivery of antiviral therapeutics, DNA, siRNA • Multivalent surface	• Cytotoxicity • The therapeutic index is low	[2, 5, 9]

Sr. no.	Types of nanomaterials used in antiviral therapeutics	Advantages	Limitations	Ref.
6	**Nanoparticles**: lipids, proteins, inorganic materials			
	Polymeric Nanoparticles: Natural or synthetic polymers like poly(lactic acid), poly(glycolic acid), poly(lactic-co-glycolic acid), cyclodextrin, polycaprolactone, alginate, cyclodextrin, and hyaluronic acid	• Biocompatible • Nontoxic & no leachable impurities • Increasing tissue compatibility and reducing cytotoxicity • Specific chemical composition • The rate of permeability, degradation, erosion, dissociation, etc. can be controlled.	• Biodegradable	[2]
	Inorganic Nanoparticles: surface modification of metal oxides (AuNPs, AgNPs, etc.) which provide several shapes, sizes, stability, and solubility. e.g., **Silver Nanoparticles (AgNPs)**: Silver (Ag$^+$) ions interact with biomolecules such as DNA, RNA, proteins, phosphorus, and sulfur	• Possess catalytic, magnetic, electronic, and optical properties • Directly affect various phases of the viral replication and protein synthesis	• Immunogenic	[9] [5] [11] [12–18]
	Gold Nanoparticles (AuNPs): delivery systems in immunosensor, nanorods, nanogold protein chip, etc.	• Detection of DNA sequences for Hepatitis B virus (HBV) • Analysis and detection of HBV	• Compatibility with antibodies • Evenness and stability	
	Lipid Nanoparticles: Solid at body temperature	• Carrier for drug delivery, Treatment of Hepatitis B	–	[5]
	Metal Oxide NPs: ZnO NPs: Concanavalin (Con A) and zinc oxide nanoparticles (ZnO NPs) in conjugation with EDC-NHS, i.e., Ethyl (dimethyl aminopropyl) carbodiimide–N-hydroxysulfosuccinimide sodium salt	• Detection of arbovirus	Biosensing	[19–20]

(Continued)

TABLE 8.1 (Continued)

Sr. no.	Types of nanomaterials used in antiviral therapeutics	Advantages	Limitations	Ref.
7	**Natural polymer**: active biological material can be encapsulated, entrapped, or dissolved in natural polymers, viz. gelatin, albumin, chitosan, cellulose, alginate, etc.	• Mild immunogenic	Biodegradable Varied in Physicochemical composition	[9]

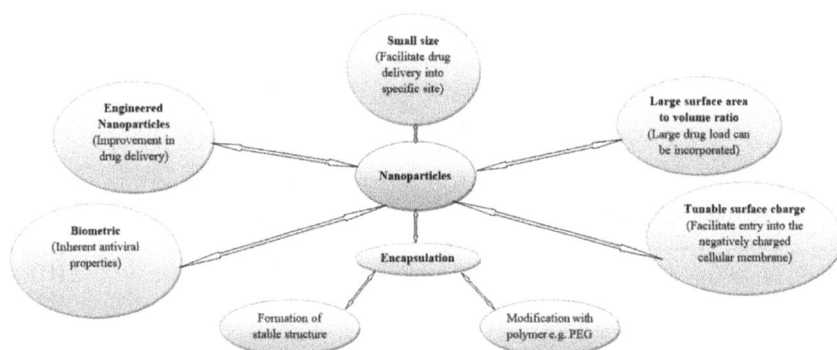

FIGURE 8.2 Schematic presentation of nanoparticles.

8.4 TYPES OF NANOMATERIALS USED IN ANTIVIRAL THERAPY

8.4.1 LIPOSOME

Hydrophilic therapeutic agents capable of being introduced inside the aqueous core. The liposome is the first commercialized nanostructure introduced in 1965, and it is mainly used as a drug delivery system. Liposome consists of at least one lipid bilayer (natural of synthetic phospholipids), and inside is an aqueous core [9]. There are many types of liposomes, viz. multilamellar vesicles, unilamellar vesicles, large unilamellar vesicles, etc. Usually, liposomes vary from 40 nm to 10 µm as per their synthesis. However, lipophilic agents are formed in the lipid bilayer, and their efficiency depends on hydrophobicity and membrane fluidity. The spleen phagocytic cells recognize liposomes rapidly after introduction in the body. However, the engulfment of liposomes by the phagocytic cells can be reduced with the help of polyethylene glycol (PEG) through chemical modification of liposomes [5–6]. There are some disadvantages of liposome nanostructure, viz. poor stability *in vivo* and *in vitro*, high production cost, and low efficacy of therapeutics in the lipid bilayer and aqueous core [5, 9]. The cellular translocation enhancement through the transactivator of transcription of HIV, i.e., TAT peptide, was achieved by introducing it into the liposome [10, 32].

8.4.2 MICELLES

Micelles are in the colloidal form with the size of 5–100 nm, and they are amphiphilic. The core of the micelle is made up of hydrophobic fragments, and its outer layer forms hydrophilic fragments. Micelles are used as a carrier for antiviral therapeutic in aqueous media. It carries lipophilic drugs in the core, whereas surfaces bind to polar molecules. Polymeric micelle shows more excellent stability in vivo. Viruses use lectin receptors for getting entry into the host cell [20]. Carbohydrate binding proteins, viz. lectins are also efficiently used for receptor-mediated targeting for drug delivery against Hemagglutinin type 5 and neuraminidase type 1 (H5N1) of influenza virus [20, 33]. Micelles consisting of polyethylene glycol (PEG) polylactide copolymer surface altered with galactose. This galactose residue interacts with lectins [5, 9].

8.4.3 MICROSPHERES

These are biocompatible spherical microparticles made up of biodegradable polymers, and these are mainly used as carriers for drug delivery. These are prepared from biodegradable poly-D,L-lactide, and poly(D,L-lactide-co-glycolide) and compacted with antiviral drug acyclovir, which has been recommended intraocular (in the eye). There are two types of microspheres, viz. matrix and capsular (Figure 8.3). Many drugs can be incorporated into microspheres.

Poly(D,L-lactide-co-glycolide) and vitamin 'A' Palmitate, along with acyclovir drug, increases acyclovir loading, resulting in prolonged drug release. However, mucoadhesive microspheres prepared from 'thiolated chitosan' retain the therapeutic in the upper gastrointestinal tract (UGT). Microspheres specially encapsulated with 'interferon α' have been designed for oral delivery. These are used as a carrier for vaccine delivery to maintain immunological challenges. The microspheres are prepared with encapsulated acyclovir and cross-linked malonyl chitosan, collectively increasing the drug concentration in the epidermis [5].

8.4.4 DENDRIMERS

Dendrimers are branched polymeric nanostructures that can bind different ligands and can be used as carriers for drug delivery [6]. The diameter is lower than 100 nm.

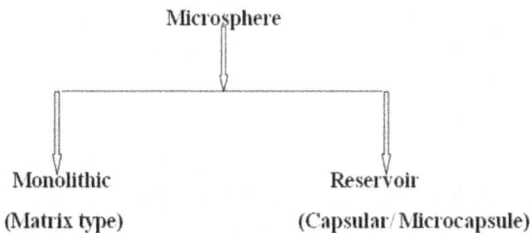

Microsphere

Monolithic   Reservoir
(Matrix type)   (Capsular/Microcapsule)

FIGURE 8.3 Types of microspheres.

It consists of three parts, viz. core, inner, and outer shell. However, branches coming out from the core part, and it looks like three-dimensional trees. Every element possesses distinct characteristics such as solubility and combining with ligand. Dendrimers are widely used to deliver antiviral therapeutics, DNA, siRNA, etc., e.g., VivaGel dendrimer (mucoadhesive gel) is prepared from divalent benzhydylamine amide of l-lysine, and it consists of 32 sodium 1-(carboxymethoxy)naphthalene-3,6-disulfonate as a terminal functional group. This formulation helps to remain active for a prolonged duration, and it is used for antiviral therapy [2, 5, 9].

8.4.5 POLYMERIC NANOPARTICLES

Several materials like lipids, proteins, and inorganic materials are used to prepare nanoparticles capable of using intravenously. The polymeric nanoparticles (NPs) are from natural or synthetic biodegradable and biocompatible polymers like poly(lactic acid), poly(glycolic acid), poly(lactic-co-glycolic acid), cyclodextrin, polycaprolactone, alginate, cyclodextrin, and hyaluronic acid. These polymers are effective for increasing tissue compatibility and reducing cytotoxicity. Active molecules of therapeutics can be adsorbed, encapsulated, dissolved, or conjugated within the NPs. In contrast, phagocytosis of NPs is avoided by adding hydrophilic elements such as polyethylene glycol (PEG) chain on the surface [2]. The polymeric nanoparticles prepared from poly(isobutyl cyanoacrylate), methacrylate, polylactide, chloromethyl methacrylate, and poly(ethyl acrylate) incorporated acyclovir lead to increasing bioavailability and activity of acyclovir drug [5, 9].

8.4.6 LIPID NANOPARTICLES

Lipid nanoparticles are in solid-state at body temperature, used as a carrier for drug delivery (Figure 8.4). Lipid nanoparticles are more advantageous when compared to liposomes. Adefovir dipivoxil was previously known as bis-POM PMEA, prepared with lipid nanoparticles, and is used to treat the Hepatitis B virus [5].

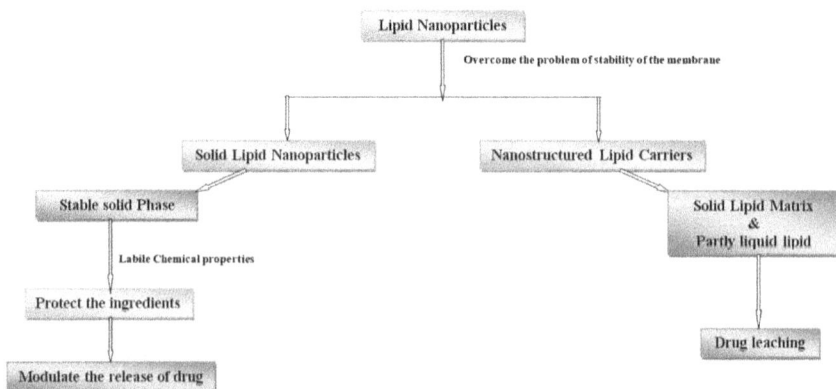

FIGURE 8.4   Lipid nanoparticles as carrier for drug delivery.

Albumin polymer protein nanoparticles are prepared for delivery of Ganciclovir and antisense oligonucleotides against Cytomegalovirus infections. The antisense oligonucleotides ('Vitravene®') are used as therapeutic agents against the treatment of ocular cytomegalovirus retinitis [34–36].

Silver nanoparticles (AgNPs): Several studies reported that AgNPs are effective against the human immunodeficiency virus, i.e., HIV, H3N2 influenza virus [6, 21–24], respiratory syncytial virus [25], Hepatitis B virus [26], H1N1 influenza A virus [27–28], monkey poxvirus [29], Tacaribe virus [30], herpes simplex virus type 1 [31], etc.

Silver (Ag+) ions interact with biomolecules such as DNA, RNA, proteins, phosphorus, and sulfur. Consequently, AgNPs have antiviral potential [2, 9, 21]. However, it is proved that AgNPs directly affect through various phases of viral replication, viz. addition of virus to the host cell membrane, access of virus to cell, DNA and RNA duplication process, and protein production process [5, 11]. The nanocomposite composed from graphene oxide (GO) sheet and AgNPs exhibited antiviral activity against feline coronavirus, i.e., FCov (enveloped) and Infectious Bursal disease virus, i.e., IBDV (non-enveloped). However, only GO sheets can inhibit enveloped virus infection [6, 24].

Gold nanoparticles (AuNPs): AuNPs are widely used in the diagnostic field. These are biocompatible and have optical [6, 16].

The detection of DNA sequences for the Hepatitis B virus (HBV) is carried out by 'Gold enhanced nanoformulation with conjugation of magnetic beads.' This technique is based on an electrochemical method [14, 37]. The electric potential shown by immunosensors is directly proportional to the Hepatitis B virus [12]. Gold AuNPs are compatible with antibodies under which these are used as delivery systems for Immunosensor [16]. The detection and analysis of antibodies associated with Hepatitis B and C can be achieved using nano-sized 'Gold protein chips' [13]. However, AuNPs-Quantum Dot (AuNP-QD) successfully diagnose the Hepatitis B virus [38]. The active replication of HBV (Hepatitis B Virus) was detected by using gold nanorods (Au NRs) biosensor based on localized surface plasmon resonance (LSPR) technique [17–18]. The fluorescence resonance energy transfer technique is used for the detection of DNA hybridization. In this technique, Hepatitis B virus sequences were detected by a Fluorescent biosensor with gold nanorods and FAM-single-stranded DNA as a probe DNA [17–18].

The diagnosis of Hemagglutinin type 5 and Neuraminidase type 1, i.e., the H5N1 virus, was successfully diagnosed by colorimetric signals created by AuNPs deposition at gold nanopyramids [39–41].

The magnetic nanozyme-linked immunosorbent assay, i.e., MagLISA technique, is successfully used to detect Influenza 'A' virus. Influenza 'A' disease is proven to be an acute infectious disease. However, it is seen by Antibody-conjugated magnetic nanobeads, i.e., MagNB-Abs and gold nanozymes (AnNZ-Abs) (MagNBs) techniques [15, 42]. The detection of arbovirus through biosensing by using lectin-NPs conjugation technique was reported by [19]. Concanavalin (Con A) and zinc oxide nanoparticles (ZnO NPs) in conjugation with EDC-NHS, i.e., Ethyl (dimethyl aminopropyl) carbodiimide-*N*-Hydroxysulfosuccinimide sodium salt was efficiently detecting arbovirus [20]. The plant-based nanocomposite derived from lignin is loaded with ascorbic acid (bioactive agent) to treat HSV-1, i.e., Herpes Simplex virus type 1 [43–44].

8.5 SITE-SPECIFIC DELIVERY OF ANTIVIRAL THERAPEUTICS

The NPs show intrinsic properties such as lipophilicity, different sizes ranging between 1 and 100 nm, and drug incorporated within surface nanoparticulates. There are three essential strategies for targeting drugs to sites, viz. passive targeting, active targeting, and direct injection of therapeutic to the precise location. The systematic process of passive targeting site-specific drug delivery through NPs is shown in Figure 8.5.

8.5.1 PASSIVE TARGETING

The surface characteristics and small size of NPs enable them for taking up by lymphatic tissues, more specifically by Peyer's patches (M cells). Then, lymph vessels transport them into lymphocytes. In this way, drugs are absorbed after oral administration. Furthermore, nanoparticles are accumulated in lymph nodes and targeting the lymphatic system (Figure 8.5). Eventually, this type of nanoparticles can get in lymphatic tissues and be utilized against viral reservoirs [2, 5].

8.5.2 ACTIVE TARGETING

Surface alterations carry out active targeting through a particular ligand-receptor system. It incorporated different strategies, viz. monoclonal antibodies for antigens communicated on desired cells of tissues, stimuli sensitive nanocarriers, etc. However, stimuli-sensitive nanocarriers are susceptible to intracellular organelles or pathological sites such as abnormal temperature, pH, temperature, and magnetic field. These internal and external stimuli amend to nanoparticles and result in the release of carried drugs in the desired region. The pH-sensitive nanocarriers such as liposomes, polymeric micelles, and nanogels promote the intracellular release of drugs. The pH-sensitive carriers are remaining unchanged at the physiological

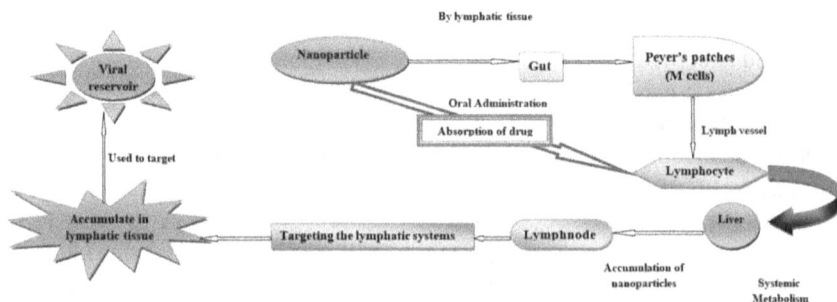

FIGURE 8.5 Passive targeting drug delivery through NPs.

pH level. However, in an acidic environment such as in liposomes, it becomes unstable and releases its aqueous content in the intracellular space [5].

8.5.3 LYMPHATIC TARGETING

Lymphatic targeting and nanoparticles in injectable systems can be obtained using small-sized particles to disperse through the interstitium and enough large-sized particles (10–100 nm) to drain through lymph vessels. Eventually, hydrophilic nanoparticles can be cleared rapidly than hydrophobic nanoparticles [2, 5].

8.6 CONCLUSIONS

Infectious viral diseases are rapidly spreading worldwide, leading to increased mortality rates and severe health concerns for society. Therefore, the development of antiviral drugs by using nanotechnology is a novel approach in the biomedical field to avoid the constraints of typical antiviral drugs. Though the basic steps for antiviral drug development are identical, many engineered nanomaterials have emerged to target-specific disease sites. These nanomaterials are liposomes, micelles, microspheres, dendrimers, polymeric nanoparticles, silver and gold nanoparticles, etc., which are easy to synthesize and cost-effective. These antiviral-based nanomaterials products should be commercialized for the benefit of the weaker section of society.

REFERENCES

1. Saxena, Shailendra K., Shailja Saxena, Rakhi Saxena, M.L. Arvinda Swamy, Ankur Gupta, and Madhavan P.N. Nair. 2010. "Emerging Trends, Challenges and Prospects in Antiviral Therapeutics and Drug Development for Infectious Diseases." *Electronic Journal of Biology* 6 (2): 26–31.
2. Singh, Lavanya, Hendrik G. Kruger, Glenn E.M. Maguire, Thavendran Govender, and Raveen Parboosing. 2017. "The Role of Nanotechnology in the Treatment of Viral Infections." *Therapeutic Advances in Infectious Disease* 4 (4). Sage Publications: 105–131. doi:10.1177/2049936117713593.
3. World Health Organization Regional Office for South-East Asia. 2005. *Combating Emerging Infectious Diseases in the South-East Asia Region*. World Health Organization Regional Office for South-East Asia, New Delhi, SEA-CD-139 February 2005.
4. Nikaeen, Ghazal, Sepideh Abbaszadeh, and Saeed Yousefinejad. 2020. "Application of Nanomaterials in Treatment, Anti-Infection and Detection of Coronaviruses." *Nanomedicine* 15 (15). Future Medicine Ltd.: 1501–1512. doi:10.2217/nnm-2020-0117.
5. Milovanovic, Marija, Aleksandar Arsenijevic, Jelena Milovanovic, Tatjana Kanjevac, and Nebojsa Arsenijevic. 2017. "Nanoparticles in Antiviral Therapy." In *Antimicrobial Nanoarchitectonics: From Synthesis to Applications*, 383–410. Elsevier Inc. doi:10.1016/B978-0-323-52733-0.00014-8.
6. Gurunathan, Sangiliyandi, Muhammad Qasim, Youngsok Choi, Jeong Tae Do, Chankyu Park, Kwonho Hong, Jin Hoi Kim, and Hyuk Song. 2020. "Antiviral Potential of Nanoparticles – Can Nanoparticles Fight Against Coronaviruses?" *Nanomaterials* 10 (9): 1–29. doi:10.3390/nano10091645.
7. Lakshmi, Badireddi Subathra, Mohan Latha Abillasha, and Pandjassarame Kangueane. 2019. "Emerging Technologies for Antiviral Drug Discovery." In *Global Virology III: Virology in the 21st Century*, 59–71. Springer. doi:10.1007/978-3-030-29022-1_3.

8.   Singh, Kshitij R.B., Vanya Nayak, Tanushri Sarkar, and Ravindra Pratap Singh. 2020. "Cerium Oxide Nanoparticles: Properties, Biosynthesis and Biomedical Application." *RSC Advances.* Royal Society of Chemistry. doi:10.1039/d0ra04736h.

9.   Mahajan, Supriya D., Ravikumar Aalinkeel, Wing Cheung Law, Jessica L. Reynolds, Bindukumar B. Nair, Donald E. Sykes, Ken Tye Yong, Indrajit Roy, Paras N. Prasad, and Stanley A. Schwartz. 2012. "Anti-HIV-1 Nanotherapeutics: Promises and Challenges for the Future." *International Journal of Nanomedicine.* doi:10.2147/IJN.S25871.

10. Jain, Akhlesh Kumar, and Umesh Gupta. 2020. "Nanomaterials Used for Delivery of Bioactives." In *Nanomaterials and Environmental Biotechnology*, 381–405. Springer. doi:10.1007/978-3-030-34544-0_19.

11. Iqbal, Mohammed Shariq, Akhilesh Kumar Singh, Satarudra Prakash Singh, and Mohammad Israil Ansari. 2020. "Nanoparticles and Plant Interaction with Respect to Stress Response." In *Nanomaterials and Environmental Biotechnology*, 1–15. Springer. doi:10.1007/978-3-030-34544-0_1.

12. Tang, D. P., R. Yuan, Y. Q. Chai, X. Zhong, Y. Liu, J. Y. Dai, and L. Y. Zhang. 2004. "Novel Potentiometric Immunosensor for Hepatitis B Surface Antigen Using a Gold Nanoparticle-Based Biomolecular Immobilization Method." *Analytical Biochemistry* 333 (2). Academic Press Inc.: 345–350. doi:10.1016/j.ab.2004.06.035.

13. Duan, Lianlian, Yefu Wang, Shawn Shun Cheng Li, Zhixiang Wan, and Jianxin Zhai. 2005. "Rapid and Simultaneous Detection of Human Hepatitis B Virus and Hepatitis C Virus Antibodies Based on a Protein Chip Assay Using Nano-Gold Immunological Amplification and Silver Staining Method." *BMC Infectious Diseases* 5 (July). doi:10.1186/1471-2334-5-53.

14. Hanaee, H., H. Ghourchian, and A. A. Ziaee. 2007. "Nanoparticle-Based Electrochemical Detection of Hepatitis B Virus Using Stripping Chronopotentiometry." *Analytical Biochemistry* 370 (2). Academic Press Inc.: 195–200. doi:10.1016/j.ab.2007.06.029.

15. Sharma, Chandni, Shanka Walia, and Amitabha Acharya. 2020. "Nanomaterials for Point of Care Disease Detection." In *Nanomaterial – Based Biomedical Applications in Molecular Imaging, Diagnostics and Therapy*, 55–77. Springer. doi:10.1007/978-981-15-4280-0_4.

16. Radwan, Sarah H., and Hassan M.E. Azzazy. 2009. "Gold Nanoparticles for Molecular Diagnostics." *Expert Review of Molecular Diagnostics.* doi:10.1586/erm.09.33.

17. Cheng, Keyi, Jianguo Zhang, Liping Zhang, Lun Wang, and Hongqi Chen. 2017. "Aptamer Biosensor for *Salmonella typhimurium* Detection Based on Luminescence Energy Transfer from Mn^{2+}-Doped NaYF4:Yb, Tm Upconverting Nanoparticles to Gold Nanorods." *Spectrochimica Acta – Part A: Molecular and Biomolecular Spectroscopy* 171 (January). Elsevier B.V.: 168–173. doi:10.1016/j.saa.2016.08.012.

18. Elahi, Narges, Mehdi Kamali, and Mohammad Hadi Baghersad. 2018. "Recent Biomedical Applications of Gold Nanoparticles: A Review." *Talanta.* Elsevier B.V. doi:10.1016/j.talanta.2018.02.088.

19. Simão, Estefani P., Dammyres B.S. Silva, Marli T. Cordeiro, Laura H.V. Gil, Cesar A.S. Andrade, and Maria D.L. Oliveira. 2020. "Nanostructured Impedimetric Lectin-Based Biosensor for Arboviruses Detection." *Talanta* 208 (February). Elsevier B.V.: 120338. doi:10.1016/j.talanta.2019.120338.

20. Verma, Mohini, Ashish K. Shukla, and Amitabha Acharya. 2020. "Lectin Nanoconjugates for Targeted Therapeutic Applications." In *Nanomaterial – Based Biomedical Applications in Molecular Imaging, Diagnostics and Therapy*, 103–127. Springer. doi:10.1007/978-981-15-4280-0_6.

21. Albrecht, Matthew A., Cameron W. Evans, and Colin L. Raston. 2006. "Green Chemistry and the Health Implications of Nanoparticles." *Green Chemistry* 8 (5). The Royal Society of Chemistry: 417–432. doi:10.1039/b517131h.

22. Elechiguerra, Jose Luis, Justin L. Burt, Jose R. Morones, Alejandra Camacho-Bragado, Xiaoxia Gao, Humberto H. Lara, and Miguel Jose Yacaman. 2005. "Interaction of Silver Nanoparticles with HIV-1." *Journal of Nanobiotechnology* 3 (June). doi:10.1186/1477-3155-3-6.

23. Lara, Humberto H., Nilda V. Ayala-Nuñez, Liliana Ixtepan-Turrent, and Cristina Rodriguez-Padilla. 2010. "Mode of Antiviral Action of Silver Nanoparticles against HIV-1." *Journal of Nanobiotechnology* 8 (1). BioMed Central: 1. doi:10.1186/1477-3155-8-1.

24. Chen, Yi Ning, Yi Huang Hsueh, Chien Te Hsieh, Dong Ying Tzou, and Pai Ling Chang. 2016. "Antiviral Activity of Graphene – Silver Nanocomposites Against Non-Enveloped and Enveloped Viruses." *International Journal of Environmental Research and Public Health* 13 (4). MDPI AG. doi:10.3390/ijerph13040430.

25. Sun, Lova, Ankur K. Singh, Komal Vig, Shreekumar R. Pillai, and Shree R. Singh. 2008. "Silver Nanoparticles Inhibit Replication of Respiratory Syncytial." *Journal of Biomedical Nanotechnology* 4 (2): 149–158. doi:10.1166/jbn.2008.012.

26. Lu, Lei, Raymond Wai Yin Sun, Rong Chen, Chee Kin Hui, Chi Ming Ho, John M. Luk, George K.K. Lau, and Chi Ming Che. 2008. "Silver Nanoparticles Inhibit Hepatitis B Virus Replication." *Antiviral Therapy* 13 (2): 252–262. http://europepmc.org/article/med/18505176.

27. Mehrbod, P., N. Motamed, M. Tabatabaian, R. Soleimani Estyar, E. Amini, M. Shahidi, and M. T. Kheiri. 2009. "In Vitro Antiviral Effect of 'nanosilver' on Influenza Virus." *Daru* 17 (2): 88–93.

28. Mori, Yasutaka, Takeshi Ono, Yasushi Miyahira, Vinh Quang Nguyen, Takemi Matsui, and Masayuki Ishihara. 2013. "Antiviral Activity of Silver Nanoparticle/chitosan Composites against H1N1 Influenza A Virus." *Nanoscale Research Letters* 8 (1). Springer Nature: 93. doi:10.1186/1556-276x-8-93.

29. Rogers, James V., Christopher V. Parkinson, Young W. Choi, Janice L. Speshock, and Saber M. Hussain. 2008. "A Preliminary Assessment of Silver Nanoparticle Inhibition of Monkeypox Virus Plaque Formation." *Nanoscale Research Letters* 3 (4). Springer: 129–133. doi:10.1007/s11671-008-9128-2.

30. Speshock, Janice L., Richard C. Murdock, Laura K. Braydich-Stolle, Amanda M. Schrand, and Saber M. Hussain. 2010. "Interaction of Silver Nanoparticles with Tacaribe Virus." *Journal of Nanobiotechnology* 8 (1). BioMed Central: 19. doi:10.1186/1477-3155-8-19.

31. Baram-Pinto, Dana, Sourabh Shukla, Nina Perkas, Aharon Gedanken, and Ronit Sarid. 2009. "Inhibition of Herpes Simplex Virus Type 1 Infection by Silver Nanoparticles Capped with Mercaptoethane Sulfonate." *Bioconjugate Chemistry* 20 (8). American Chemical Society: 1497–1502. doi:10.1021/bc900215b.

32. Rudolph, Carsten, Ulrike Schillinger, Aurora Ortiz, Kerstin Tabatt, Christian Plank, Rainer H. Müller, and Joseph Rosenecker. 2004. "Application of Novel Solid Lipid Nanoparticle (SLN)-Gene Vector Formulations Based on a Dimeric HIV-1 TAT-Peptide in Vitro and in Vivo." *Pharmaceutical Research* 21 (9). Springer: 1662–1669. doi:10.1023/B:PHAM.0000041463.56768.ec.

33. Ting, S., R. Simon, Gaojian Chen, and Martina H. Stenzel. 2010. "Synthesis of Glycopolymers and Their Multivalent Recognitions with Lectins." *Polymer Chemistry.* The Royal Society of Chemistry. doi:10.1039/c0py00141d.

34. Toub, N., C. Malvy, E. Fattal, and P. Couvreur. 2006. "Innovative Nanotechnologies for the Delivery of Oligonucleotides and siRNA." *Biomedicine and Pharmacotherapy* 60 (9). Elsevier Masson SAS: 607–620. doi:10.1016/j.biopha.2006.07.093.

35. Orr, R. M. 2001. "Technology Evaluation: Fomivirsen, Isis Pharmaceuticals Inc/CIBA Vision." *Current Opinion in Molecular Therapeutics* 3 (3): 288–294. https://europepmc.org/article/med/11497353.

36. Roehr, B. 1998. "Fomivirsen Approved for CMV Retinitis." *Journal of the International Association of Physicians in AIDS Care* 4 (October).

37. Parveen, Shama, Neera Yadav, and Monisha Banerjee. 2020. "Nano-Based Drug Delivery Tools for Personalized Nanomedicine." In *Nanomaterials and Environmental Biotechnology*, 189–199. Springer. doi:10.1007/978-3-030-34544-0_11.

38. Draz, Mohamed Shehata, Binbin Amanda Fang, Lanjuan Li, Zhi Chen, Yingjie Wang, Yuhong Xu, Jun Yang, Kevin Killeen, and Fanqing Frank Chen. 2012. "Hybrid Nanocluster Plasmonic Resonator for Immunological Detection of Hepatitis B Virus." *ACS Nano* 6 (9). American Chemical Society: 7634–43. doi:10.1021/nn3034056.

39. Pooja, Sarthak Sharma, Avnesh Kumari, and Amitabha Acharya. 2020. "Critical Overview of the Subject: Current Scenario and Future Prospects." In *Nanomaterial – Based Biomedical Applications in Molecular Imaging, Diagnostics and Therapy*, 185–203. Springer. doi:10.1007/978-981-15-4280-0_9.

40. Xu, Shaohua, Wenjun Ouyang, Peisi Xie, Yi Lin, Bin Qiu, Zhenyu Lin, Guonan Chen, and Longhua Guo. 2017. "Highly Uniform Gold Nanobipyramids for Ultrasensitive Colorimetric Detection of Influenza Virus." *Analytical Chemistry* 89 (3). American Chemical Society: 1617–1623. doi:10.1021/acs.analchem.6b03711.

41. Xu, Hui, Lihua Wang, and Chunhai Fan. 2012. "Bioanalysis and Bioimaging with Fluorescent Conjugated Polymers and Conjugated Polymer Nanoparticles." In *Functional Nanoparticles for Bioanalysis, Nanomedicine, and Bioelectronic Devices Volume 1*, 1112: 81–117. American Chemical Society. doi:10.1021/bk-2012-1112.ch004.

42. Oh, Sangjin, Jeonghyo Kim, Van Tan Tran, Dong Kyu Lee, Syed Rahin Ahmed, Jong Chul Hong, Jaewook Lee, Enoch Y. Park, and Jaebeom Lee. 2018. "Magnetic Nanozyme-Linked Immunosorbent Assay for Ultrasensitive Influenza A Virus Detection." *ACS Applied Materials and Interfaces* 10 (15). American Chemical Society: 12534–12543. doi:10.1021/acsami.8b02735.

43. Lopez, Blanca Silvia Gonzalez, Masaji Yamamoto, Katsuaki Utsumi, Chiaki Aratsu, and Hiroshi Sakagami. 2009. "A Clinical Pilot Study of Lignin-Ascorbic Acid Combination Treatment of Herpes Simplex Virus." *In Vivo* 23 (6): 1011–1016.

44. Abidi, Syed M. S., Aqib Iqbal Dar, and Amitabha Acharya. 2020. "Plant-Based Polymeric Nanomaterials for Biomedical Applications." In *Nanomaterial – Based Biomedical Applications in Molecular Imaging, Diagnostics and Therapy*, 129–158. Springer. doi:10.1007/978-981-15-4280-0_7.

9 Antimicrobial/Antiviral Nano-TiO$_2$ Coatings for Medical Applications

Jariyavadee Sirichantra

CONTENTS

DOI: 10.1201/9781003143093-9

9.1   INTRODUCTION

Titanium dioxide (titania, TiO_2) is a well-known material in the form of white oxide ceramic. There are three crystalline forms: rutile, anatase, and brookite, as shown in Figure 9.1 [1]. Anatase structure has often been material selection to apply in several industries for many years. The photocatalytic activity of TiO_2 is an outstanding property in many applications, such as the removal of organic contaminants and the production of self-cleaning glass. In addition, there has been a great interest in the applications of photocatalysis in disinfection, which is the ability to kill a wide range of gram-negative and gram-positive bacteria, filamentous and unicellular fungi, algae, protozoa, mammalian viruses, and bacteriophage by TiO_2 [2]. In many recent years, nanotechnology has been increasing interest, which offers substantial advantages in several fields. TiO_2 is the most widely used nanoparticle, which is of various particle sizes. The ultrafine particles are less than 100 nm, and the fine particles are 0.1–3 µm [3]. This chapter focuses on recent advances in antimicrobial/antiviral nanoparticle titanium dioxide coatings for medical applications. Firstly, we give the backgrounds of photocatalytic mechanisms and photocatalytic action on microbial and viral TiO_2. Then, the study of nanoparticle titanium dioxide (nano-TiO_2) coating for medical application focuses on either characteristics or properties; for example, the particle size analysis by using dynamic light scattering (DSC) and the ability to kill microorganisms and viruses. We also provide some results to show the safety of nano-TiO_2 on animals. In addition, the effect of dispersion state and interfacial adhesion of the nano-TiO_2 coating on various substrates, which are built in the interior of ambulances such as glass fiber reinforced polymer (GFRP), stainless steel, and polyvinylchloride (PVC), is investigated to extend into the pilot scale for using the medical application.

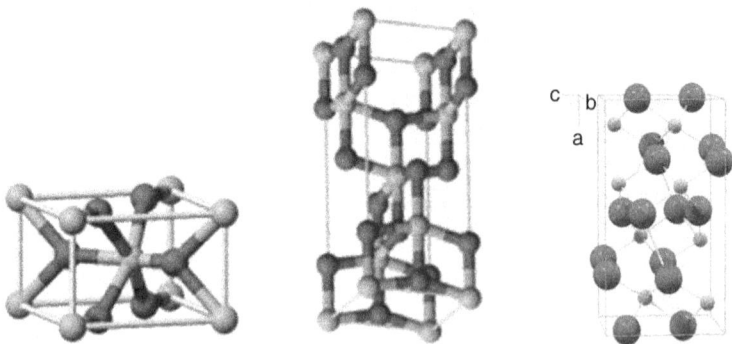

FIGURE 9.1   Tetragonal structures of crystalline forms of rutile, anatase, and brookite TiO_2 NPs (spheres: red—O_2, grey—Ti).

Source: Based on Ben [4], Benjah [5] and Krizu [6]

9.2 PHOTOCATALYTIC MECHANISM

The photocatalytic TiO$_2$ is an essential property for antimicrobial and antiviral that there is a mechanism describing a semiconductor. Firstly, the absorption of a photon with appropriate energy by TiO$_2$ encourages electrons from the valence band (e_{vb}^-) to the conduction band (e_{cb}^-), which leaves a positively charged hole in the valence band (h_{vb}^+) as shown in Eq. (9.1). The bandgap energy (energy required to encourage an electron) of anatase is approximately 3.2 eV. It means that photons can activate photocatalysis with a wavelength of roughly 385 nm, which is the wavelength of UVA. Then, the electrons are free to migrate in the conduction band, and an electron from an adjacent molecule may fill the holes. It is a repetitive process many times; therefore, holes are mobiles as well. Electrons and holes may recombine either a non-productive reaction or a reactive oxygen species (ROS) on the surface, such as O$_2^-$ (see in Eq. 9.2) and ·OH (see in Eq. 9.3).

Furthermore, these reactions can give H$_2$O$_2$, hydroxyl, and hydroperoxyl radicals, as shown in Eqs. (9.4), (9.5), and (9.6), respectively. Then, the response of radicals with organic compounds shown in Eq. (9.7) affects mineralization. Indeed, these processes are not efficient properly due to bulk recombination. Therefore, electric fields are applied to enhance charge separation, which is a term of photo/electrocatalysis [2, 7].

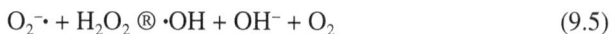

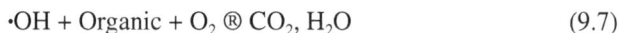

$$TiO_2 + hn \circledR e_{cb-} + h_{vb}^+ \tag{9.1}$$

$$O_2 + e_{cb}^- \circledR O_2^{-}\cdot \tag{9.2}$$

$$h_{vb}^+ + H_2O \circledR \cdot OH + H^+_{aq} \tag{9.3}$$

$$\cdot OH + \cdot OH \circledR H_2O_2 \tag{9.4}$$

$$O_2^{-}\cdot + H_2O_2 \circledR \cdot OH + OH^- + O_2 \tag{9.5}$$

$$O_2^{-}\cdot + H^+ \circledR \cdot OOH \tag{9.6}$$

$$\cdot OH + Organic + O_2 \circledR CO_2, H_2O \tag{9.7}$$

9.3 PHOTOCATALYTIC ACTION ON MICROBIAL AND VIRAL TITANIUM DIOXIDE

There are many studies to refer to photocatalytic surfaces or suspensions as being self-disinfection rather than self-sterilizing. Photocatalytic TiO$_2$ is the ability to kill microorganisms and viruses. We give a summary review of antimicrobial and antiviral for many exciting applications. Then, some results of antimicrobial and antiviral nanoparticle titanium dioxide coatings have been shown here.

9.3.1 GRAM-NEGATIVE BACTERIA

There are several formations and usabilities for killing gram-negative bacteria by photocatalytic disinfection on TiO$_2$, for example, suspension, coating, film, and nanoparticle. There were many studies in effective photocatalytic disinfection of TiO_2 on *Escherichia coli* and *E. coli* strains as follows: *E. coli* [8], *E. coli* NCIMB-4481 [9], *E. coli* IFO 3301 [10–11], *E. coli* ATCC 25922 [12–13], *E. coli* JM109 and *E. coli* XL1 Blue MRF [14], *E. coli* K12 [15], *E. coli* CCRC 10675 [16], *E. coli* IM303 [17], *E. coli* 078 [18], *E. coli* K12 ATCC10798 [19], and *E. coli* CAH57 (ESBL) [20]. Furthermore, there were some studies in other organisms killed by photocatalytic disinfection on TiO_2, for example, *Coliforms* [21], *Salmonella choleraesuis* and *Vibrio parahaemolyticus* [22], *Carotovora* and *Pseudomonas syringae* pv tomato [23], *Microcystis [24], Pseudomonas tolaasi [25], Acinetobacter* [26], *Enterobacter cloacae* [27], *Porphyromonas gingivalis* [28], *Bacteroides fragilis* [29], *Erwinia carotovora* subsp. *Flavobacterium* sp. [30], *Legionella pneumophila* ATCC 33153 and *Pseudomonas aeruginosa [31]*, and *Shigella flexneri* [32]. From the aforementioned information, TiO_2 can kill gram-negative bacteria by photocatalytic disinfection [2].

9.3.2 GRAM-POSITIVE BACTERIA

Many studies show that gram-positive bacteria were more resistant to photocatalytic disinfection on TiO_2 than gram-negative bacteria due to differences in the cell wall structure. Gram-positive bacteria have a thicker peptidoglycan layer and no outer membrane, whereas gram-negative bacteria have three layers of the cell wall; an inner membrane, a thin peptidoglycan layer, and an outer membrane [16, 22, 33–38]. There are some examples of gram-positive bacteria killed by photocatalytic disinfection on TiO_2. For example, TiO_2 suspension was studied to kill gram-positive bacteria as follows: *Lactobacillus acidophilus* [39–43], *Listeria monocytogenes* [22], *Bacillus cereus* [44], MRSA and *Staphylococcus saprophyticus* [45]. For TiO_2 thin film application, there were some examples of studies as follows: *Clostridium perfringens* spores NCIMB 6125 [9], *Staphylococcus aureus* [46], *Lactococcus lactis* 411 [38], and *Bacillus thuringiensis* [47]. In addition, there were few TiO_2 coating applications for killing organisms, for example, *Actinobacillus actinomycetemcomitans* [48] and *Streptococcus iniae* [49]. Nagame and colleagues [50] studied in killed *Streptococcus cricetus* by Kobe Steel TiO_2 99.98% anatase. Tsuang and colleagues [29] studied the effect of TiO_2 on orthopedic implants, and they found that TiO_2 was the ability to kill *Enterococcus hirae*. TiO_2 can kill gram-positive bacteria by photocatalytic disinfection [2].

9.3.3 FUNGI, ALGAE, AND PROTOZOA

Many studies were able to kill fungi, algae, and protozoa of photocatalytic disinfection on TiO_2. We give some examples of fungi, algae, and protozoa killed by photocatalytic disinfection. Firstly, there were many studies about killed fungi by either TiO_2 coating or TiO_2 thin film as follows: *Candida albicans* [51], *Aspergillus niger* [33], *Penicillium expansum* [52], fungi from spinach *[53], Candida vini [54], A. niger* AS3315 [32] *Cladosporium cladospoiroides, Epicoccum nigrum*, and *Penicillium oxalicum* [55]. Secondly, there were very few studies about killed algae by TiO_2. Linkous and colleagues [56] studied photocatalytic disinfection of *Oedogonium* sp. by TiO_2-covered concrete. Peller and colleagues [57] studied photocatalytic disinfection of *Cladophora* sp. by TiO$_2$-covered glass beads. Lastly, some studies found TiO$_2$ suspension was the effective photocatalytic disinfection of *Acanthamoeba polyphaga* environmental isolate and *Tetrahymena pyriformis* [58–59]. Navalon and colleagues [60] (2009) found that *Giardia* sp. was killed by the fibrous ceramic TiO$_2$ filter. TiO$_2$ can kill fungi, algae, and protozoa [2].

9.3.4 VIRUSES

Most studies showed *E. coli* bacteriophages in suspension, showing for icosahedral ssRNA viruses (MS2 and Qb), filamentous ssRNA virus (fr), ssDNA (FX174), and dsDNA viruses (l and T4) [61–73, 37, 74]. In addition, we give two more hosts for some important viruses, which were killed by TiO$_2$ photocatalytic disinfection. Influenza (avian) A/H5N2 was an important virus by birds. [75] found that TiO$_2$ photocatalytic disinfection could kill Influenza (avian) A/H5N2. Finally, a human was the host of serious viruses, which were destroyed by TiO$_2$ photocatalytic disinfection. In this section, we give some studies as follows: *Norovirus* [21], *Poliovirus Type 1 (ATCC VFR-192)* [76], *Influenza A/H3N2* [77], *HBsAg* [78], *Hepatitis B virus surface antigen* [79], *Influenza A/H1N1* [47], and SARS coronavirus Vaccinia [47]. As described already, many studies showed that TiO$_2$ photocatalytic disinfection was an effective antivirus [2].

Some backgrounds of photocatalytic mechanism and photocatalytic action on microbial and viral titanium dioxide were described in Sections 9.2 and 9.3, respectively. Then, the recently advanced nanoparticle titanium dioxide will be subsequently described in nanoparticle size analysis, antimicrobial and antiviral. In addition, the acute oral toxicity and skin sensitization on animals will also be described in the following.

9.4 NANOPARTICLE TITANIUM DIOXIDE (NANO-TIO₂)

Nanotechnology has been increasing the capabilities of medical applications. TiO$_2$ is the most widely used nanoparticle in several consumer goods and products of daily use, such as food, drugs, cosmetics, paints, textiles, paper, and plastics. There are two classifications for the size of nanoparticle titanium dioxide (nano-TiO$_2$). The ultrafine particles are less than 100 nm, and the fine particles are 0.1–3 μm. In this study, nanoparticle titanium dioxide for medical application was obtained from Infinite Purity Coating Co., Ltd. (Thailand) and Titanium World Technology Sdn Bhd (Malaysia). They were tested to get their characteristics and their killing abilities to microorganisms and viruses. In addition, they have also evaluated the acute oral toxicity on rats and the skin sensitization in the guinea pigs.

9.4.1 NANOPARTICLE SIZE ANALYSIS OF NANO-TIO₂

Nano-TiO$_2$ obtained from Infinite Purity Coating Co., Ltd. are the sample name as 'PCO-001-IPC.' The characteristic of PCO-001-IPC was measured the nanoparticle size analysis by using the dynamic light scattering (DSC) technique with Zetasizer Nano series (Malvern Instrument, UK) in the laboratory of National

TABLE 9.1

The Average of Diameters, Polydispersity Index (PI), and Count Rate of PCO-001-IPC

Sample name	Hydrodynamic diameters (nm)	Hydrodynamic diameters (nm) ± SD	Polydispersity index	Polydispersity index ± SD	Mean count rate kilo count per second (kcps)
PCO-001-IPC	37.38		0.245		139
		37.30±0.13		0.237±0.012	
PCO-001-IPC	37.36		0.242		138
PCO-001-IPC	37.15		0.223		140

Source: Data from National Nanotechnology Center (NANOTEC), NSTDA, Thailand [81]

Nanotechnology Center (NANOTEC), NSTDA, Thailand. The significant factors of the testing method are following as shown here. The refraction index of the sample is 0.1. The refraction index of solvent is 1.33. The viscosity of the solvent was 0.8872. The wavelength of the laser was 632.8 nm, and the light scattering angle was 173°. As shown in Table 9.1, the result of PCO-001-IPC is the average of diameters, polydispersity index (PI), and count rate. The result shows that the average of PCO-001-IPC is 37.30±0.13 nm, assuming that it is nano-TiO_2 in the classification of the ultrafine particles.

9.4.2 Killing Microorganisms of Nano-TiO_2

Nano-TiO_2 has tested the ability to kill microorganisms. There are three laboratories for testing microorganisms as the following here. Firstly, the result of the tested microorganism by SGS (Thailand) Limited is shown in Table 9.2, which shows two microorganisms: *S. aureus* (ATCC 6538) and *E. coli* (ATCC 8739). The testing method is based on JIS Z 2801:2000. Secondly, the result of tested microorganisms by Intertek Testing Services Hong Kong Ltd. is shown in Table 9.3, which has five microorganisms: *E. coli* (ATCC 10536), *S. aureus* (ATCC 6538), *Salmonella typhimurium* (ATCC 14028), *L. monocytogenes* (ATCC 15313), and *Klebsiella pneumonia* (ATCC 4352). The criteria of the testing method are according to EN 1040. Lastly, the result of tested microorganisms by the Quality Assurance Project (Microbiology), Faculty of Medical Technology, Mahidol University is shown in Table 9.4, which has two microorganisms: *S. aureus* (ATCC 6538) and *S. choleraesuis* (ATCC 10708). The testing method is based on a one-step cleaner disinfectant following AOAC OFFICIAL METHOD OF ANALYSIS [80] AOAC Official Methods 961.02, Germicidal Spray Product as disinfectants with distance 30 cm and time 10 seconds for spray coating. From Table 9.4, nano-TiO_2 called 'Infinite Purity Coating' efficiently killed *S. aureus* and *S. choleraesuis* on hard surface carriers with an exposure time of 30 minutes.

TABLE 9.2

Ability of Nanoparticle Titanium-Dioxide-Tested Microorganism by SGS (Thailand) Limited

Tested Microorganism	% Reduction
S. aureus (ATCC 6538)	>99.99
E. coli (ATCC 8739)	>99.99

Source: Data from SGS (Thailand) Limited [82]

TABLE 9.3

Ability of Nanoparticle Titanium-Dioxide-Tested Microorganism by Intertek Testing Service Hong Kong Ltd

Tested Microorganism	Initial suspension (N) (CFU/ml) Criteria: 1.5×10^8 £ N £ 5×10^8	Final count (CFU/ml)	R (% Reduction) Criteria: R ^{3} 99.999	Assessment
E. coli (ATCC 10536)	3.2×10^8	<140	99.9999	Satisfactory
S. aureus (ATCC 6538)	3.2×10^8	<140	99.9999	Satisfactory
S. typhimurium (ATCC 14028)	3.4×10^8	<140	99.9999	Satisfactory
L. monocytogenes (ATCC 15313)	3.2×10^8	<140	99.9999	Satisfactory
K. pneumoniae (ATCC 4352)	4.6×10^8	<140	99.9999	Satisfactory

Source: Data from Intertek Testing Service Hong Kong Ltd. [83]

TABLE 9.4

Ability of Nano-TiO$_2$-Tested Microorganism by Quality Assurance Project (Microbiology), Faculty of Medical Technology, Mahidol University

Tested microorganism	Exposure time	Bacteria/fungal growth after exposure of 60 soil-load contaminated carriers to infinite purity coating
S. aureus (ATCC 6538)	30 minutes	0/60
S. choleraesuis (ATCC 10708)	30 minutes	0/60

Source: Data from Faculty of Medical Technology, Mahidol University [84]

9.4.3 KILLING VIRUSES OF NANO-TiO$_2$

In 2009, the Office of the Ministry of Health, Malaysia reported that Product TiO$_2$ Photo Catalyst was able to kill the virus (H1N1). In 2018, Titanium World Technology Sdn Bhd, Malaysia studied the virucidal hard surface efficacy test Coxsackievirus

(Non-GLP). The test substance names are 'SmartCoat Plus' and 'Armor8 Plus.' This study was tested by Microbac Laboratories Inc., USA. For the experimental method, the active ingredient is nano-TiO_2 + Ag. The challenge organism is Coxsackievirus, Type B6, Strain: Schmitt, ATCC VR-155, loading 5% serum in the viral inoculum. The host cell line is LLC-MK2 cells, ATCC CCL-7.1, and the used neutralizers are minimum essential medium (MEM) + 2% fetal bovine serum (FBS) + 0.5% polysorbate 80 + 1 mM EDTA. For experimental conditions, the exposure temperature and the incubation temperature are 20 °C ± 2 °C with actual 21 °C and 36 °C ± 2 °C with 5% ± 3% CO_2, respectively. The contact time is 30 minutes and 60 minutes. For the tested results, the neutralizer effectiveness/viral interference and cytotoxicity controls—Armor8 Plus—and the viral reduction—are shown in Tables 9.5 and 9.6, respectively. In conclusion, Microbac stated that 'Titanium World Technology's SmartCoat Plus and Armor8 Plus' were evaluated for the ability to inactivate Coxsackievirus. Microbac personnel performed the inactivation procedure using Coxsackievirus. Samples were titrated by 50% tissue culture infectious dose ($TCID_{50}$) endpoint assay using LLC-MK2 cells. The viral reductions for the test substances are presented in Table 9.6. All controls met the criteria for a valid test. These conclusions are based on observed data.

As coronavirus (COVID-19) pandemic, the determination of the virucidal activity of nano-TiO_2 was tested by Viroxy Sdn Bhd, Malaysia in 2020. The exciting results showed that nano-TiO_2 was the ability to kill coronavirus significantly. The sample name of nano-TiO_2 is 'Infinite Purity Coating.' The test method is according to EN 14476:2013+A1:2015 (E): Chemical disinfectants and antiseptics—quantitative suspension test for the evaluation of virucidal activity in the medical area—test method and requirements (phase 2, step 1). For the experimental conditions, the test organism is *Human coronavirus*, strain 229E, ATCC VR-740. The concentration and contact time are 100% and 60 minutes, respectively. The loading is 0.30 g/L bovine albumin solution. The test temperature is 20 °C ± 1 °C, and the incubation period is 5 days with 36 °C ± 1 °C. For the test method and its validation, the testing method is a quantal test, and the inactivation method is immediate dilution—molecular sieving using MicroSpin™ S 400 HR (for formaldehyde only). For the test results, the

TABLE 9.5
Neutralizer Effectiveness/Viral Interference and Cytotoxicity Controls—Armor8 Plus

Dilutions*	Neutralizer effectiveness/viral interference and cytotoxicity control	Cytotoxicity Control
10^{-1}	Cytotoxicity observed; viral CPE could not be evaluated	Cytotoxicity observed
10^{-2}	Virus detected in all inoculated wells	No cytotoxicity observed
10^{-3}	Virus detected in all inoculated wells	No cytotoxicity observed

* Dilution refers to the fold of the dilution from the neutralized sample

Source: Data from Microbac Laboratories Inc., USA, [85]

TABLE 9.6

Viral Reduction of SmartCoat Plus and Armor8 Plus

Test substance	Contact time	Replicates	Initial load (log$_{10}$TCID$_{50}$)*	Output load (log$_{10}$TCID$_{50}$)	Log$_{10}$ reduction	Reduction (%)
SmartCoat Plus	30 minutes	Rep 1	6.03	£ 2.28	³ 3.75	³ 99.98
		Rep 2		£ 2.28	³ 3.75	³ 99.98
	60 minutes	Rep 1		£ 2.28	³ 3.75	³ 99.98
		Rep 2		£ 2.28	³ 3.75	³ 99.98
Armor8 Plus	30 minutes	Rep 1		£ 2.28	³ 3.75	³ 99.98
		Rep 2		£ 2.28	³ 3.75	³ 99.98
	60 minutes	Rep 1		£ 2.28	³ 3.75	³ 99.98
		Rep 2		£ 2.28	³ 3.75	³ 99.98

* The average of the two replicates of the VRC was used as the initial load.

Source: Data from Microbac Laboratories Inc., USA[85]

TABLE 9.7

Evaluation of the Virucidal Activity of Infinite Purity Coating on Test Strains According to EN 14476

Product: Infinite Purity Coating
Loading: 0.30 g/L bovine albumin solution
Test strain: *Human coronavirus* ATCC VR-740

Virus control, V_c	Cytotoxicity effect (CE)
V_{c1}: 6.25 ± 0.33	CE$_1$: 1.50 ± 0.00
V_{c2}: 6.00 ± 0.38	CE$_2$: 1.50 ± 0.00

Test concentration (%)/ contact time (min)	First assay, N$_{a1}$	Second assay, N$_{a2}$	Average reduction
100.00*/30	N$_{a1}$: £1.50 ± 0.00	N$_{a2}$: £1.50 ± 0.00	I$_g$ R: £4.63± 0.36
	I$_g$ R$_1$: £4.75± 0.33	I$_g$ R$_2$: £4.50± 0.38	
100.00*/60	N$_{a1}$: £1.50 ± 0.00	N$_{a1}$: £1.50 ± 0.00	I$_g$ R: £4.63± 0.36
	I$_g$R$_1$: £4.75± 0.33	I$_g$ R$_1$: £4.50± 0.38	

Source: Data from Viroxy lab, Malaysia [86]

evaluation of the virucidal activity of Infinite Purity Coating on test strains according to EN 14476 is stated in Table 9.7. The control tests and method validation for Table 9.7 are shown in Table 9.8. The summary of the log reductions of the quantitative suspension test according to EN 14476 is shown in Table 9.9. The validation test results in Tables 9.7–9.9 proved the viability of the method in all cases. The Viroxy labs concluded that

TABLE 9.8
Control Tests and Method Validation for Table 9.11

Test strain	Cell susceptibility control	Suppression efficiency control	Reference test for virus inactivation
Human coronavirus	A: 5.75 ± 0.33	B: 5.50 ± 0.00	C_{30} ³$4.00 \pm 0.00$
ATCC VR-740	A_{PBS}: 5.50 ± 0.00	V_C: 5.88 ± 0.37	C_{60} ³$4.00 \pm 0.00$

Note

V_C: $\log_{10}$ $TCID_{50}$ per ml in the viral test suspension at the beginning and at the maximum contact time

CE: The morphological alteration of cells caused by the cytotoxicity effect of the product test solution

N_a: $\log_{10}$ $TCID_{50}$ per ml in the test mixture at the end of the contact time

A: $\log_{10}$ $TCID_{50}$ per ml in the cell susceptibility control as compared to PBS

B: $\log_{10}$ $TCID_{50}$ per ml in the suppression efficiency control as compared to the virus control

C: $\log_{10}$ $TCID_{50}$ per ml in the reference test for virus inactivation after 30 and 60 minutes (5 and 15 minutes for vaccinia virus)

Source: Data from Viroxy lab, Malaysia [86]

TABLE 9.9
Summary of the Log Reductions of the Quantitative Suspension Test According to EN 14476

Test strain	Test concentration (%)/ contact time (min)	Log reduction ($TCID_{50}$/ml)	Associated risk**
Human coronavirus	100.00*/30	£4.63 ± 0.36	Minimal risk of false acceptance
ATCC VR-740	100.00*/60	£4.63 ± 0.36	Minimal risk of incorrect acceptance

*The product can only be tested at 80.00% concentration or more minor, as some dilution always occurs when test organisms and interfering substances are added.

** The laboratory's decision rule has been determined, and the client agrees with it before testing. The acceptance rule is not to guard the band and up to 50% risk of false acceptance or rejection.

Source: Data from Viroxy lab, Malaysia [86]

INFINITE PURITY COATING showed the required virus reduction of ³$4.0$ $\log_{10}$ against test strain *Human coronavirus*, strain 229E, ATCC VR-740 in according with 14476:2013+A1:2015 (E) at 100.00% concentration after 30 and 60 minutes under the stated condition. According to the simple acceptance decision rule, there is a minimal risk of false acceptance.

9.4.4 ACUTE ORAL TOXICITY STUDY OF NANO-TiO₂ COATINGS

Nano-TiO_2 coatings called 'Smart Coat' were evaluated in the acute oral toxicity study on rats from a single dose by the oral route, tested by Industrial Biotechnology Research Centre (SIRIM BERHAD). The acute oral toxicity up-and-down procedure

(UDP)–limit test is a sequential test that uses five animals. For the method of evaluation in acute oral toxicity, animals are dosed in sequential behavior. They have received the same dose if the first animal survives with a limited dose. A 2000 mg/kg starting dose is selected based on a BALB/c 3T3 NRU cytotoxicity test recommendation. In this study, the Smart Coat was prepared in reverse osmosis water freshly prepared before being processed to five rats. Then, the acute oral toxicity was performed on the first female rat with the single-dose at 2000 mg/kg body weight, and the first rat survived a 48-hour observation. Therefore, the adding four rats were sequentially dosed at about 48-hour intervals. All five rates were tested to observe individually for mortality, signs of gross toxicity, and behavioral changes once during the first 30 minutes after dosing. Then, they were mainly observed again during the first 4 hours, periodically during 48 hours post-dosing, and daily for 14 days. In addition, the body weights were recorded before and after dosing on day 7 and day 14 (termination). The result showed that all animals gained bodyweight and appeared normal. They did not also demonstrate any abnormal behavior during the observation period. 'Smart Coat' showed that a median lethal oral dose (LD50) was more significant than 2000 mg/kg body weight. Thus, it was classified as Category 5 according to the Globally Harmonised System to classify chemicals.

9.4.5 SKIN SENSITIZATION STUDY (CLOSED-PATCH TEST) OF NANO-TiO$_2$ COATINGS

Nano-TiO$_2$ coatings called 'Armor8' were determination the potential of skin sensitization by using closed-patch test (Buehler test) in guinea pigs, which was studied by Industrial Biotechnology Research Centre (SIRIM BERHAD). The test method is according to International Organization for Standardization 10993: Biological Evaluation of Medical Devices, Part 10: Tests for Irritation and Sensitisation. Ten guinea pigs were patched for testing items for the test method, and five guinea pigs were negative control groups without testing things. The gauze was cut into approximately 2.5 cm × 2.5 cm patches. Then, it was soaked with the test item, and it was applied on the test site by covering a double-layer gauze swab. The patches were wrapped into the trunk of each animal with surgical tape and securing with self-adherent wrap. After that, the patches were removed after 6±0.5 hours of exposure. This procedure was repeated three times a week for three weeks. It was nine applications. There were 14 ±1 days for the rest period after the final induction patch. For observation, the dermal patch sites were tested for erythema and edema by 24±2 hours and by 48±2 hours after patch removal. Each animal was evaluated for skin sensitization response based on the dermal scores. To compare, there were no reactions in the negative control group. Industrial Biotechnology Research Centre (SIRIM BERHAD) concluded that 'Armor8' did not induce sensitization in ten guinea pigs.

9.5 NANOPARTICLE TITANIUM DIOXIDE COATING (NANO-TiO$_2$ COATING)

There are different techniques for nano-TiO$_2$ coatings, such as a pump sprayer, trigger sprayer, and electrostatic sprayer. In this study, the electrostatic sprayer was selected for the nano-TiO$_2$ layer because it provided better coverage. With better coverage, it can save time and cost. The electrostatic sprayer applies an electrical charge to a coating material as it is sprayed through the nozzle. The charged droplets are attracted to the spray target that they can wrap around objects. They are also able to be overcome gravity and give through the coating. To compare coverage, each white construction paper sheet was sprayed by using black ink. To determine the amount of ink applied, each sheet was weighed before and after spraying. Figure 9.2 shows the coverage comparison

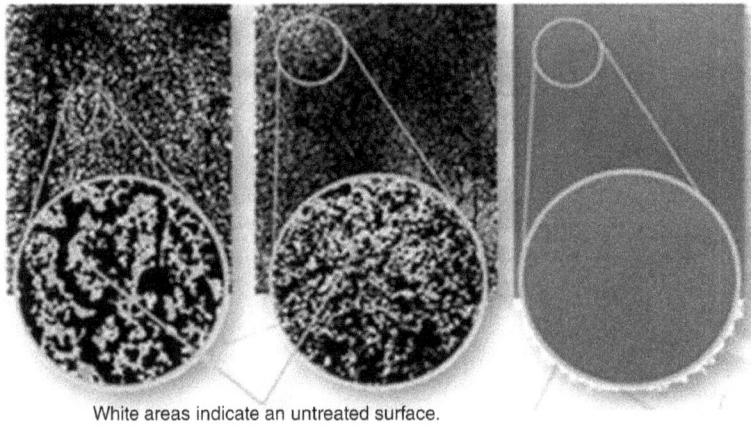

White areas indicate an untreated surface.

FIGURE 9.2 Comparison of surface covered for nano-TiO$_2$ with different techniques: (a) pump sprayer, (b) trigger spray, and (c) electrostatic sprayer.

Source: Adapted from ESS [87]

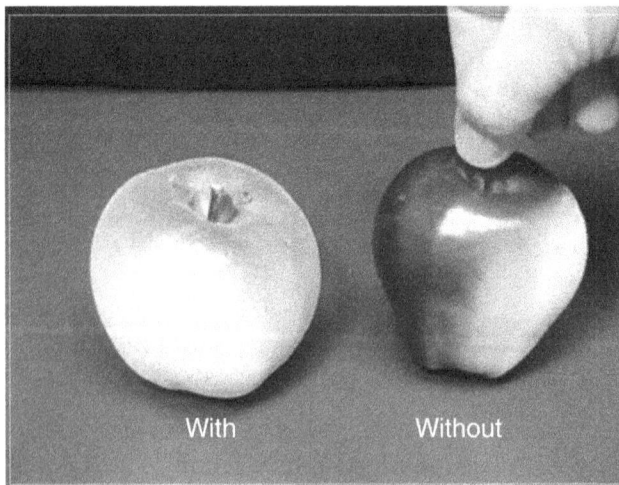

FIGURE 9.3 Comparison through coating between with and without electrostatic sprayer on two apples.

Source: Adapted from ESS [88]

between (a) pump sprayer, (b) trigger spray, and (c) electrostatic sprayer. The results showed that the pump sprayer used 1.68 g of black ink, and the coverage was 70% of the surface covered. The trigger sprayer used 1.18 g of black ink, and the coverage was 65% of the surface covered. The electrostatic sprayer used 0.58 g of black ink, and the coverage was 100% of the surface sprayer. In addition, the potential of through coating was investigated by comparison through layer between with and without electrostatic sprayer on two apples as shown in Figure 9.3. As described already, the electrostatic sprayer is suitable to spray nano-TiO₂ on materials for medical application.

9.6 NANO-TIO₂ COATING FOR MEDICAL APPLICATION: AMBULANCE INTERIORS

In recent two years, the research institute and private companies in Thailand have concentrated on research and development in antimicrobial and antiviral nano-TiO₂ coatings for medical application, especially in the ambulance interiors. The cooperation of research and development in Thailand consisted of the Department of Science Service, Ministry of Higher Education, Science, Research and Innovation, TKD Fiber Co., Ltd. (Carryboy), and Infinite Purity Coating Co., Ltd. Generally, a box body ambulance is made from a sandwich-structured composite. In this study, glass fiber reinforced polymer (GFRP) was used to be panels for a sandwich-structured composite. GFRP panels were coated by the automotive interior car paint called '2K' and 'Solid.' The aims of this project consist of three main objectives. Firstly, the surface analysis of nano-TiO₂ coating on GFRP panels is investigated by using scanning electron microscope (SEM): JEOL, JSM-6610LV, Mode BEC with 20 keV, and then the accumulation of nano-TiO₂ is tested by dispersive X-ray spectrometer (EDS): OXFORD INCA X-act with 20 keV and Model INCA 350 program. Secondly, the aggregation of nano-TiO₂ coating on GFRP panels coated with the car paint is developed to be dispersion well using cellulose nanofibril. Thirdly, expansion of the application of cellulose nanofibril is set to use for other materials in the interior of ambulances. The efficiency of nano-TiO₂ adhesive bonding on materials in the ambulance interiors is investigated by using SEM and EDS.

9.6.1 OBSERVATION OF NANO-TIO₂ COATING AGGLOMERATION

GFRP laminates coated with '2K' and 'Solid' interior car paints were fabricated by TKD Fiber Co., Ltd. (Carryboy), Thailand. Then, the panels were coated nano-TiO₂ with the electrostatic sprayer serviced by Infinite Purity Coating Co., Ltd. (Thailand). The observation of agglomeration of nano-TiO₂ coating on boards using SEM and EDS was studied by the Department of Science Service, Ministry of Higher Education, Science, Research and Innovation, Thailand. In this study, eight samples were separated into two groups by coating interior car paint. The first group was GFRP panels coated with '2K,' which were four samples: (1) without nano-TiO₂ coating, (2) with the nano-TiO₂ coating, (3) with nano-TiO₂ coating and cleaning 5 times, and (4) with nano-TiO₂ coating and cleaning 10 times. The second group was GFRP panels coated with 'Solid,' which were four samples: (1) without nano-TiO₂ coating, (2) with the nano-TiO₂ coating, (3) with nano-TiO₂ coating and cleaning 5 times, and (4) with nano-TiO₂ coating and cleaning 10 times. The recommendations of cleaning samples from Infinite Purity Coating Co., Ltd. (Thailand) were as follows: washing with the deionized water and then wiping with a clean cloth. The images of surface analysis on GFRP panels coated '2K' and 'Solid' samples with SEM (magnification 50×) are shown in Figures 9.4 and 9.5, respectively. As seen in Figures 9.4 and 9.5,

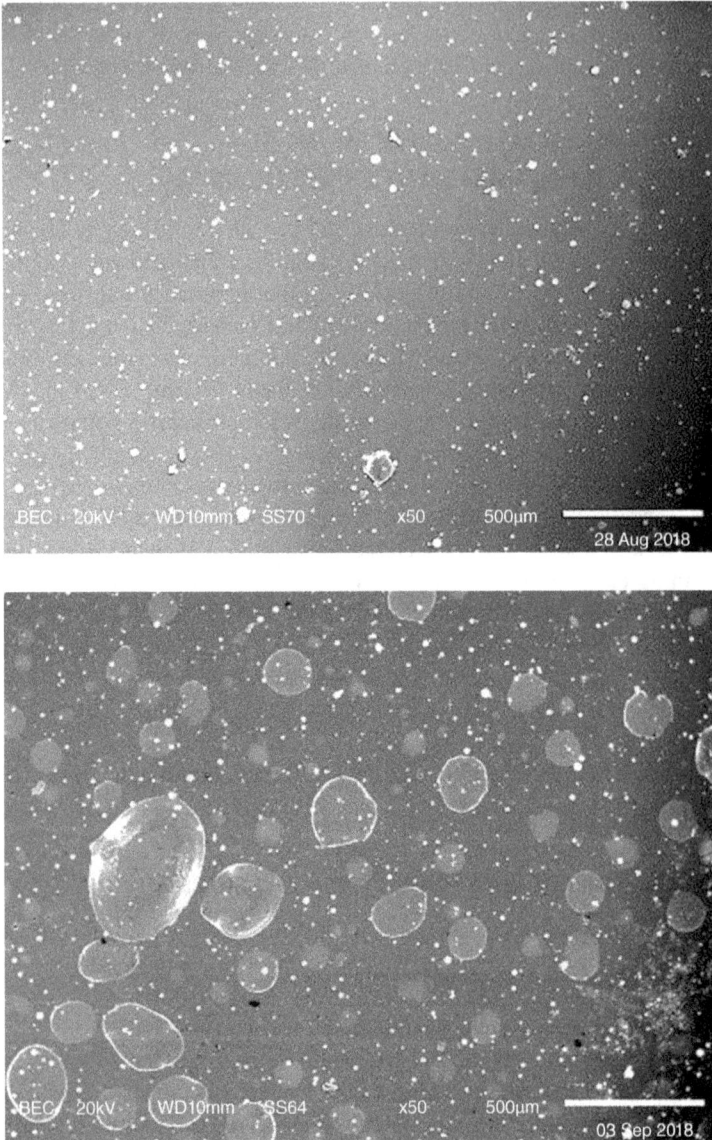

FIGURE 9.4 Images of surface analysis on GFRP panels coated '2K' by SEM (magnification 50×): (a) without nano-TiO$_2$ coating, (b) with the nano-TiO$_2$ coating, (c) with nano-TiO$_2$ coating and cleaning 5 times, and (d) with nano-TiO$_2$ coating and cleaning 10 times.

Source: Department of Science Service, Ministry of Higher Education, Science, Research and Innovation, Thailand [89]

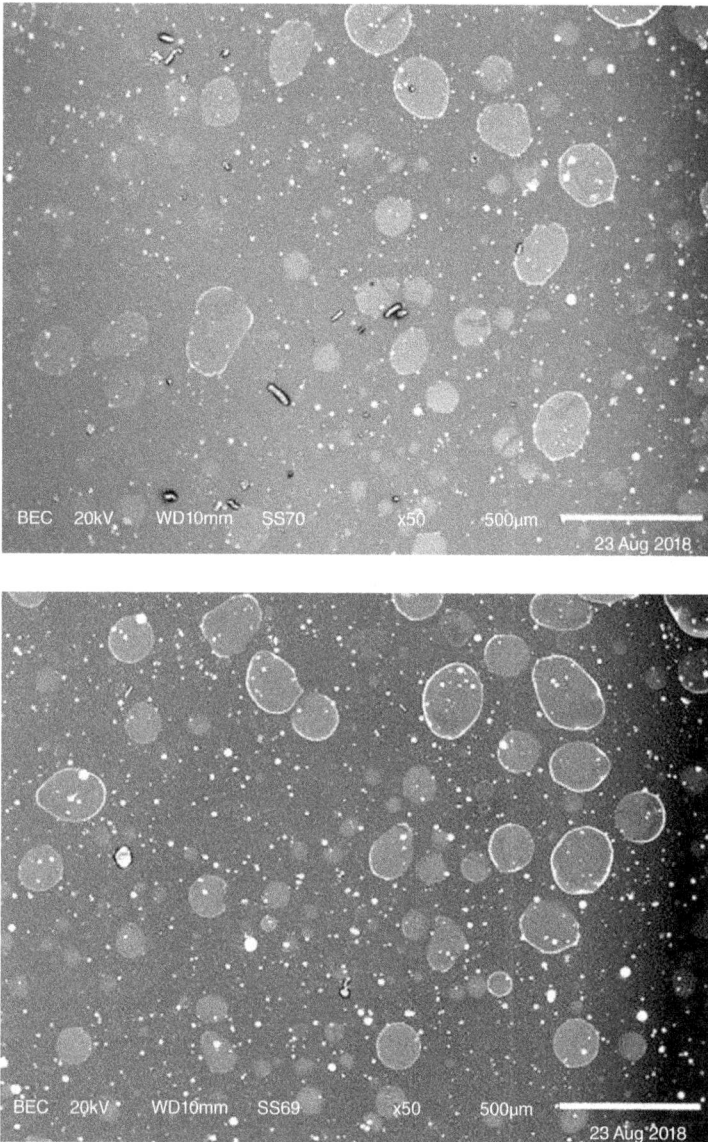

FIGURE 9.4 (Continued)

the formation of oval and circle shapes appears in Figures 9.4(b–d) and 9.5(b–d), but it does not appear in Figures 9.4(a) and 9.5(a). The appearance of shapes may be the accumulation of nano-TiO₂, especially at the edge of each form. To prove this appearance, SEM and EDS were used to observe and analyze the collection of nano-TiO₂. Figure 9.6 shows the surface analysis of nano-TiO₂ coating on GFRP panels coated '2K' by SEM (magnification 200×). As seen in Figure 9.6, the different areas of spectrum (1)–(4) are tested to compare the quantitative element analysis of nano-TiO₂ by

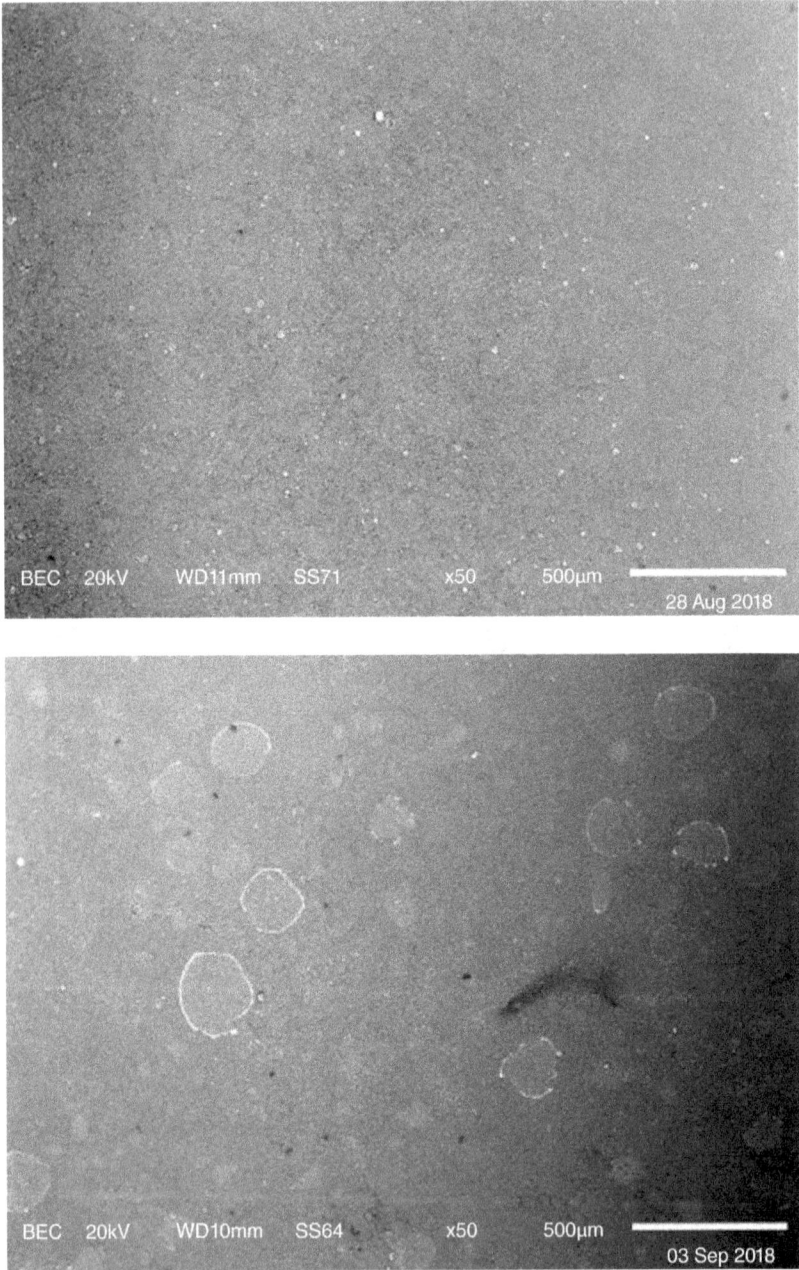

FIGURE 9.5 Images of surface analysis on GFRP panels coated 'Solid' by SEM (magnification 50×): (a) without nano-TiO$_2$ coating, (b) with a nano-TiO$_2$ coating, (c) with nano-TiO$_2$ coating and cleaning 5 times, and (d) with nano-TiO$_2$ coating and cleaning 10 times.

Source: Department of Science Service, Ministry of Higher Education, Science, Research and Innovation, Thailand [89]

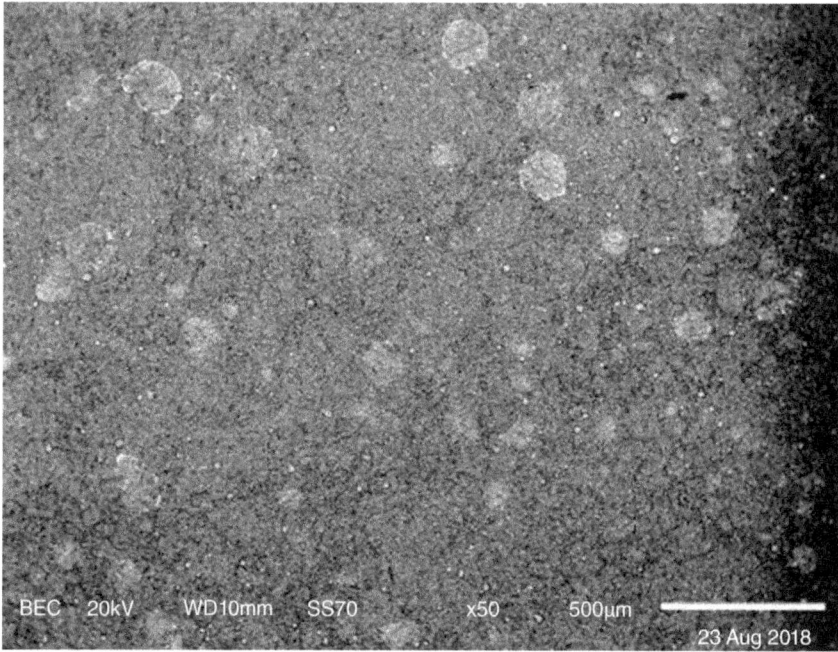

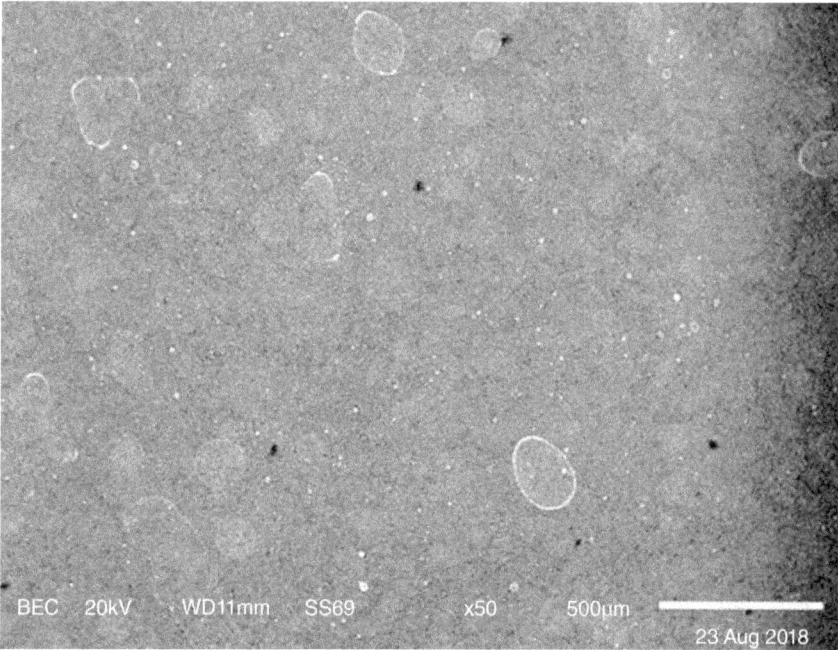

FIGURE 9.5   (Continued)

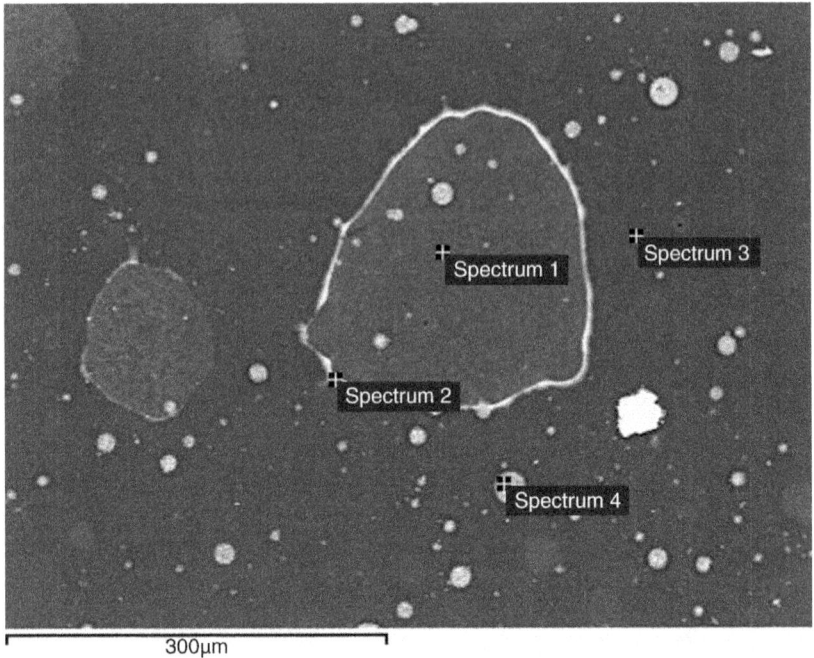

FIGURE 9.6   Images of surface analysis of nano-TiO_2 coating on GFRP panels coated '2K' by SEM (magnification 200×).

Source: Department of Science Service, Ministry of Higher Education, Science, Research and Innovation, Thailand [89]

the EDS technique. The results are shown in Table 9.10. This study focuses on only the quantitative element analysis of titanium (Ti) in Table 9.10, which assumes the accumulation of nano-TiO_2 coating on GFRP panels coated '2K.' From Figure 9.6 and Table 9.10, the results show that the area of the spectrum (4) is the highest percent of Ti (19.46%), and the site of the spectrum (2) is the second-highest percent of Ti (10.80%). On the other hand, the area of the spectrum (1) is very few percent of Ti (1.59%), and the location of the spectrum (3) is not detected any percent of Ti (0%). It was found that the areas of spectrum (4) and (2) were the white areas; there were around the edge of liked droplet water and a small circle. It may be assuming that they were an aggregation of nano-TiO_2. In addition, the surface analysis of nano-TiO_2 coating on GFRP panels coated 'Solid' was observed by SEM (magnification 200×) as seen in Figure 9.7. Then, the different areas of spectrum (1)–(4) are tested to compare the quantitative element analysis of nano-TiO_2 by the EDS technique. The results are shown in Table 9.11. In this project, we only concentrate on the quantitative element analysis of titanium (Ti) in Table 9.11, assuming the accumulation of nano-TiO_2 coating on GFRP panels coated 'Solid.' From Figure 9.7 and Table 9.11, the results show that the area of the spectrum (2) is the highest percent of Ti (26.80%). The size of the spectrum (1) is the second-highest percent of Ti (23.53%). The third-highest percent

TABLE 9.10
Quantitative Element Analysis of Nano-TiO$_2$ by EDS Technique: 1–4 Spectrum Areas from Figure 9.6

Element	Spectrum 1 %	Spectrum 2 %	Spectrum 3 %	Spectrum 4 %
C	82.01	51.71	81.53	49.98
O	7.60	32.22	11.12	25.56
Al	0	0	0	0.62
Si	0	0.16	0	0.25
Ca	0	0.26	0	0
Ti	1.59	10.80	0	19.46
Zn	0	0.28	0	0
Au	8.80	4.57	7.35	4.14

Source: Data from Department of Science Service, Ministry of Higher Education, Science, Research and Innovation, Thailand [89]

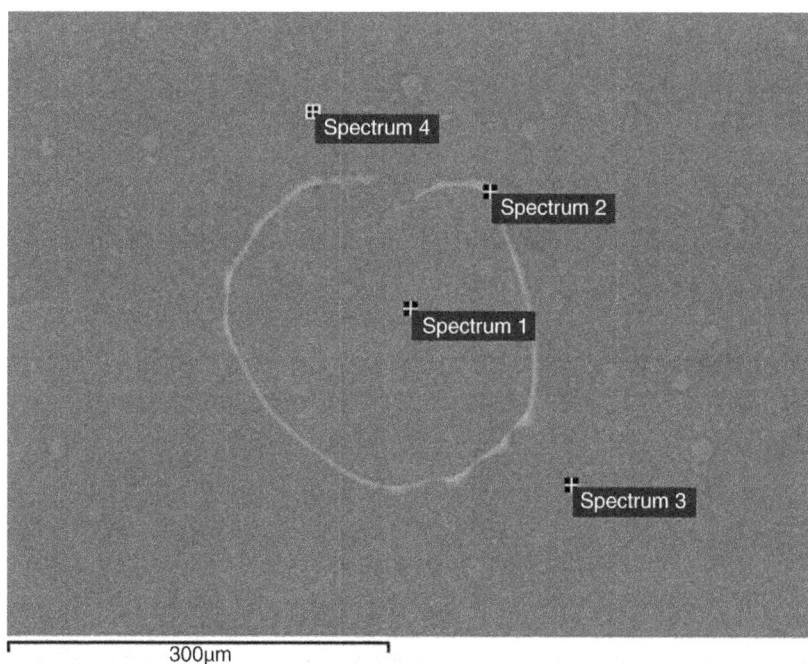

FIGURE 9.7   Images of surface analysis of nano-TiO$_2$ coating on GFRP panels coated 'Solid' by SEM (magnification 200×).

Source: Department of Science Service, Ministry of Higher Education, Science, Research and Innovation, Thailand [89]

TABLE 9.11
Quantitative Element Analysis of Nano-TiO$_2$ by EDS Technique: 1–4 Spectrum Areas from Figure 9.7

Element	Spectrum 1 %	Spectrum 2 %	Spectrum 3 %	Spectrum 4 %
C	45.93	32.43	51.14	49.03
O	25.00	34.88	28.15	22.27
Al	0.75	0.55	0.51	0.68
Si	0.28	0.41	0.21	0.27
Ca	0	0.33	0	0
Ti	23.53	26.80	15.44	21.69
Au	4.51	4.61	4.55	6.07

Source: Data from Department of Science Service, Ministry of Higher Education, Science, Research and Innovation, Thailand [89]

of Ti (21.69%) in the area of the spectrum (4), whereas the size of the spectrum (3) is the lowest percent of Ti (15.44%). It was found that all spectrum areas appeared a high percent of Ti. From the Material Safety Data Sheet of Evercoat Industries (Thailand) Co., Ltd., 'Solid' color consists of TiO$_2$, which is a reason for detecting a high percent of Ti around all spectrum areas. However, spectrum (2) was the white areas, where were around the edge of liked droplet water, which assumed that it was an aggregation of nano-TiO$_2$ due to the highest percent of Ti.

Summary: GFRP panels coated '2K' and 'Solid' are samples of coated nano-TiO$_2$ on the surface by electrostatic sprayer. The accumulation of nano-TiO$_2$ appears on their GFRP panels that SEM and EDS techniques are used to test their surface analysis and quantitative element analysis.

9.6.2 DEVELOPMENT OF NANO-TiO$_2$ COATING DEAGGLOMERATION

The results showed the accumulation of nano-TiO$_2$ coating on GFRP panels coated with the interior car paint '2K' and 'Solid' as described in Section 9.6.1. In this section, we will focus on the development of nano-TiO$_2$ coating deagglomeration on their panels. In this study, the cellulose nanofibril was used to develop the deagglomeration of nano-TiO$_2$. The preparation of samples is the same as Section 9.6.1, except for the cellulose nanofibril coating on panels before nano-TiO$_2$ coating. After that, observation of surface analysis on all boards was tested using SEM and EDS in the Department of Science Service laboratory, Ministry of Higher Education, Science, Research and Innovation, Thailand. The images of surface analysis on GFRP panels coated either '2K' or 'Solid' and cellulose nanofibril samples with SEM (magnification 50×) are shown in Figures 9.8 and 9.9, respectively. Comparing Figures 9.4 and 9.8, the images of surface analysis on all GFRP panels coated '2K' and cellulose nanofibril significantly reduces the accumulation of nano-TiO$_2$. If also comparing between Figures 9.5 and 9.9, the images of surface analysis on all GFRP panels

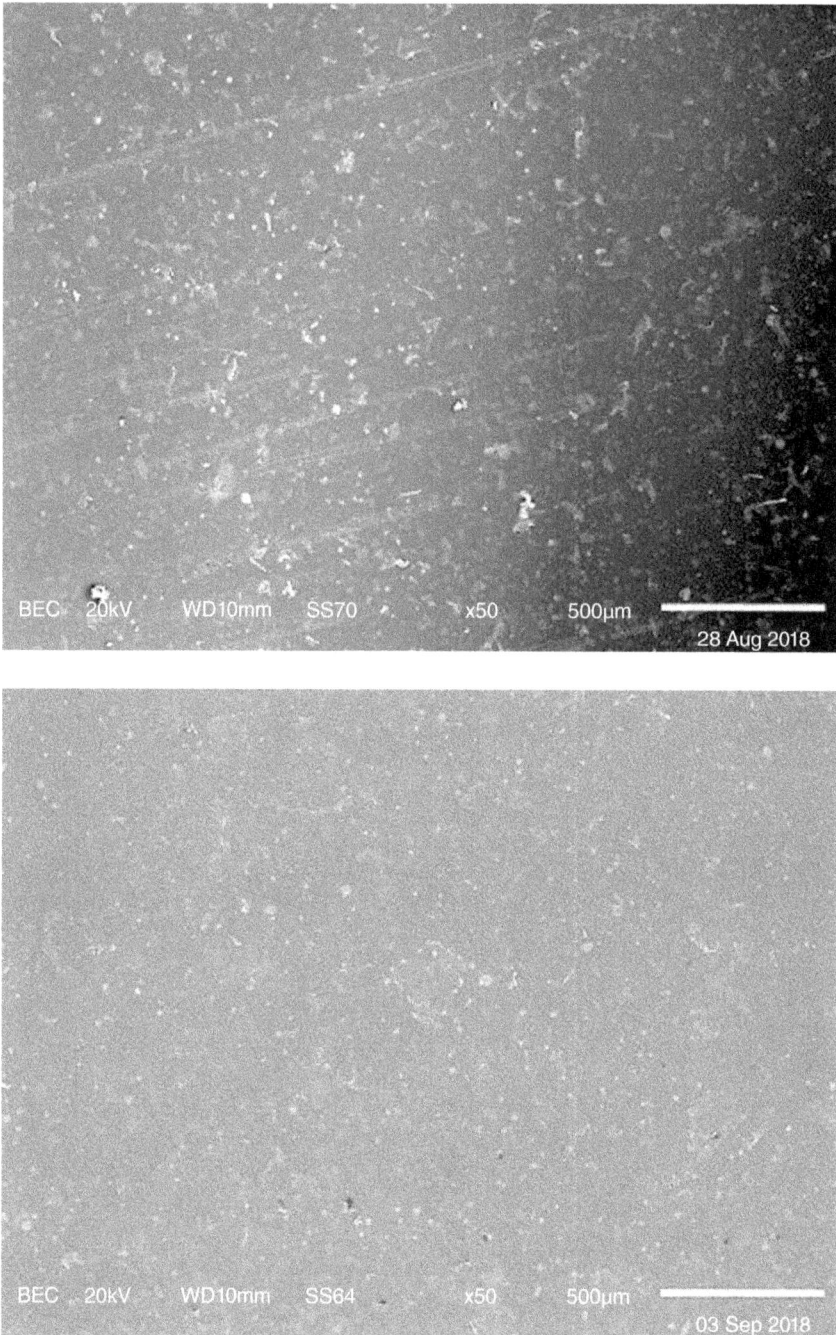

FIGURE 9.8 Images of surface analysis on GFRP panels coated '2K' and cellulose nanofibril (a) without nano-TiO₂ coating, (b) with the nano-TiO₂ coating, (c) with nano-TiO₂ coating and cleaning 5 times, and (d) with nano-TiO₂ coating and cleaning 10 times.

Source: Department of Science Service, Ministry of Higher Education, Science, Research and Innovation, Thailand [89]

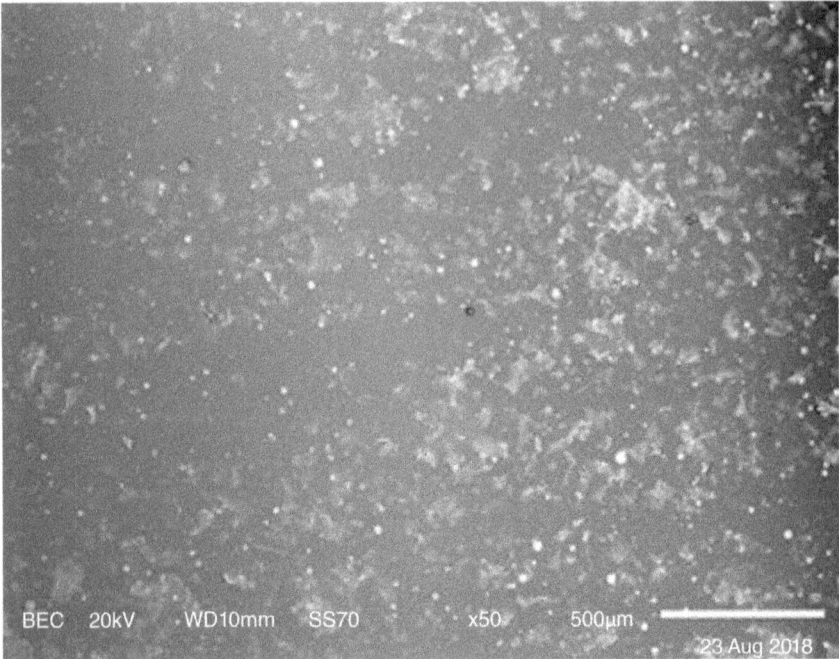

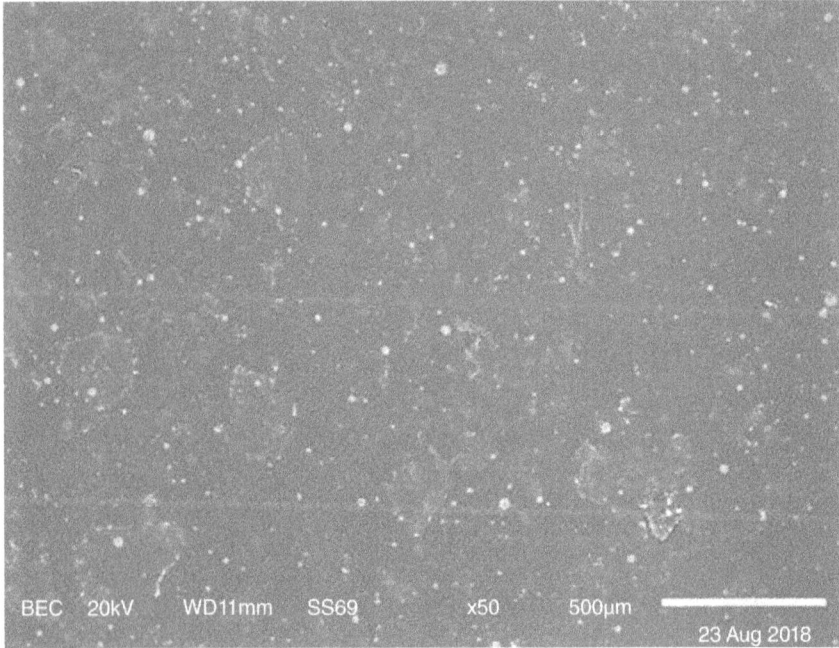

FIGURE 9.8   (Continued)

FIGURE 9.9   Images of surface analysis on GFRP panels coated 'Solid' and cellulose nano-fibril (a) without nano-TiO$_2$ coating, (b) with the nano-TiO$_2$ coating, (c) with nano-TiO$_2$ coating and cleaning 5 times, and (d) with nano-TiO$_2$ coating and cleaning 10 times.

Source: Department of Science Service, Ministry of Higher Education, Science, Research and Innovation, Thailand [89]

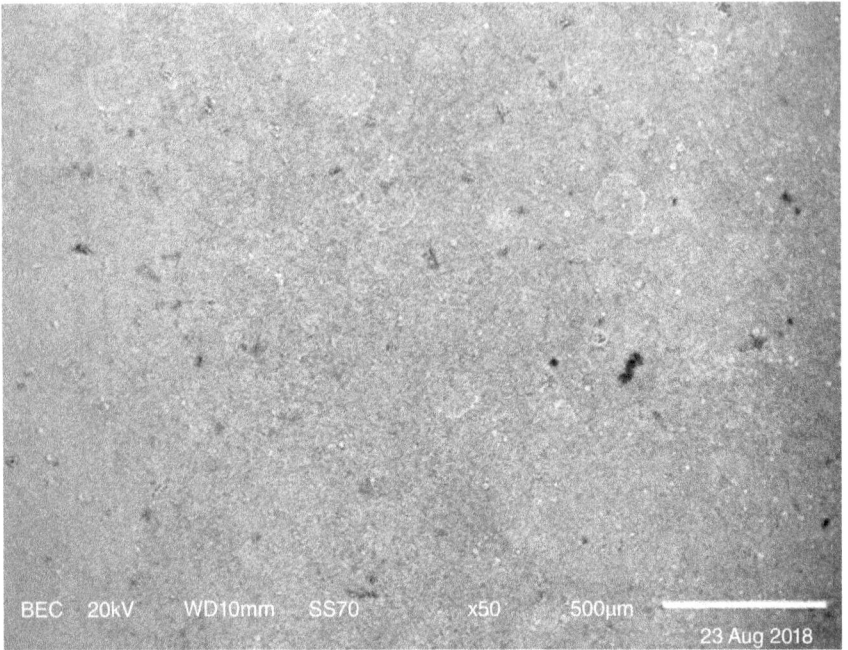

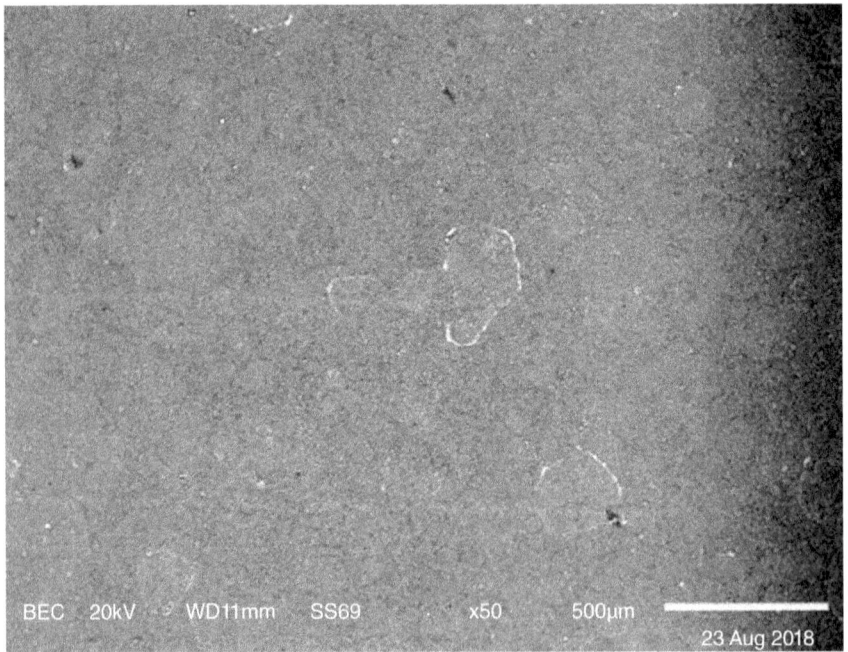

FIGURE 9.9 (Continued)

coated 'Solid' and cellulose nanofibril significantly reduce the aggregation of nano-TiO_2. To confirm their results, the surface analysis by SEM (magnification 200×) of nano-TiO_2 coating on GFRP panels coated either '2K' or 'Solid' and cellulose nanofibril was tested as seen in Figures 9.10 and 9.11, respectively. In addition, the quantitative element analysis by EDS was tested to analyze in terms of the percent of Ti as shown in Tables 9.12 and 9.13, respectively. Figure 9.10 and Table 9.12, the spectrum (2) which liked small droplet water is the highest percent of Ti (17.82%), whereas there were few percent of Ti for other areas. This result may be the reduction of accumulation by applying cellulose nanofibril, which agrees with the comparison of images between Figures 9.4 and 9.8.

Furthermore, from Figure 9.11 and Table 9.13, the spectrum (2) area at the edge of liked circle shape is the highest percent of Ti (30.61%). Other areas are not significantly different percents of Ti which are 25.51% and 26.12% for the spectrum (1) and (3), respectively. As described in 9.6.1 before, 'Solid' had the composition of TiO_2 as according to the Material Safety Data Sheet of Evercoat Industries (Thailand) Co., Ltd. Therefore, there is a reasonably high percentage of Ti from the spectrum (1), (2), and (3) in Figure 9.11. However, the adhesive bonding efficiency of nano-TiO_2 on GFRP panel coated 'Solid' and cellulose nanofibril by using EDX technique is still doubt. SEM (magnification 3,000× and 25,000×) were used to confirm the

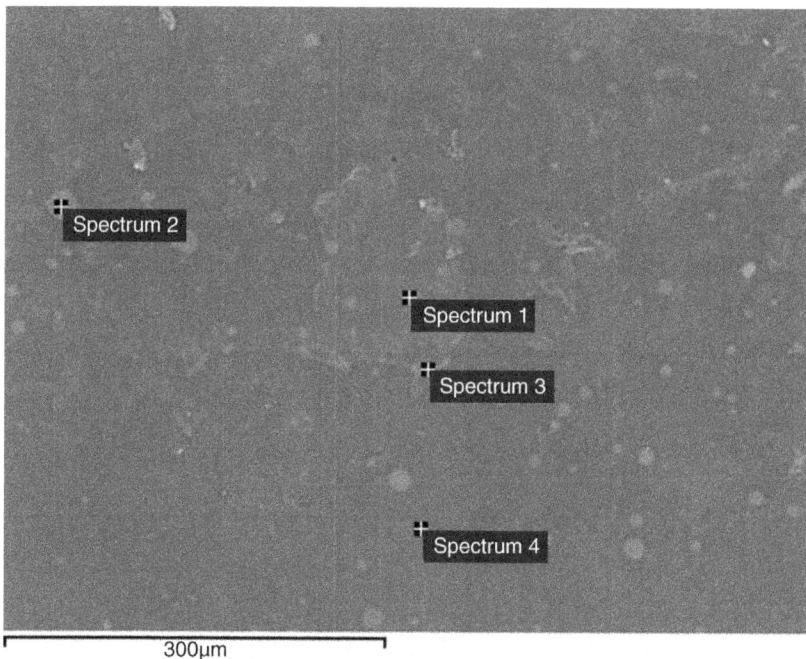

FIGURE 9.10   Images of surface analysis of nano-TiO_2 coating on GFRP panels coated '2K' and cellulose nanofibril by SEM (magnification 200×).

Source: Department of Science Service, Ministry of Higher Education, Science, Research and Innovation, Thailand [89]

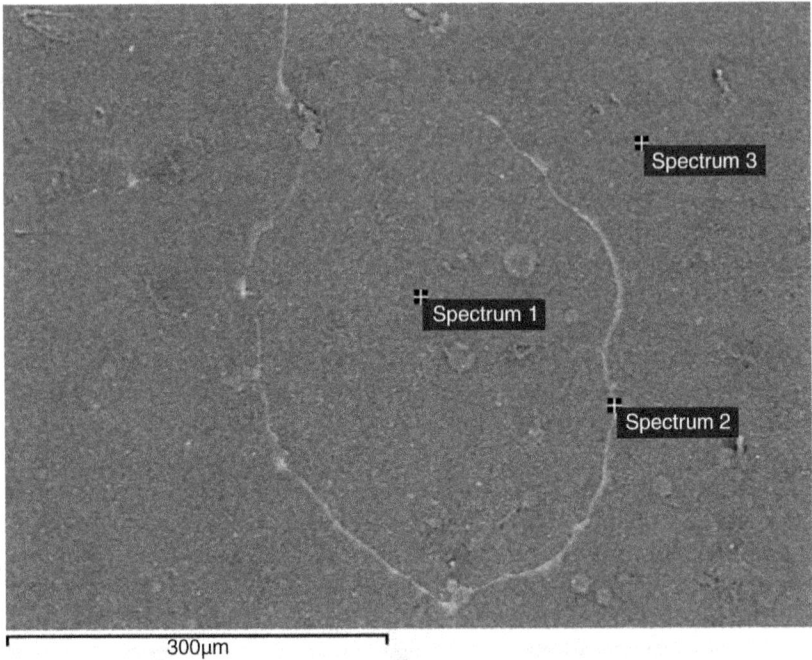

FIGURE 9.11 Images of surface analysis of nano-TiO$_2$ coating on GFRP panels coated 'Solid' and cellulose nanofibril by SEM (magnification 200×).

Source: Department of Science Service, Ministry of Higher Education, Science, Research and Innovation, Thailand [89]

TABLE 9.12
Quantitative Element Analysis of Nano-TiO$_2$ by EDS Technique: 1–4 Spectrum Areas from Figure 9.10

Element	Spectrum 1 %	Spectrum 2 %	Spectrum 3 %	Spectrum 4 %
C	67.12	53.90	62.23	80.18
O	17.11	18.96	21.95	6.39
Al	0	0.56	0	0
Si	0	0.22	0	0
Cl	0	0	0.17	0
Ti	1.89	17.82	4.59	0
Zn	0	0	0.39	0
Au	13.87	8.54	10.67	13.43

Source: Data from Department of Science Service, Ministry of Higher Education, Science, Research and Innovation, Thailand [89]

TABLE 9.13
Quantitative Element Analysis of Nano-TiO$_2$ by EDS Technique: 1–3 Spectrum Areas from Figure 9.11

Element	Spectrum 1 %	Spectrum 2 %	Spectrum 3 %
C	45.35	27.58	50.12
O	24.14	36.54	17.87
Al	0.79	0.46	0.76
Si	0.31	0.33	0.30
Ca	0	0.49	0.14
Ti	25.51	30.61	26.12
Au	3.91	3.98	4.70

Source: Data from Department of Science Service, Ministry of Higher Education, Science, Research and Innovation, Thailand [89]

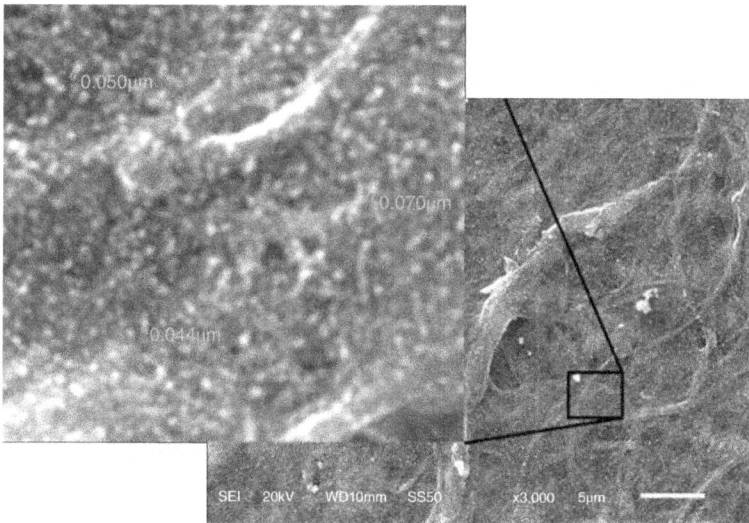

FIGURE 9.12 Image of adhesive boding nano-TiO$_2$ particles with cellulose nanofibril on GFRP panels coated 'Solid' by SEM (magnification 3000× and 25,000×).

Source: Department of Science Service, Ministry of Higher Education, Science, Research and Innovation, Thailand [89]

efficiency of adhesive bonding between nano-TiO$_2$ particles and cellulose nanofibril on GFRP panels coated 'Solid' as seen in Figure 9.12. The image shows the adhesion of nano-TiO$_2$ particles on cellulose nanofibril. This is reasonable to confirm that cellulose nanofibril and nano-TiO$_2$ coating processes can develop the deagglomeration of nano-TiO$_2$ particles on GFRP panel coated 'Solid.'

Summary: The deagglomeration of nano-TiO$_2$ on GFRP panels coated '2K' and 'Solid' by electrostatic sprayer is developed by coating cellulose nanofibril interval nano-TiO$_2$ process. In the next section, the cellulose nanofibril and nano-TiO$_2$ coating processes will be expanded to apply for other materials in the interior of ambulances to get dispersion well. In addition, the efficiency of adhesion of nano-TiO$_2$ particles for the interior ambulances will also be studied.

9.6.3 ADHESIVE EFFICIENCY OF NANO-TiO$_2$ FOR AMBULANCE INTERIORS

The process of nano-TiO$_2$ deagglomeration of GFRP coated either '2K' or 'Solid' was developed by coating cellulose nanofibril as described in Section 9.6.2. This section will apply the cellulose nanofibril and nano-TiO$_2$ coating processes in five ambulance interior materials: GFRP coated 'Solid,' PVC, stainless steel, PVC antistatic, and aluminum with checker plate as seen in Figure 9.13. In addition, the efficiency of adhesion of nano-TiO$_2$ particles for the interior ambulance materials was tested in the surface analysis by SEM before and after cleaning processes. It was also tested in the quantitative element analysis of Ti by EDS after cleaning methods. There are two cleaning processes, and the samples are separated into six groups for each method: 0, 20, 40, 60, 80, and 100 cycles. Firstly, the washing samples use deionized (DI) water. Then, the samples are wiped with a cleaning cloth, and they are dried by blowing any air called the 'first cleaning method.' Secondly, the washing samples by the

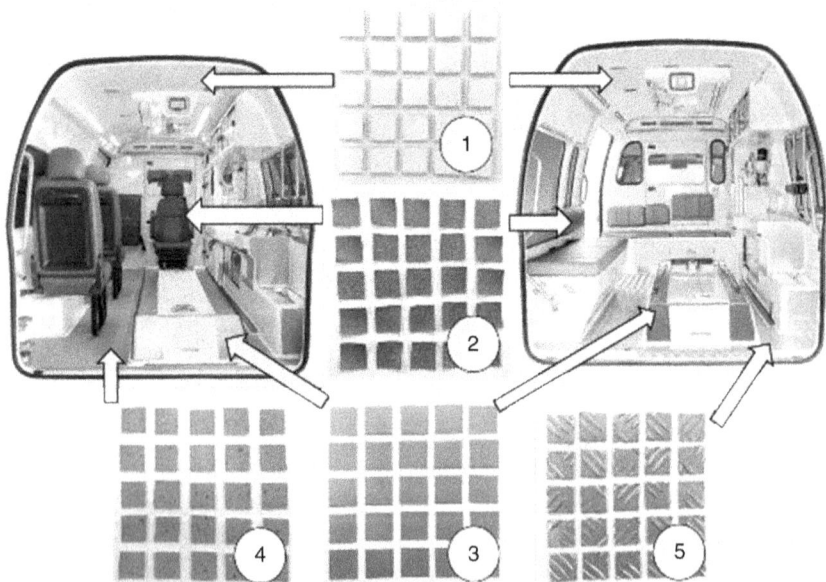

FIGURE 9.13 Cellulose nanofibril and nano-TiO$_2$ coating processes applied in five ambulance interior materials: (1) GFRP coated 'Solid,' (2) PVC, (3) stainless steel, (4) PVC antistatic, and (5) aluminum with checker plate.

Source: Department of Science Service, Ministry of Higher Education, Science, Research and Innovation, Thailand [90]

deionized water is done, and then the wiping samples by a cleaning cloth is done in this process. Then, Sporeclear™ medical device disinfectant wipes are used to clean the samples and leave them for a minute before wiping again with a cleaning cloth called the 'second cleaning method.' The adhesive efficiency of nano-TiO_2 particles for the interior ambulance materials will be described in the following sections.

9.6.3.1 GFRP Coated Solid

The first ambulance interior material is GFRP coated 'Solid,' which applied cellulose nanofibril and nano-TiO_2 coating processes. The adhesive bonding efficiency of nano-TiO_2 on this material was tested and analyzed by SEM and EDS techniques, as explained in the previous section. To begin with, the sample after first cleaning method for each cycle was observed the surface analysis by SEM (magnification 50×) with BEC mode as seen in Figure 9.14. The images from Figure 9.14 show that there are not a significant difference for 0, 20, 40, 60, 80, and 100 cleaning cycles. In addition, the sample after second cleaning method for each cycle was also observed the surface analysis by SEM (magnification 50×) with BEC mode as seen in Figure 9.15. There are not a significant difference for each cleaning cycle as well. Figure 9.16 shows the quantity of Ti by EDS techniques for both cleaning methods.

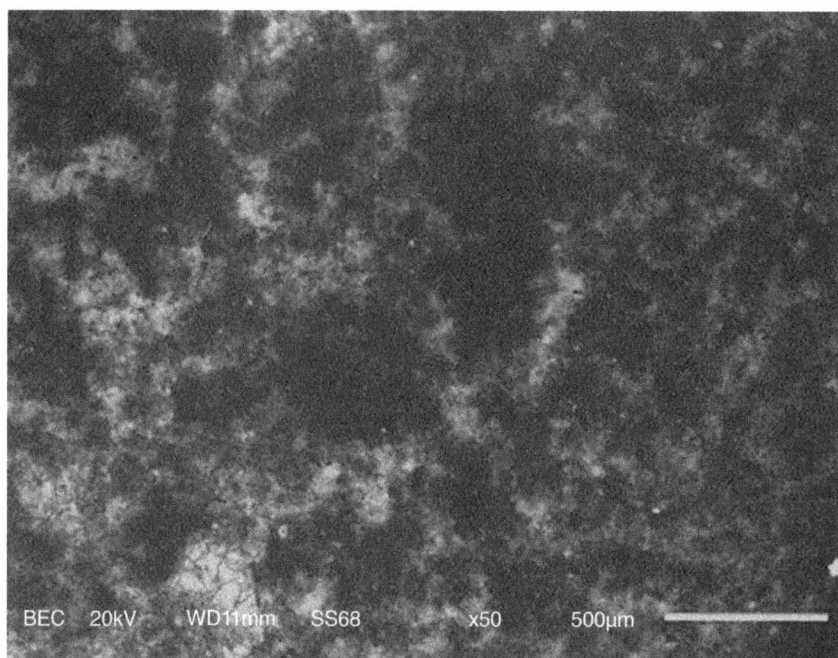

FIGURE 9.14 Images by SEM (magnification 50×) with BEC mode for cellulose nanofibril and nano-TiO_2 coating processes applied in GFRP coated 'Solid' after first cleaning method for each cycle: (a) 0, (b) 20, (c) 40, (d) 60, (e) 80, and (f) 100.

Source: Department of Science Service, Ministry of Higher Education, Science, Research and Innovation, Thailand [90]

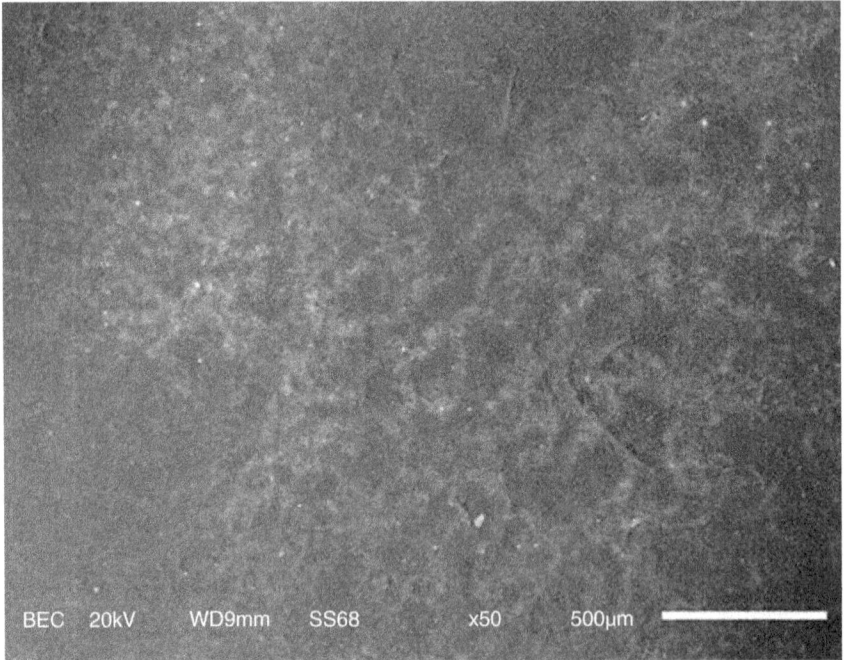

BEC   20kV   WD9mm   SS68   x50   500µm

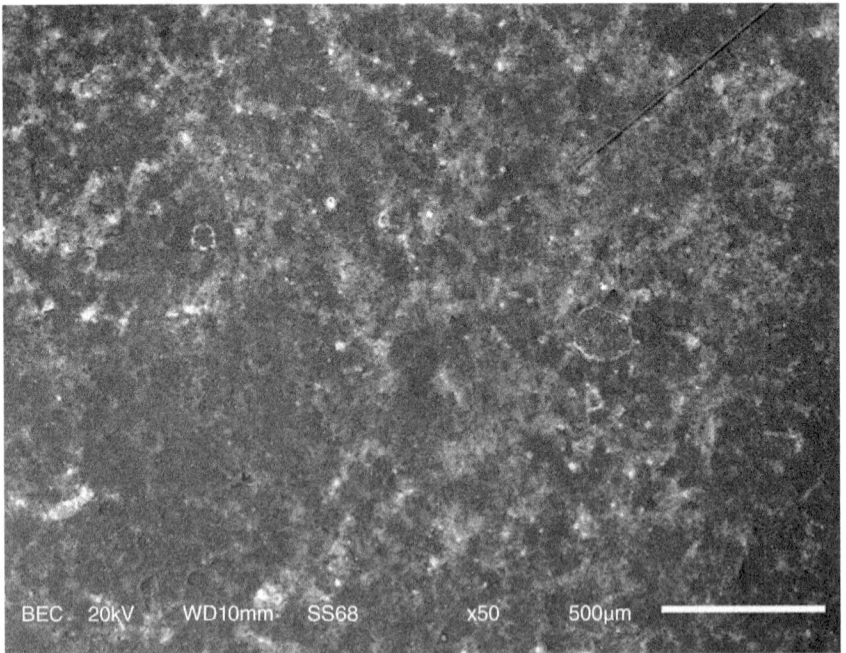

BEC   20kV   WD10mm   SS68   x50   500µm

FIGURE 9.14   (Continued)

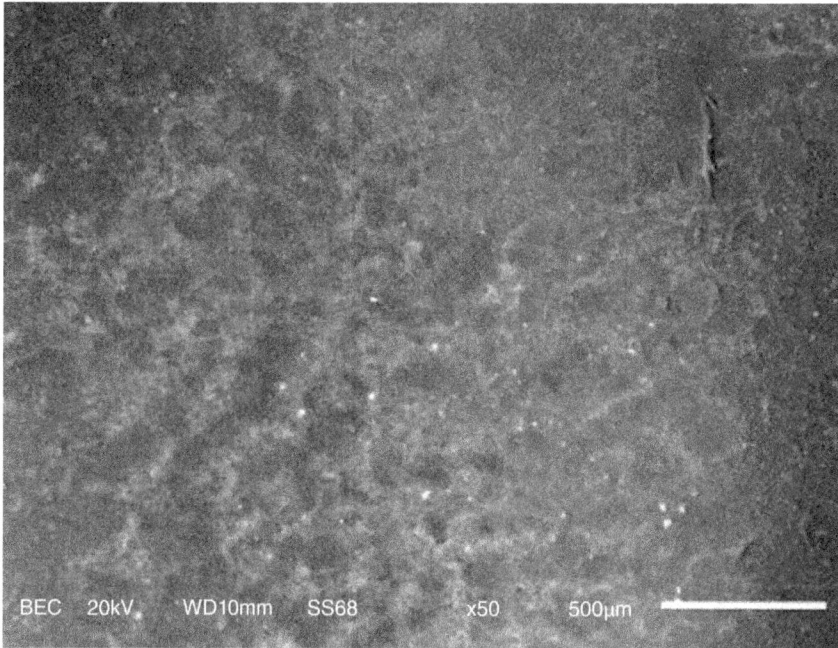

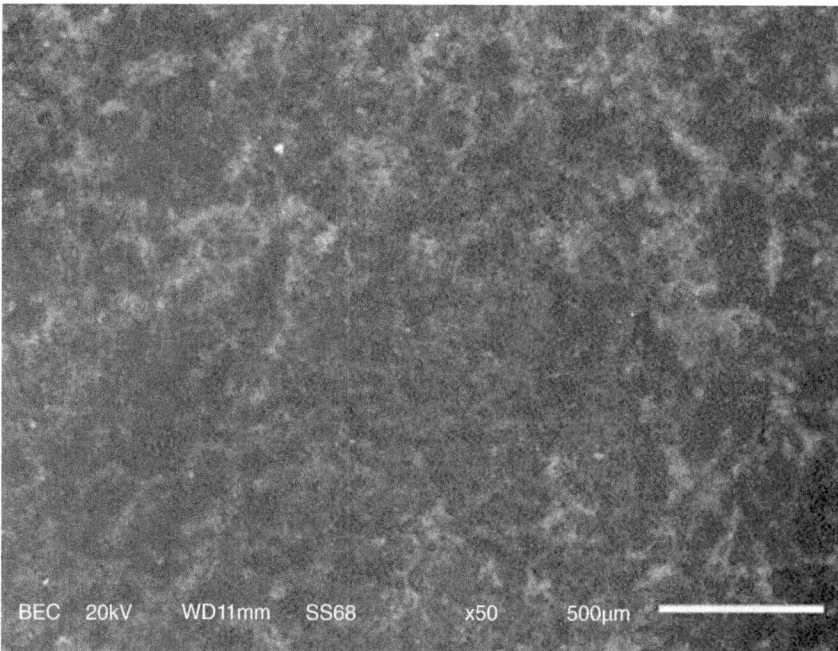

FIGURE 9.14 (Continued)

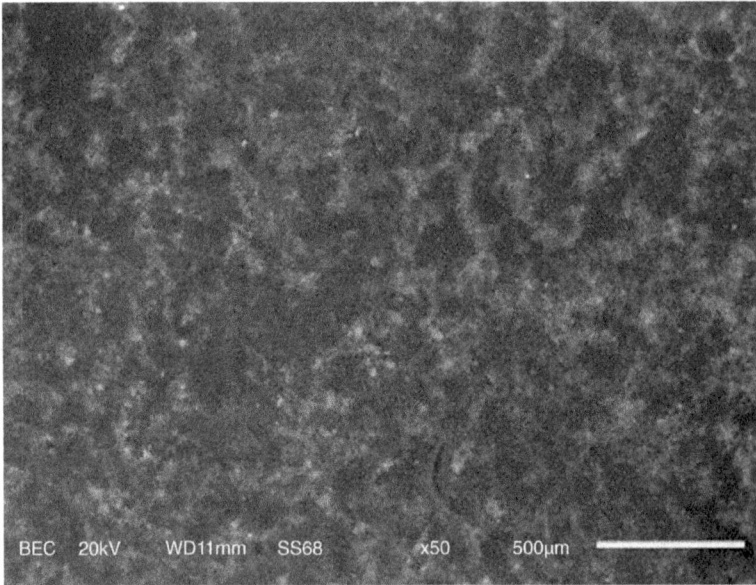

FIGURE 9.14   (Continued)

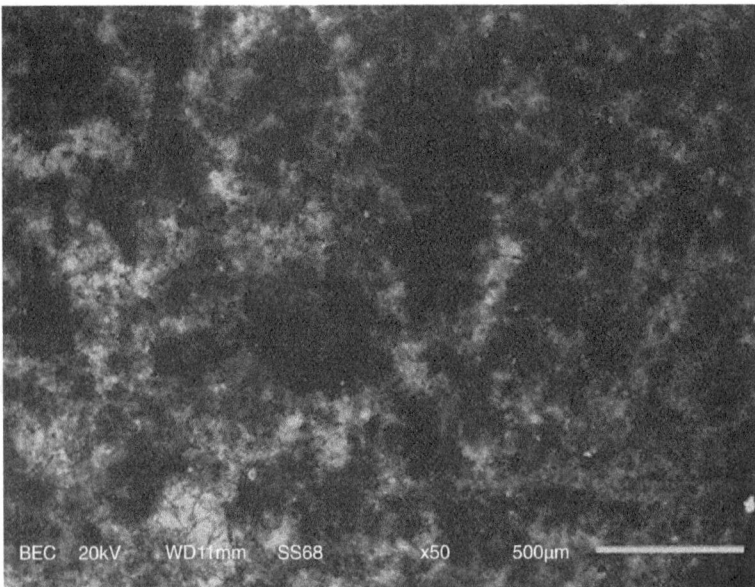

FIGURE 9.15   Images by SEM (magnification 50×) with BEC mode for cellulose nanofibril and nano-TiO$_2$ coating processes applied in GFRP coated 'Solid' after second cleaning method for each cycle: (a) 0, (b) 20, (c) 40, (d) 60, (e) 80, and (f) 100.

Source: Department of Science Service, Ministry of Higher Education, Science, Research and Innovation, Thailand [90]

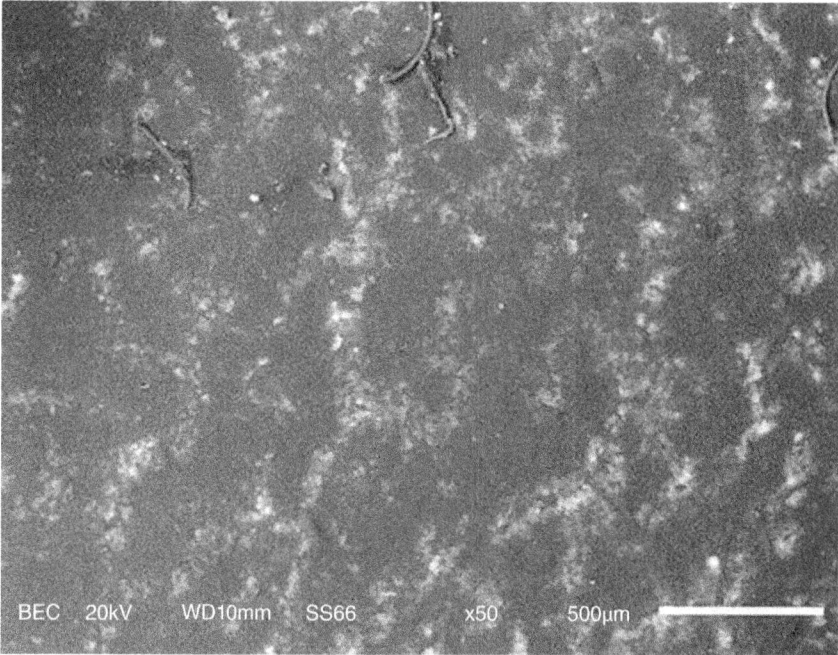

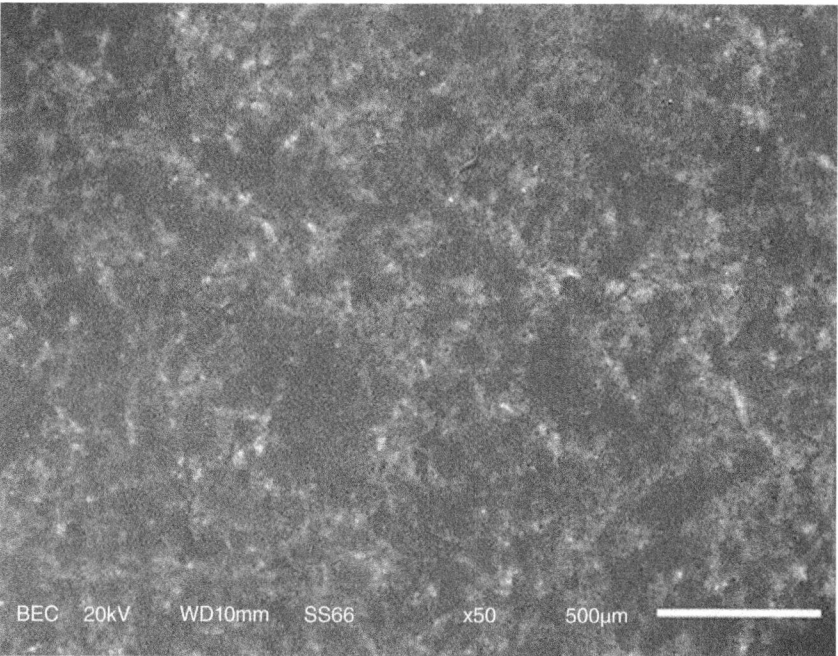

FIGURE 9.15 (Continued)

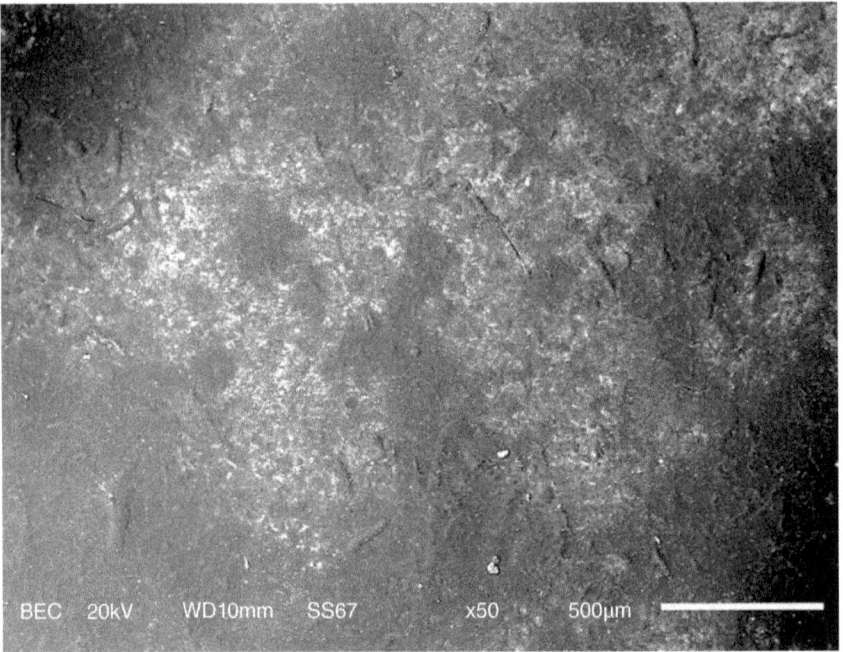

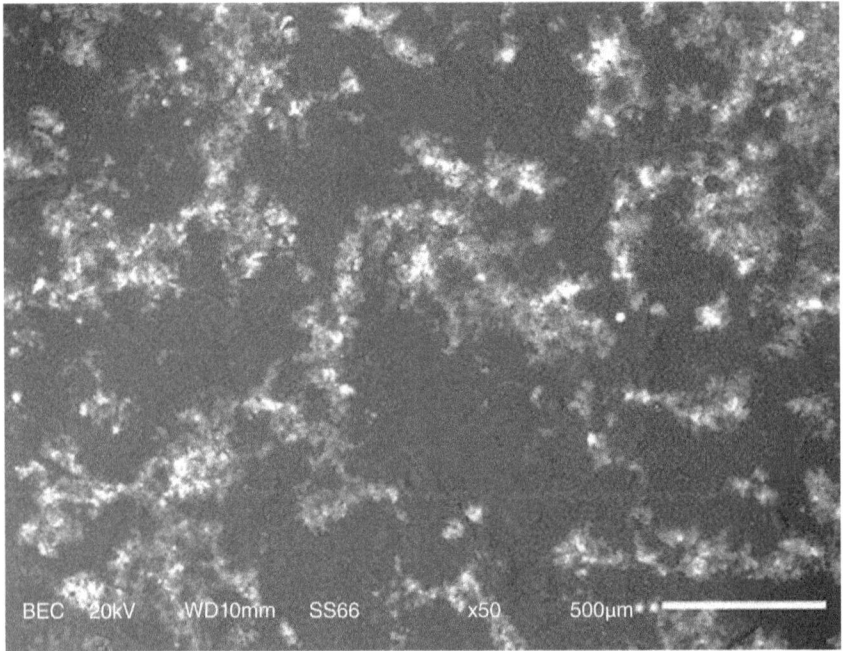

FIGURE 9.15   (Continued)

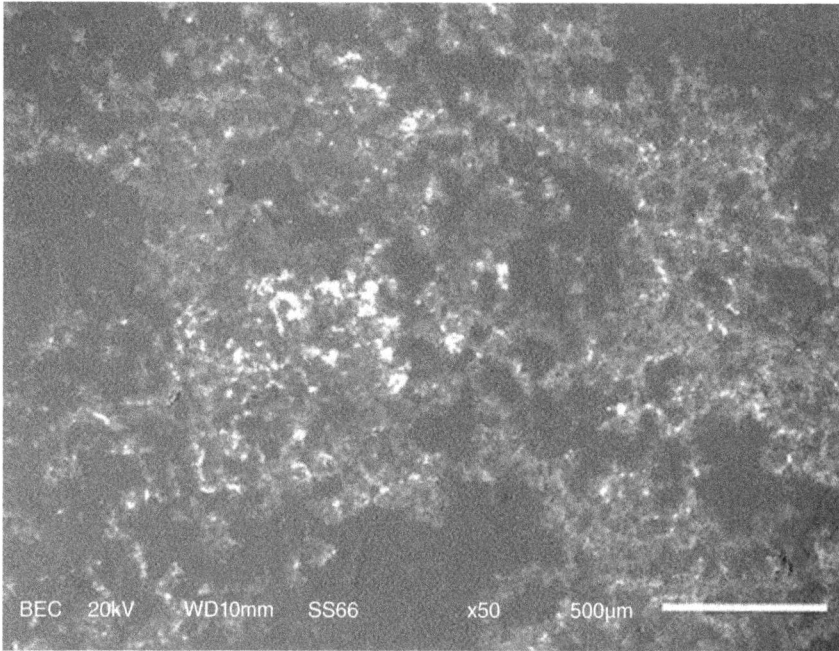

FIGURE 9.15   (Continued)

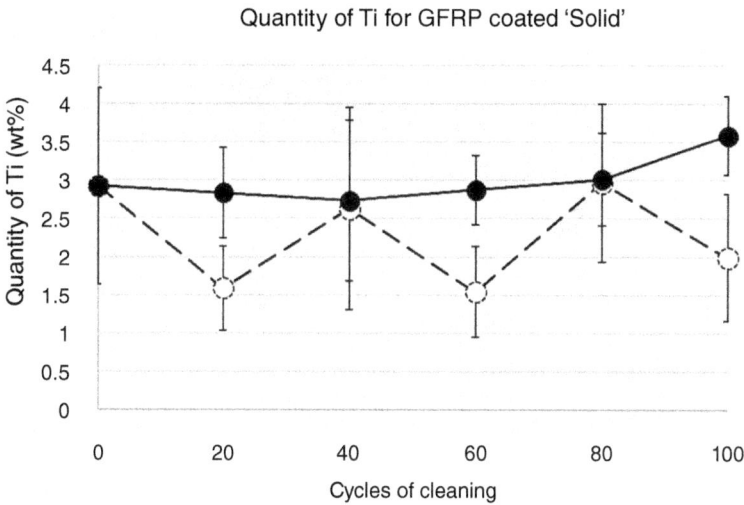

FIGURE 9.16   Graph shows the quantity of Ti for cellulose nanofibril and nano-TiO$_2$ coating processes applied in GFRP coated 'Solid' after cleaning for each cycle: (•) first cleaning method, (o) second cleaning method.

Source: Department of Science Service, Ministry of Higher Education, Science, Research and Innovation, Thailand [90]

For first cleaning method, the results show that the amounts of Ti are no significant differences for each cleaning cycle. The results for second cleaning method are not significantly different for each cleaning cycle as well. These results of images from both cleaning methods agree with the results of quantities of Ti in Figure 9.16.

Furthermore, the surface of the sample after second cleaning method for 100 cycles was tested in the microstructural observation by SEM (magnification 1000× and 5000×) with SEI mode, as seen in Figure 9.17. The image of SEM (magnification 5000×) shows many white particles on the sample's surface, assuming that particles may be nano-TiO_2. The sample was tested in the microstructural observation by SEM (magnification 25,000×) with SEI mode to confirm the result. It was measured the size of particles as seen in Figure 9.18. The image shows some particles of nano-TiO_2 on the surface of this material with dimensions from 0.049 to 0.088 μm. It means that the second cleaning method for 100 cycles cannot peel off nano-TiO_2 on the surface of the GFRP panel. With all results as described before, the adhesive bonding efficiency for cellulose nanofibril and nano-TiO_2 coating processes applied in GFRP coated 'Solid' panel is suitable for using ambulance interior materials.

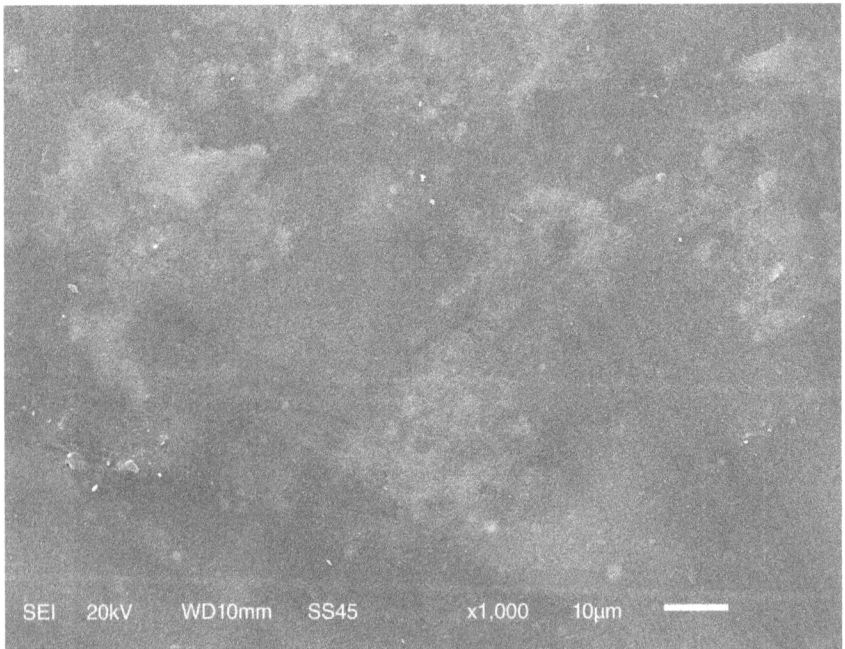

FIGURE 9.17   Images of cellulose nanofibril and nano-TiO_2 coating processes applied in GFRP coated 'Solid' after second cleaning method for 100 cycles by SEM with SEI mode: (a) magnification 1000×, (b) magnification 5000×.

Source: Department of Science Service, Ministry of Higher Education, Science, Research and Innovation, Thailand [90]

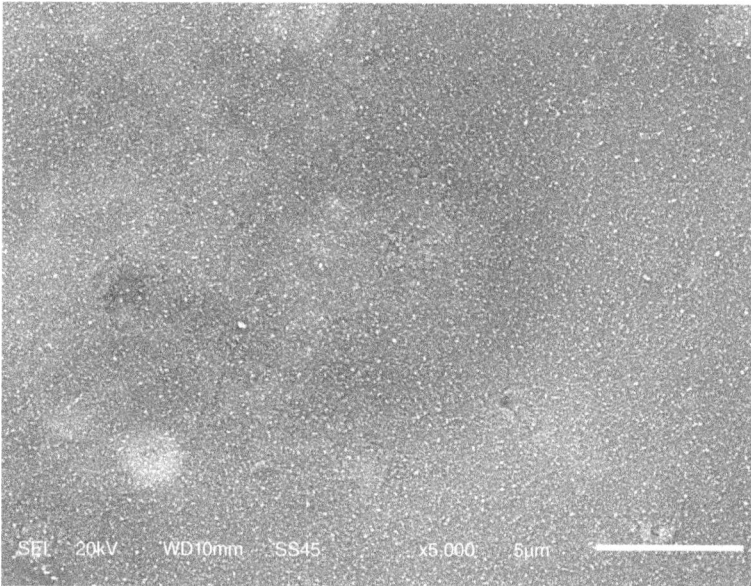

FIGURE 9.17 (Continued)

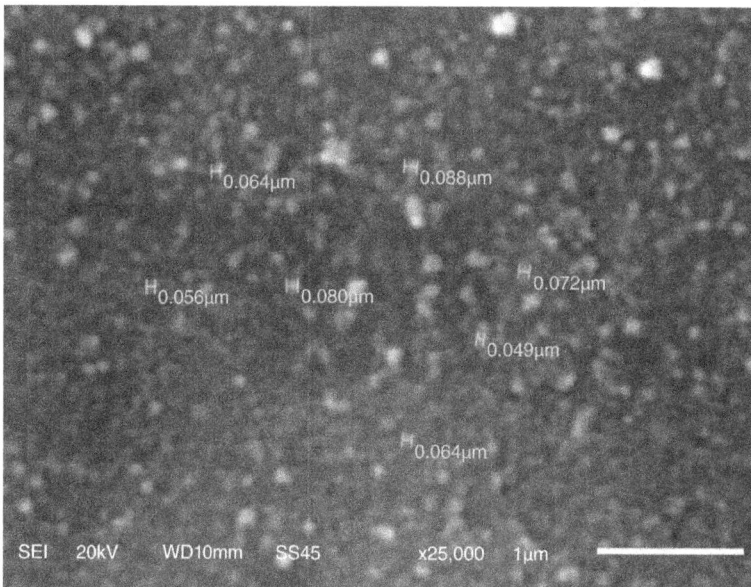

FIGURE 9.18 Particle sizes of Ti for cellulose nanofibril and nano-TiO₂ coating processes applied in GFRP coated 'Solid' after second cleaning method for 100 cycles by SEM (magnification 25,000×) with SEI mode.

Source: Department of Science Service, Ministry of Higher Education, Science, Research and Innovation, Thailand [90]

9.6.3.2 PVC

Secondly, PVC applied cellulose nanofibril and nano-TiO_2 coating processes are tested in the efficiency of adhesive bonding for nano-TiO_2 on its surface, and the methodology was described in Section 9.6.3. Figure 9.19 shows the sample after first cleaning method for each cycle, which observed the surface analysis by SEM (magnification 50×) with BEC mode. From Figure 9.19, there is a bright white in some areas, except in 20 cleaning cycles. This appearance is the charging effect from SEM because the specimens had not a smooth surface. Therefore, it does not confirm the surface observation from Figure 9.19. To solve this problem, the sample after second cleaning method for each cycle was coated a carbon on the surface for longer times. All specimens were observed the surface analysis by SEM (magnification 50×) with BEC mode as seen in Figure 9.20. It was found that there was a reduction in the charging effect. There are no significant differences for each cleaning cycle as well. Figure 9.21 shows the quantity of Ti by EDS techniques for both cleaning methods. For 1st cleaning method, the results show that the amounts of Ti are not significantly different for each cleaning cycle. The graph of the second cleaning method shows the tendency of reduction with the increasing cycles. It is possible that Sporeclear medical device disinfectant wipes can peel off some nano-TiO_2 on the surface of PVC.

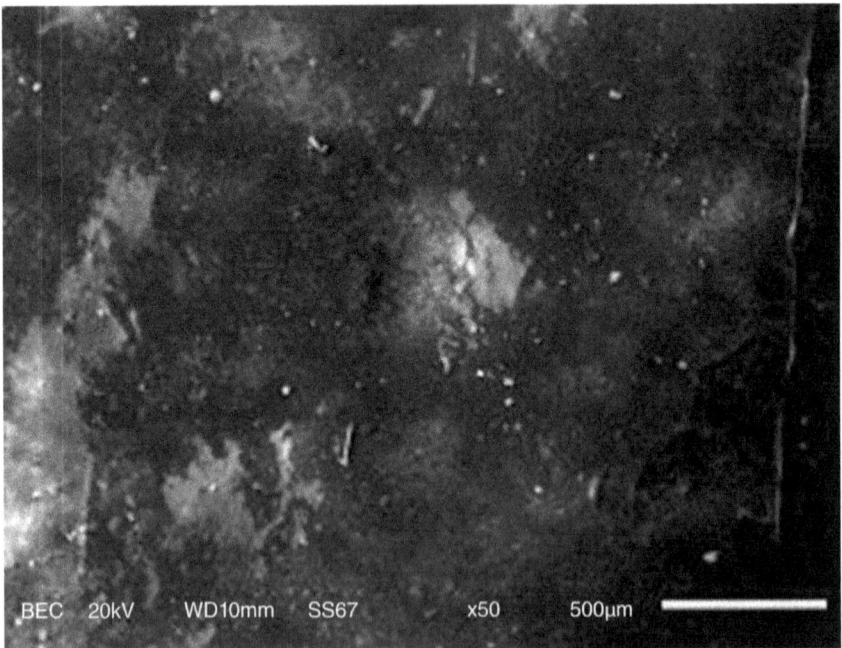

FIGURE 9.19 Images by SEM (magnification 50×) with BEC mode for cellulose nanofibril and nano-TiO_2 coating processes applied in PVC after first cleaning method for each cycle: (a) 0, (b) 20, (c) 40, (d) 60, (e) 80, and (f) 100.

Source: Department of Science Service, Ministry of Higher Education, Science, Research and Innovation, Thailand [90]

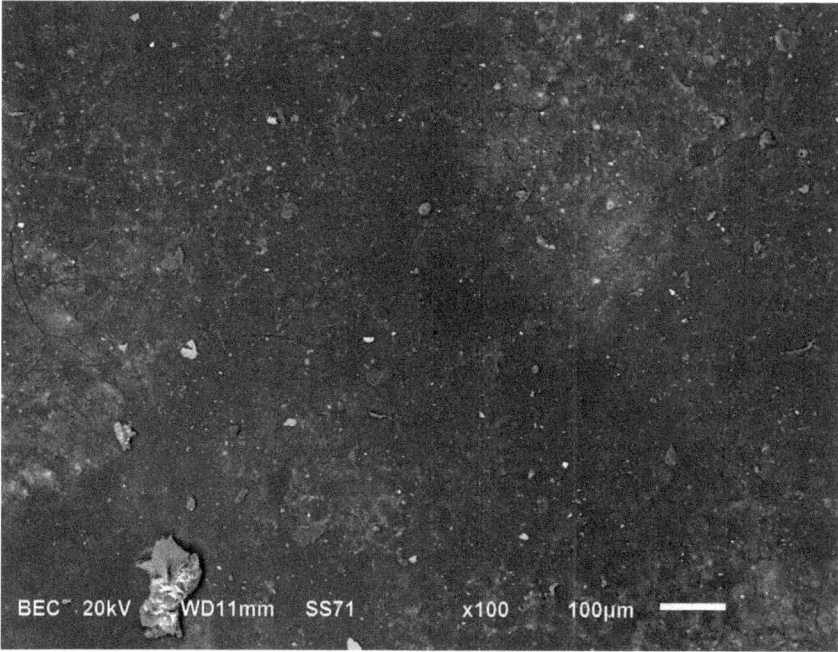

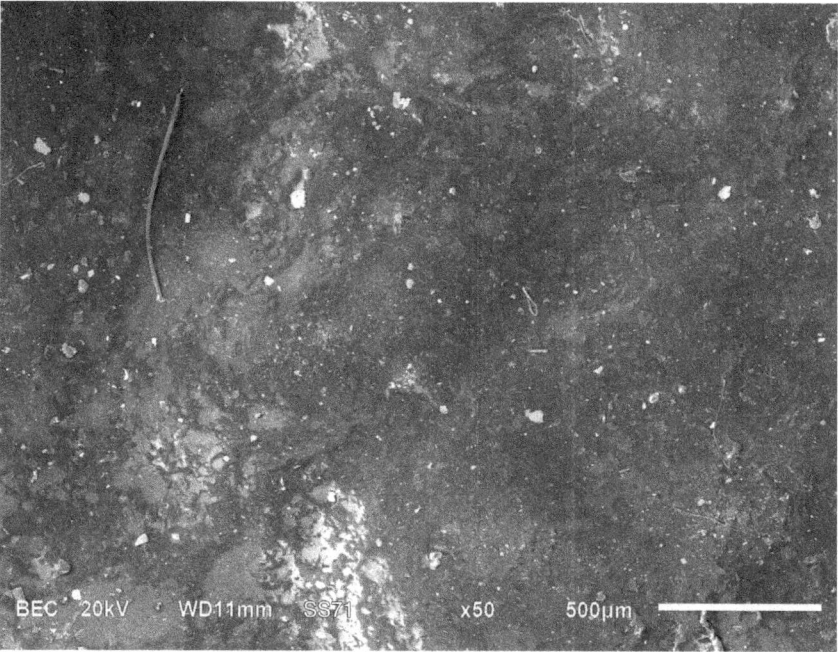

FIGURE 9.19 (Continued)

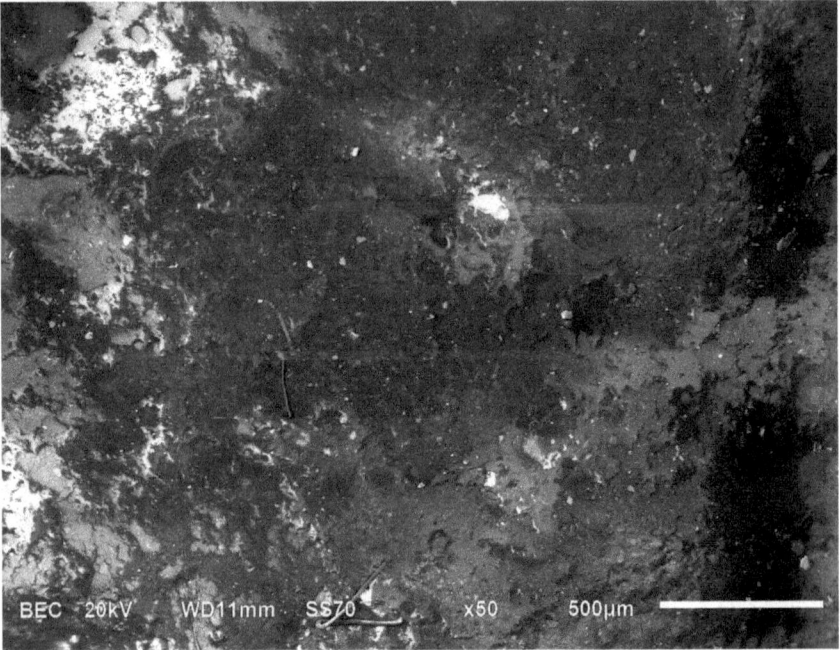

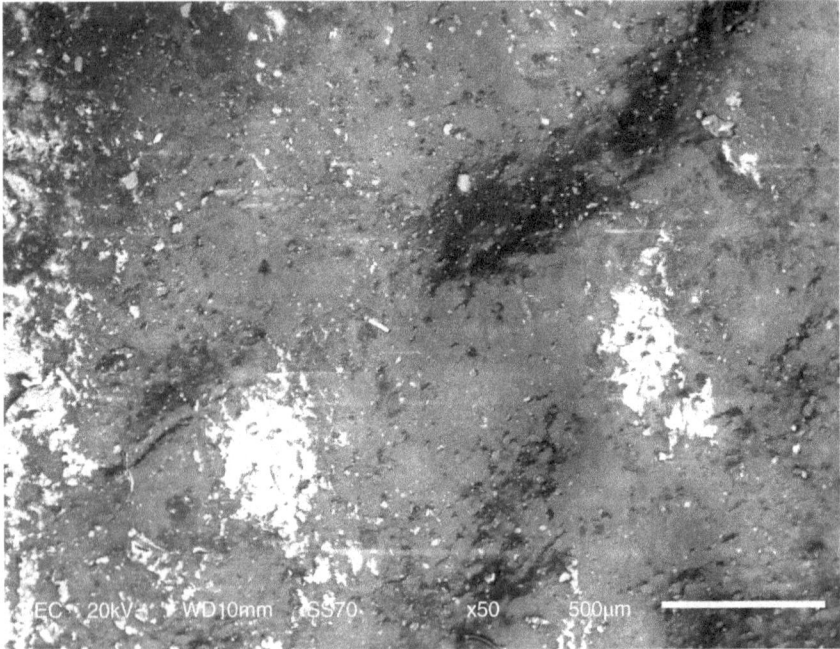

FIGURE 9.19   (Continued)

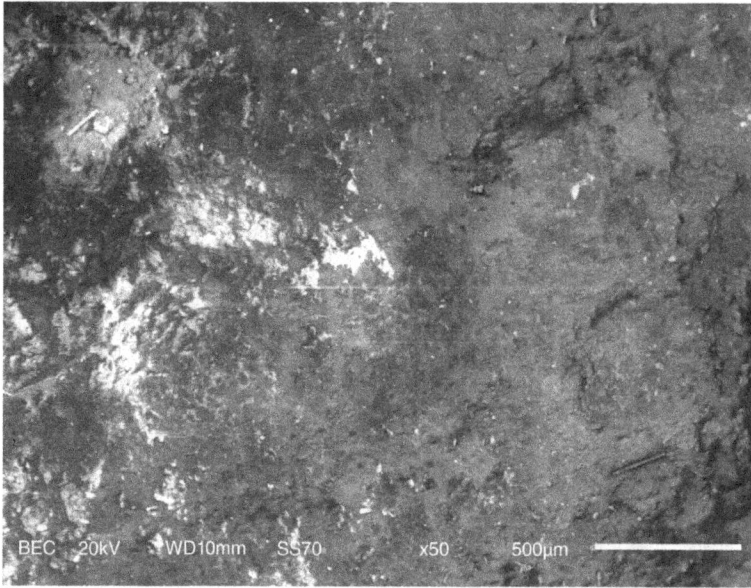

FIGURE 9.19   (Continued)

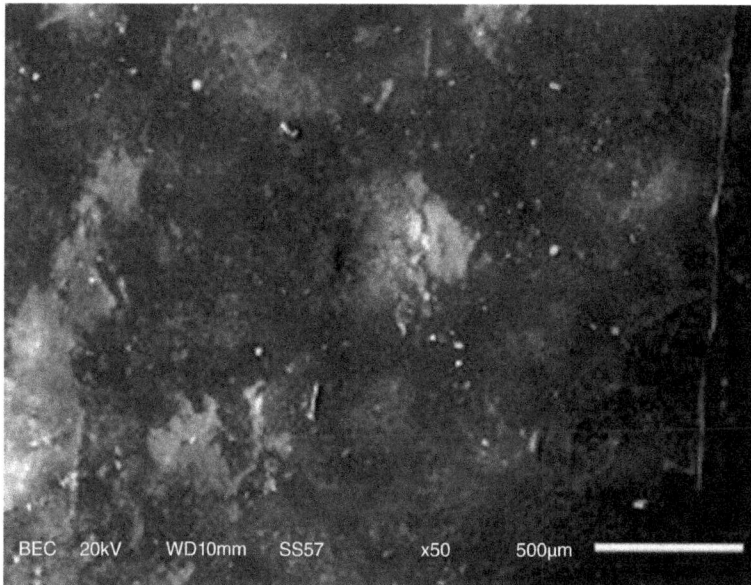

FIGURE 9.20   Images by SEM (magnification 50×) with BEC mode for cellulose nanofibril and nano-TiO$_2$ coating processes applied in PVC after second cleaning method for each cycle: (a) 0, (b) 20, (c) 40, (d) 60, (e) 80, and (f) 100.

Source: Department of Science Service, Ministry of Higher Education, Science, Research and Innovation, Thailand [90]

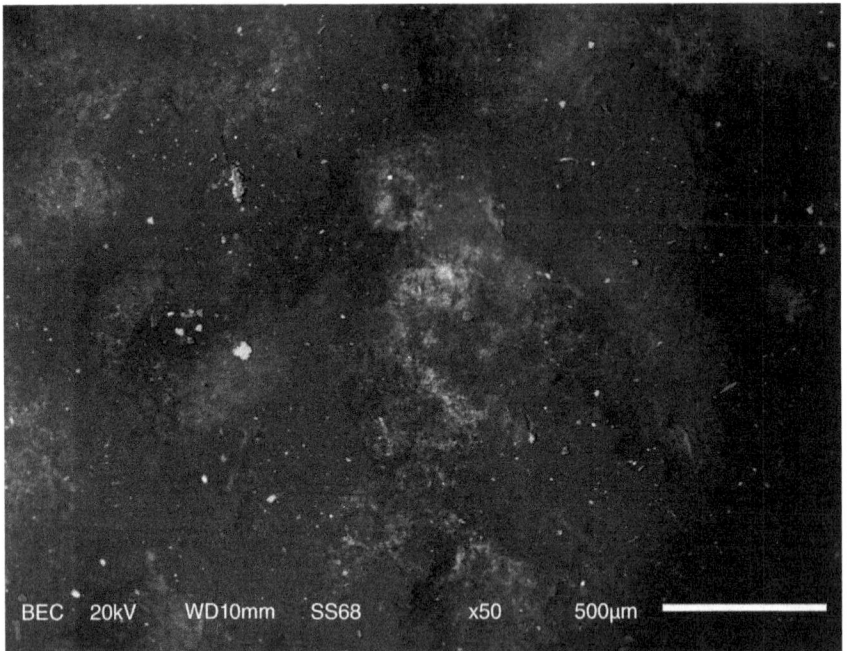

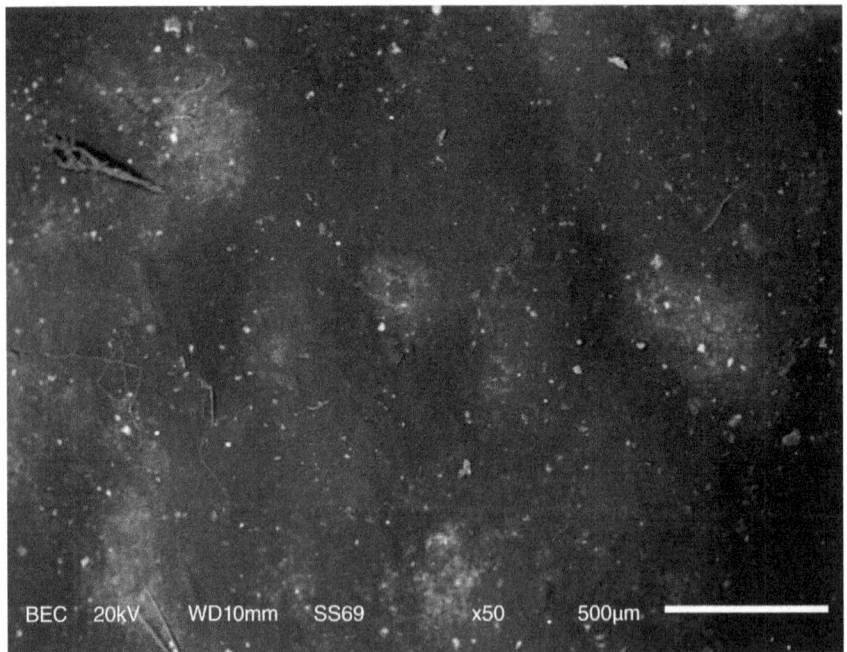

FIGURE 9.20   (Continued)

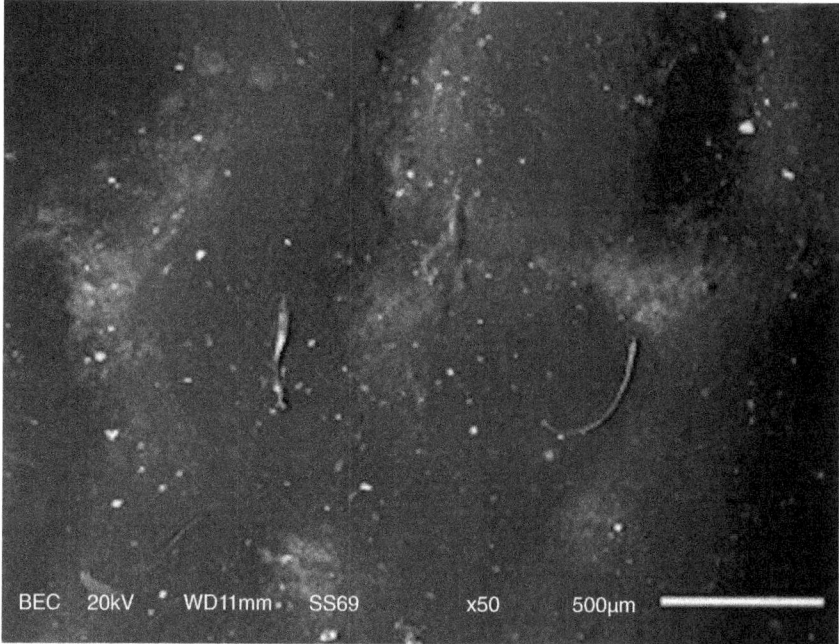

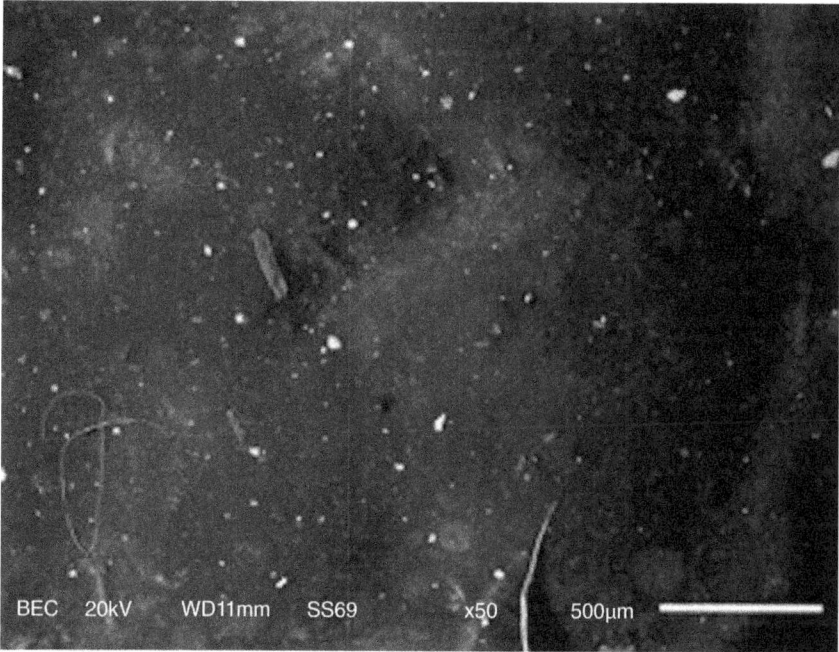

FIGURE 9.20 (Continued)

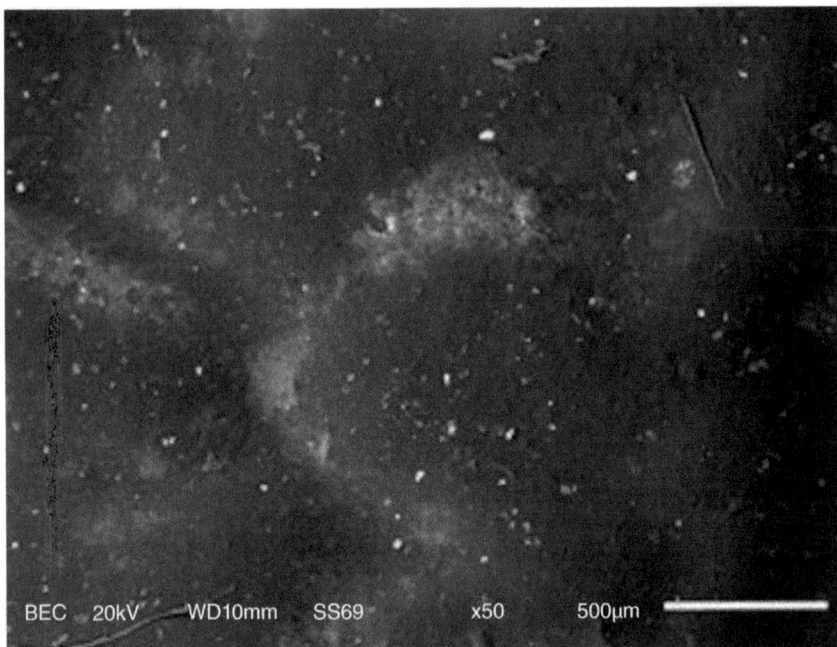

FIGURE 9.20 (Continued)

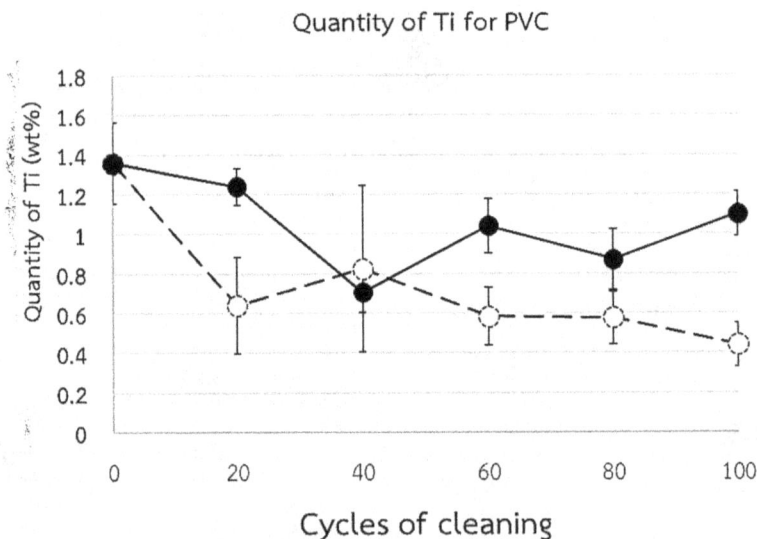

FIGURE 9.21 Graph shows the quantity of Ti for cellulose nanofibril and nano-TiO$_2$ coating processes applied in PVC after cleaning for each cycle: (•) first cleaning method, (○) second cleaning method.

Source: Department of Science Service, Ministry of Higher Education, Science, Research and Innovation, Thailand [90]

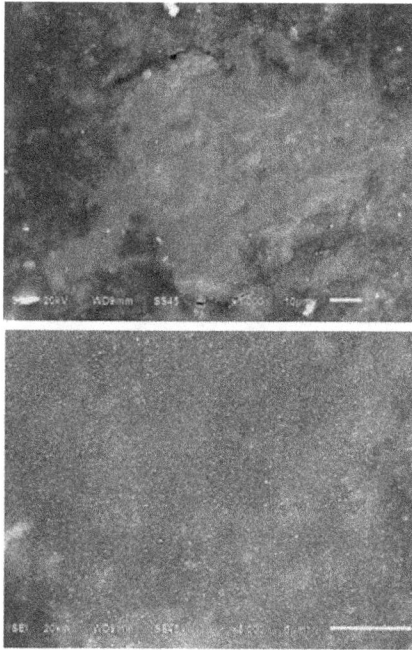

FIGURE 9.22   Images of cellulose nanofibril and nano-TiO$_2$ coating processes applied in PVC after second cleaning method for 100 cycles by SEM with SEI mode: (a) magnification 1000×, (b) magnification 5000×.

Source: Department of Science Service, Ministry of Higher Education, Science, Research and Innovation, Thailand [90]

Furthermore, the surface of the sample after second cleaning method for 100 cycles was tested in the microstructural observation by SEM (magnification 1000× and 5000×) with SEI mode, as seen in Figure 9.22. The image of SEM (magnification 5000×) shows many white particles on the sample's surface, assuming that particles may be nano-TiO$_2$. The sample was tested in the microstructural observation by SEM (magnification 25,000×) with SEI mode for confirmation of the result, as seen in Figure 9.23. The images show some white particles on the surface of this material, assuming that it may be nano-TiO$_2$ because their sizes are similar sizes to nano-TiO$_2$ in Figure 9.18. It means that the second cleaning method for 100 cycles cannot peel off nano-TiO$_2$ on the surface of PVC. There are enough remaining nano-TiO$_2$ appearing on the surface of PVC. With all results described before, the adhesive bonding efficiency for cellulose nanofibril and nano-TiO$_2$ coating processes applied in PVC is suitable for using ambulance interior materials, which is usually a part of the car seat.

9.6.3.3   Stainless Steel

Thirdly, stainless steel was applied with cellulose nanofibril and nano-TiO$_2$ coating processes. Then, an adhesive efficiency of nano-TiO$_2$ on the surface of this material was tested by the method as described before in Section 9.6.3. First of all, the specimens after the first cleaning method for each cycle were tested to observe surface

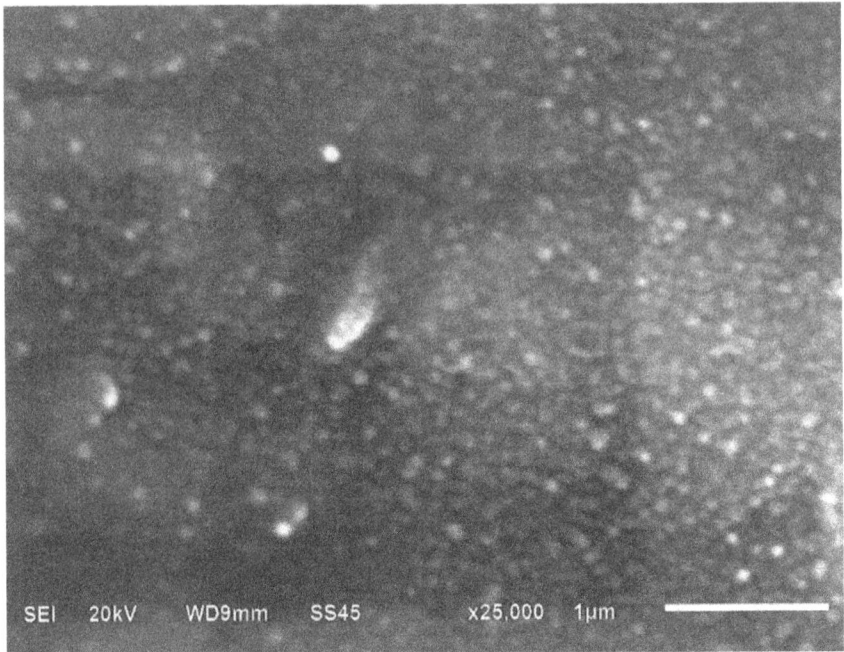

FIGURE 9.23   Image of Ti for cellulose nanofibril and nano-TiO$_2$ coating processes applied in PVC after second cleaning method for 100 cycles by SEM (magnification 25,000×) with SEI mode.

Source: Department of Science Service, Ministry of Higher Education, Science, Research and Innovation, Thailand [90]

analysis by SEM (magnification 50×) with BEC mode, as seen in Figure 9.24. It was found that the appearance of the surface was no significant difference for each cycle. In addition, the samples after second cleaning method for each cycle have also tested the observation of surface analysis by SEM (magnification 50×) with BEC mode, as seen in Figure 9.25. The images show that there were no significant differences in the appearance of the surface for each cycle. Then, EDS was used to investigate the quantity of Ti for both cleaning methods, as seen in Figure 9.26. It was found that the results of surface observation from Figures 9.24 and 9.25 are in agreement with the quantities of Ti from Figure 9.26.

Moreover, the surface of the sample after second cleaning method for 100 cycles was tested in the microstructural observation by SEM (magnification 1000× and 5000×) and (magnification 25,000×) with SEI mode as seen in Figures 9.27 and 9.28, respectively. The images of SEM (magnification 1000×, 5000×, and 25,000×) show similar results with GFRP coated 'Solid' and PVC, assuming that the white particles are nano-TiO$_2$. However, the average Ti amount for the second cleaning method is lower than the value of the first cleaning method because Sporeclear medical device disinfectant wipes may peel off some nano-TiO$_2$ on the material's surface (see Figure 9.26). Sporeclear medical device disinfectant wipes may be able to peel off

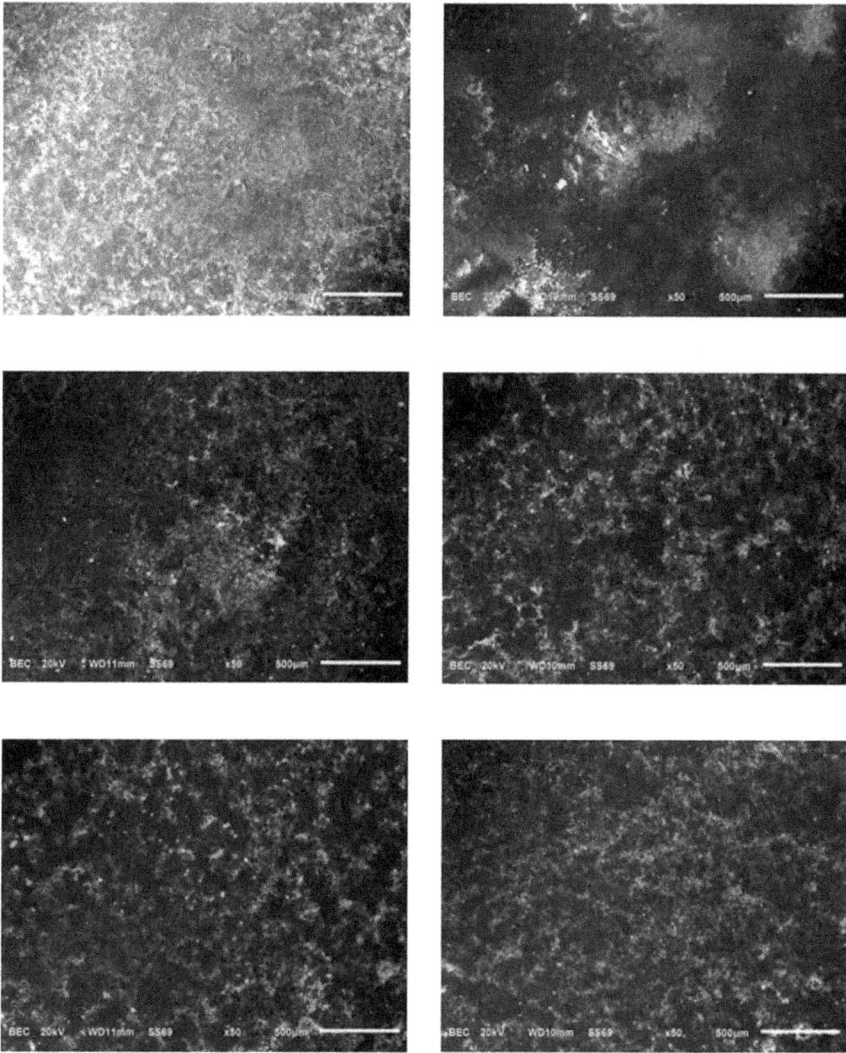

FIGURE 9.24 Images by SEM (magnification 50×) with BEC mode for cellulose nanofibril and nano-TiO₂ coating processes applied in stainless steel after first cleaning method for each cycle: (a) 0, (b) 20, (c) 40, (d) 60, (e) 80, and (f) 100.

Source: Department of Science Service, Ministry of Higher Education, Science, Research and Innovation, Thailand [90]

some nano-TiO₂ on the stainless steel's surface. However, the particles of nano-TiO₂ remain enough, and they still appear on the surface of stainless steel after 100 cycles of second cleaning method. With the results as described before, the adhesive bonding efficiency for cellulose nanofibril and nano-TiO₂ coating processes applied in the stainless steel is appropriate for applying a part of the floor in the ambulance interior.

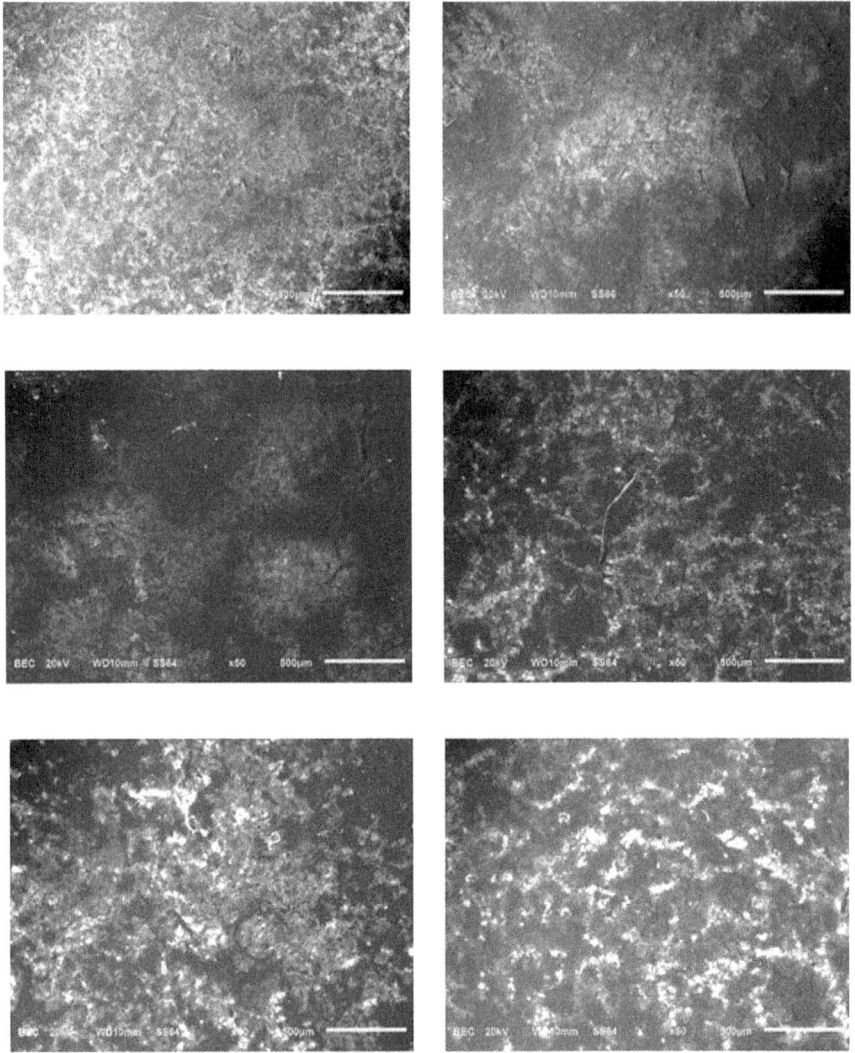

FIGURE 9.25 Images by SEM (magnification 50×) with BEC mode for cellulose nanofibril and nano-TiO$_2$ coating processes applied in stainless steel after second cleaning method for each cycle: (a) 0, (b) 20, (c) 40, (d) 60, (e) 80, and (f) 100.

Source: Department of Science Service, Ministry of Higher Education, Science, Research and Innovation, Thailand [90]

9.6.3.4 PVC Antistatic

The fourth material is PVC antistatic applied with cellulose nanofibril and nano-TiO$_2$ coating processes. The adhesive efficiency of nano-TiO$_2$ on the surface of this material was tested by the method described in Section 9.6.3. To begin with, the

Quantity of Ti for stainless steel

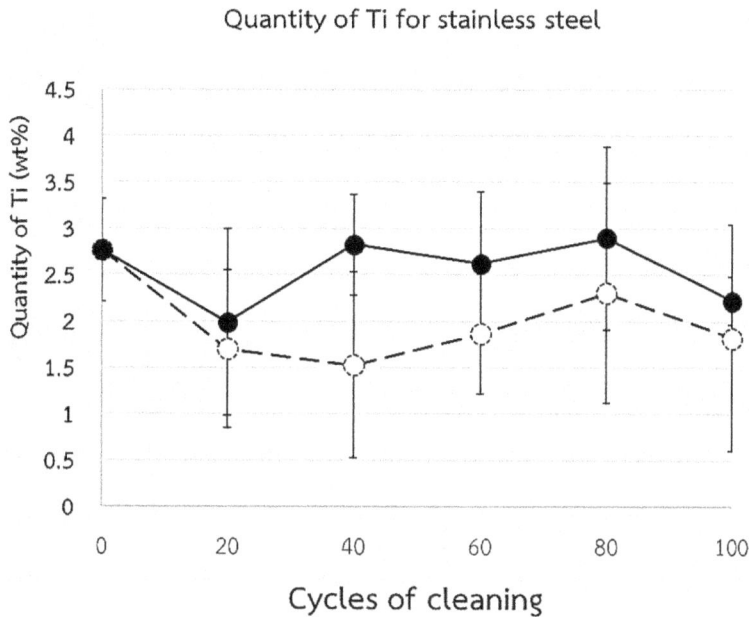

FIGURE 9.26   Graph shows the quantity of Ti for cellulose nanofibril and nano-TiO$_2$ coating processes applied in stainless steel after cleaning for each cycle: (•) first cleaning method, (○) second cleaning method.

Source: Department of Science Service, Ministry of Higher Education, Science, Research and Innovation, Thailand [90]

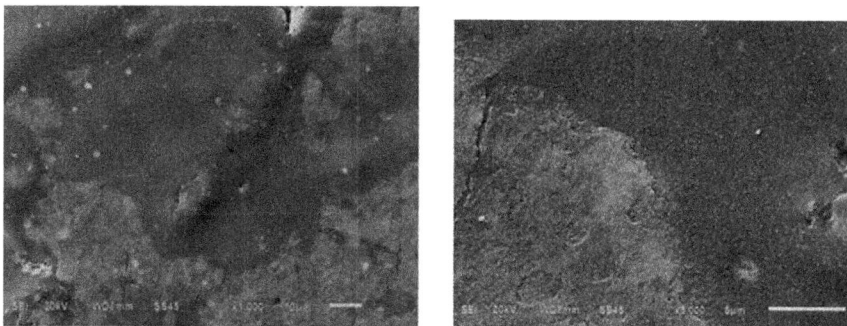

FIGURE 9.27   Images of cellulose nanofibril and nano-TiO$_2$ coating processes applied in stainless steel after second cleaning method for 100 cycles by SEM with SEI mode: (a) magnification 1000×, (b) magnification 5000×.

Source: Department of Science Service, Ministry of Higher Education, Science, Research and Innovation, Thailand [90]

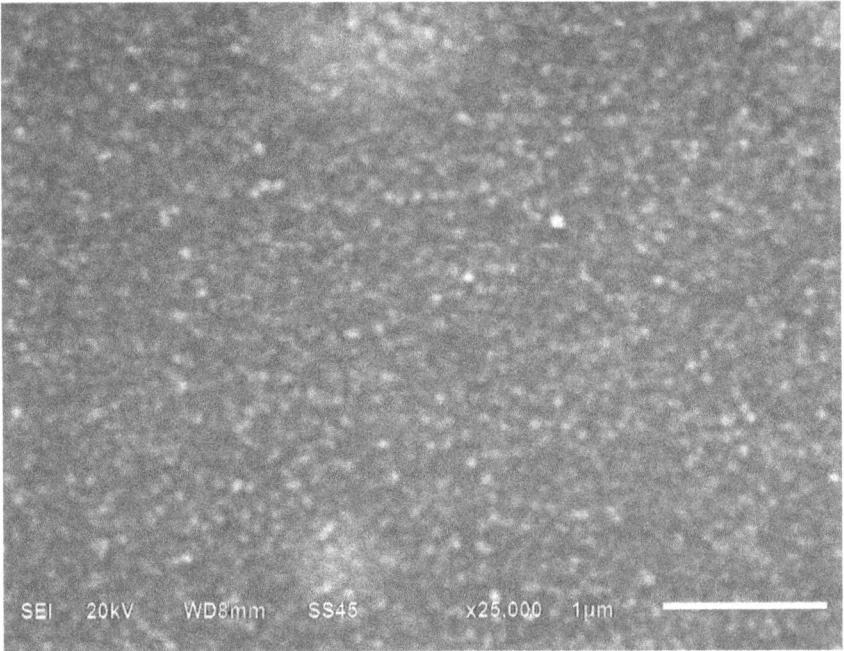

FIGURE 9.28   Image of Ti for cellulose nanofibril and nano-TiO$_2$ coating processes applied in stainless steel after second cleaning method for 100 cycles by SEM (magnification 25,000×) with SEI mode.

Source: Department of Science Service, Ministry of Higher Education, Science, Research and Innovation, Thailand [90]

observation of surface analysis by SEM (magnification 50×) with BEC model was used to observe the material after first and second cleaning methods for each cycle as shown in Figures 9.29 and 9.30, respectively. The result from Figure 9.29 shows that the appearance of the surface is not significantly different for each cycle. The result from Figure 9.30 shows that the appearances of the surface in Figure 9.30(d) and (f) are more significant than the black area, which are in agreement with the results of the EDS technique (see Figure 9.31). It was found that both graphs are the tendency of reduction as the cleaning cycles increase because of the limitation of SEM and EDS techniques for rough surfaces for this material. The average Ti amount for the second cleaning method is lower than the value of the first cleaning method because Sporeclear medical device disinfectant wipes may peel off some nano-TiO$_2$ on the material's surface. In addition, the material after second cleaning method for 100 cycles was tested in the microstructural observation by SEM (magnification 1000× and 5000×) and (magnification 20,000×) with SEI mode as seen in Figures 9.32 and 9.33, respectively. The appearances of images assume that many white particles may be nano-TiO$_2$ on the material surface, which are similar to the characteristic of GFRP coated 'Solid' in Figures 9.17 and 9.18. These results can confirm enough remaining nano-TiO$_2$ on this material surface. With the results described before, the adhesive

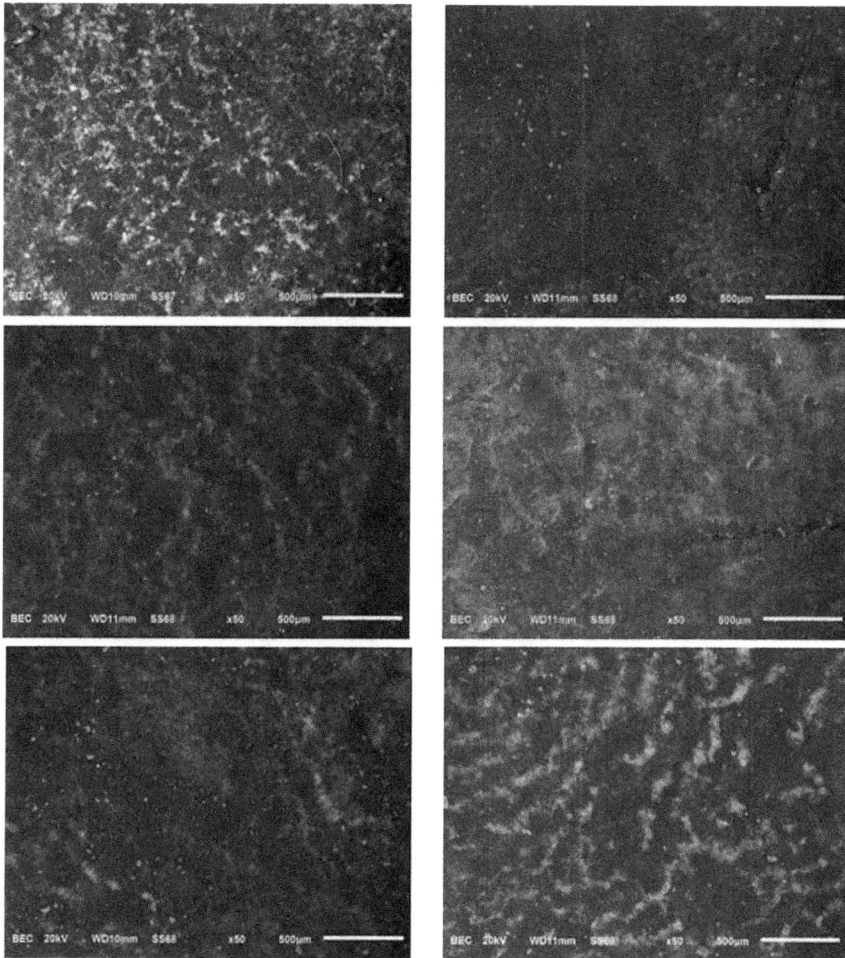

FIGURE 9.29 Images by SEM (magnification 50×) with BEC mode for cellulose nanofibril and nano-TiO$_2$ coating processes applied in PVC antistatic after first cleaning method for each cycle: (a) 0, (b) 20, (c) 40, (d) 60, (e) 80, and (f) 100.

Source: Department of Science Service, Ministry of Higher Education, Science, Research and Innovation, Thailand [90]

bonding efficiency for cellulose nanofibril and nano-TiO$_2$ coating processes applied in PVC antistatic is applicable for the ambulance interior.

9.6.3.5 Aluminum with Checker Plate

Finally, the material is aluminum with a checker plate applied with cellulose nano-fibril and nano-TiO$_2$ coating processes. The adhesive efficiency of nano-TiO$_2$ on the surface of this material was tested by the method described in Section 9.6.3. To begin with, the observation of surface analysis by SEM (magnification 50×) with BEC model was used to observe the material after first and second cleaning methods

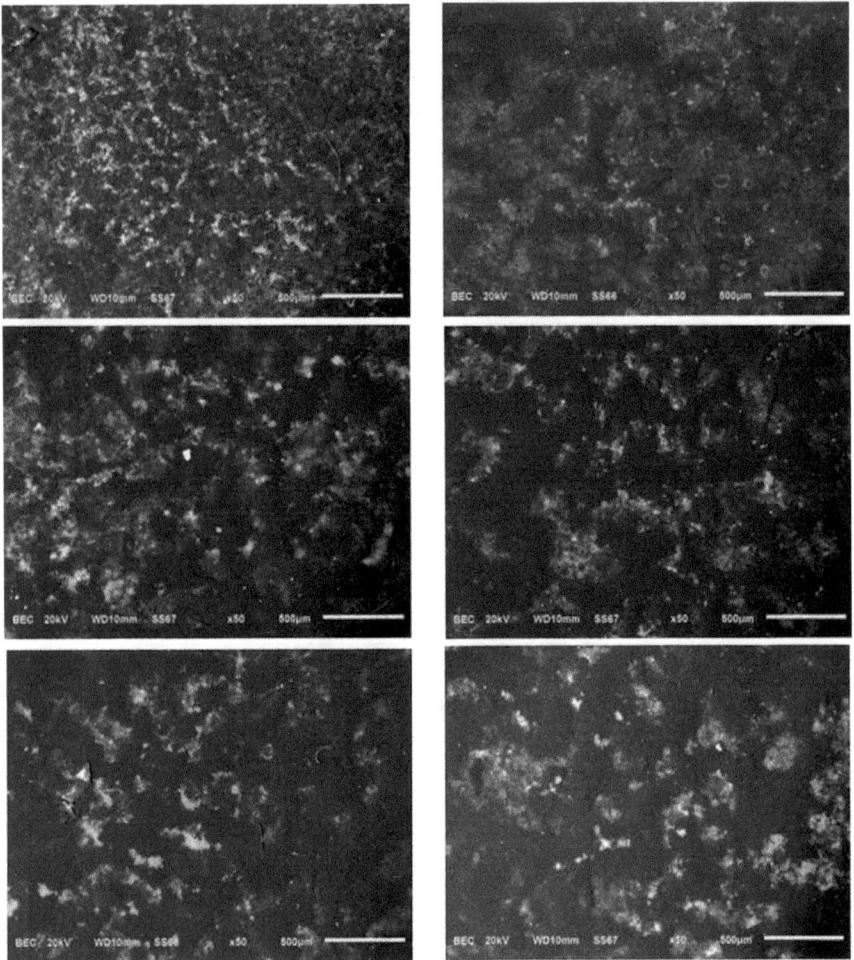

FIGURE 9.30   Images by SEM (magnification 50×) with BEC mode for cellulose nanofibril and nano-TiO$_2$ coating processes applied in PVC antistatic after second cleaning method for each cycle: (a) 0, (b) 20, (c) 40, (d) 60, (e) 80, and (f) 100.

Source: Department of Science Service, Ministry of Higher Education, Science, Research and Innovation, Thailand [90]

for each cycle as shown in Figures 9.34 and 9.35, respectively. It was found that the appearances of their samples were not a significant difference for either first or second cleaning methods with all cycles. SEM (magnification 50×) results with BEC mode agree with the Ti amount from the EDS technique, as seen in Figure 9.36. The graph shows that the average Ti amount for first cleaning method is not a significant difference for each cycle, while the average Ti amount for each cycle of second cleaning method is fluctuating, and it is lower than the average value of first cleaning method. It is assumed that Sporeclear medical device disinfectant wipes may peel off some nano-TiO$_2$ on the aluminum with checker plate. However, the average

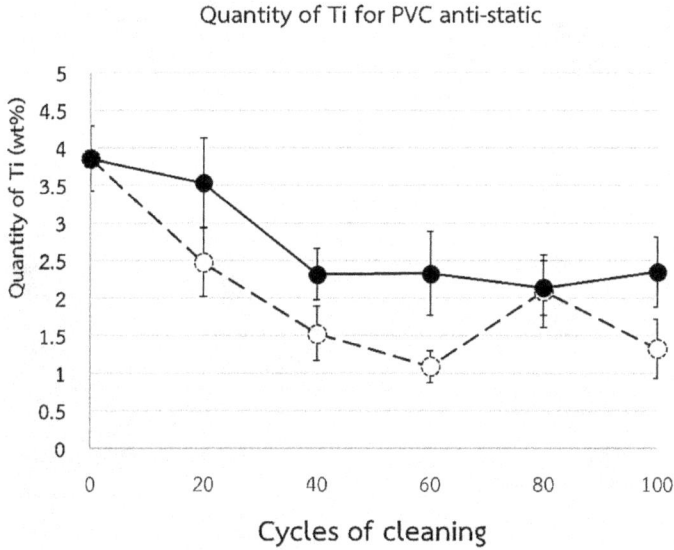

FIGURE 9.31   Graph shows the quantity of Ti for cellulose nanofibril and nano-TiO₂ coating processes applied in PVC antistatic after cleaning for each cycle: (●) first cleaning method, (○) second cleaning method.

Source: Department of Science Service, Ministry of Higher Education, Science, Research and Innovation, Thailand [90]

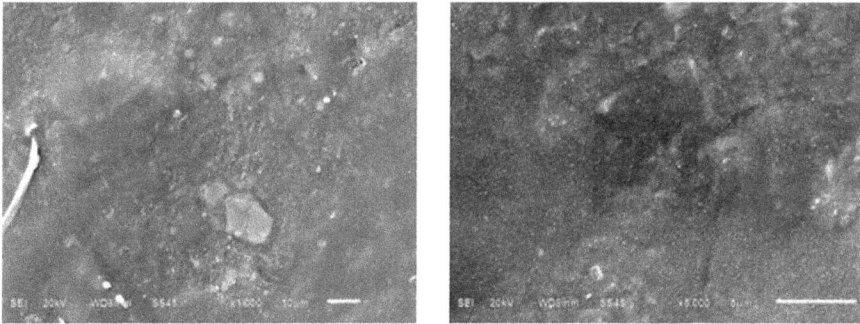

FIGURE 9.32   Images of cellulose nanofibril and nano-TiO₂ coating processes applied in PVC antistatic after second cleaning method for 100 cycles by SEM with SEI mode: (a) magnification 1000×, (b) magnification 5000×.

Source: Department of Science Service, Ministry of Higher Education, Science, Research and Innovation, Thailand [90]

values of Ti amount for both cleaning methods are not significantly different. The sample after second cleaning method for 100 cycles was tested in the microstructural observation by SEM (magnification 1000× and 5000×) and (magnification 25,000×) with SEI mode as seen in Figures 9.37 and 9.38, respectively. The images show many

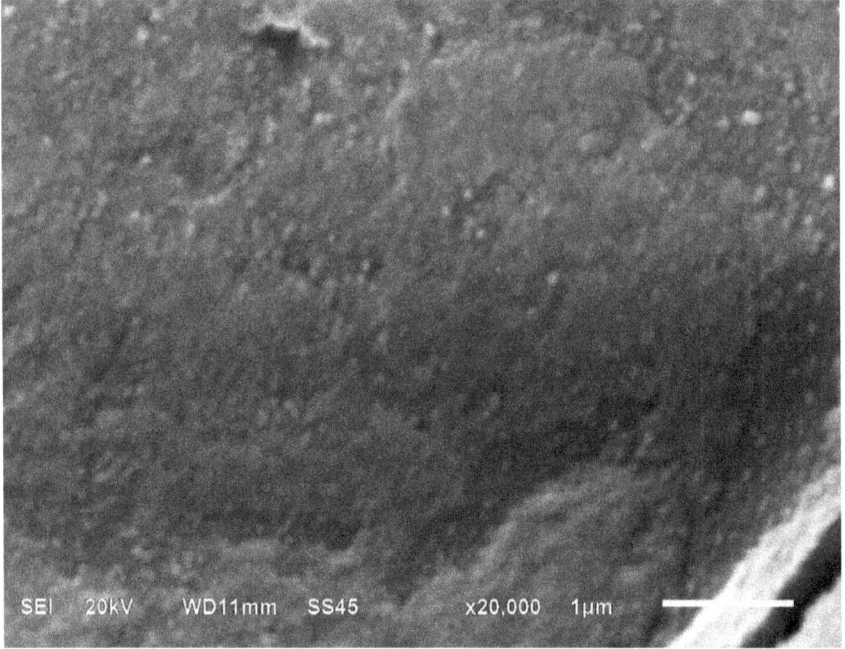

FIGURE 9.33 Image of Ti for cellulose nanofibril and nano-TiO$_2$ coating processes applied in PVC antistatic after second cleaning method for 100 cycles by SEM (magnification 20,000×) with SEI mode.

Source: Department of Science Service, Ministry of Higher Education, Science, Research and Innovation, Thailand [90]

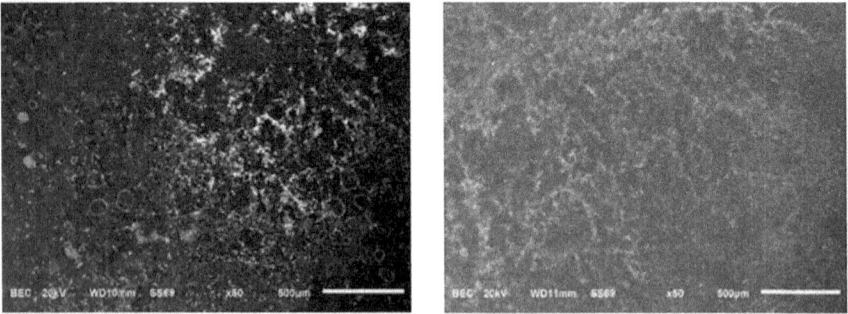

FIGURE 9.34 Images by SEM (magnification 50×) with BEC mode for cellulose nanofibril and nano-TiO$_2$ coating processes applied in aluminum with checker plate after first cleaning method for each cycle: (a) 0, (b) 20, (c) 40, (d) 60, (e) 80, and (f) 100.

Source: Department of Science Service, Ministry of Higher Education, Science, Research and Innovation, Thailand [90]

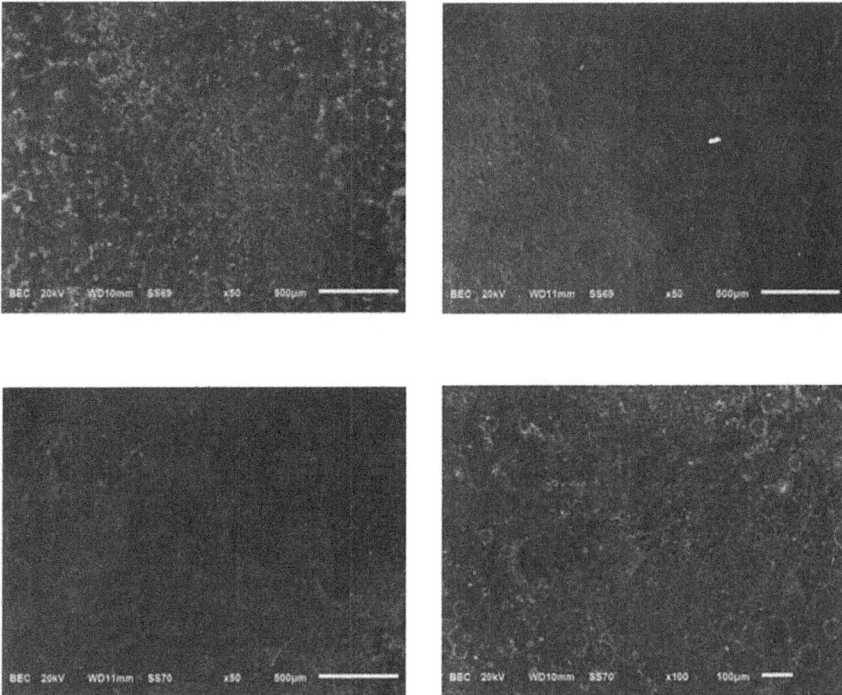

FIGURE 9.34 (Continued)

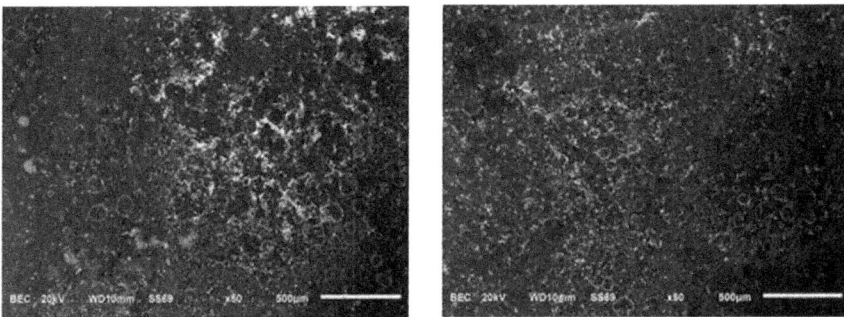

FIGURE 9.35 Images by SEM (magnification 50×) with BEC mode for cellulose nanofibril and nano-TiO$_2$ coating processes applied in aluminum with checker plate after second cleaning method for each cycle: (a) 0, (b) 20, (c) 40, (d) 60, (e) 80, and (f) 100.

Source: Department of Science Service, Ministry of Higher Education, Science, Research and Innovation, Thailand [90]

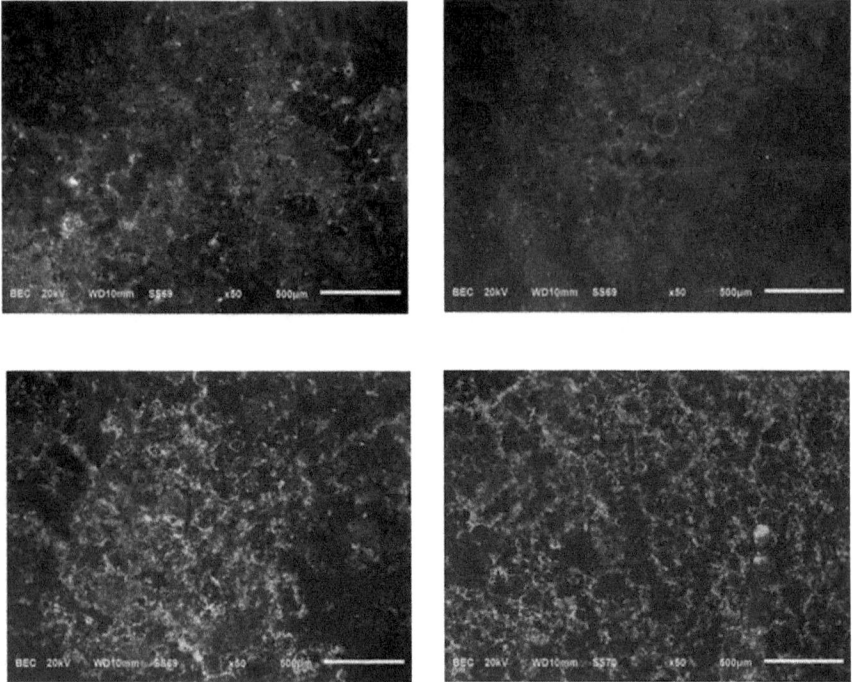

FIGURE 9.35 (Continued)

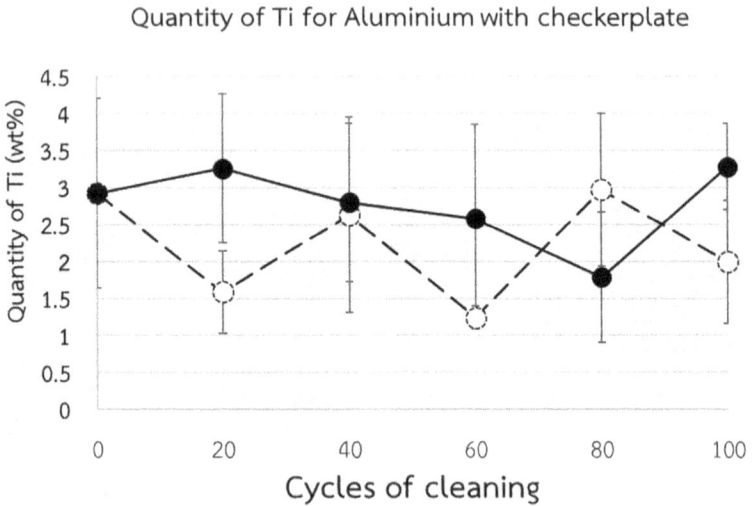

Quantity of Ti for Aluminium with checkerplate

FIGURE 9.36 Graph shows the quantity of Ti for cellulose nanofibril and nano-TiO$_2$ coating processes applied in aluminum with checker plate after cleaning for each cycle: (●) first cleaning method, (○) second cleaning method.

Source: Department of Science Service, Ministry of Higher Education, Science, Research and Innovation, Thailand [90]

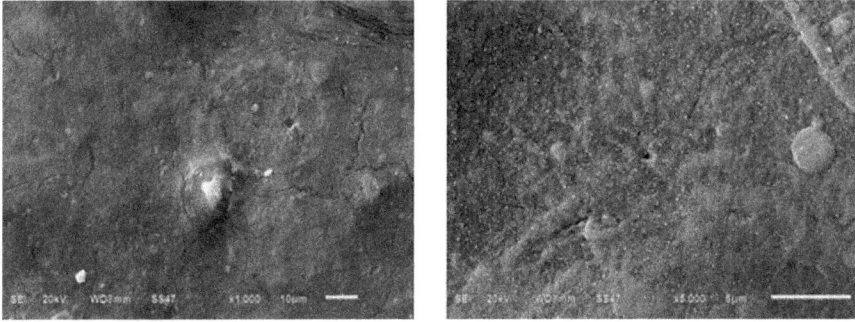

FIGURE 9.37 Images of cellulose nanofibril and nano-TiO₂ coating processes applied in aluminum with checker plate after second cleaning method for 100 cycles by SEM with SEI mode: (a) magnification 1000×, (b) magnification 5000×.

Source: Department of Science Service, Ministry of Higher Education, Science, Research and Innovation, Thailand [90]

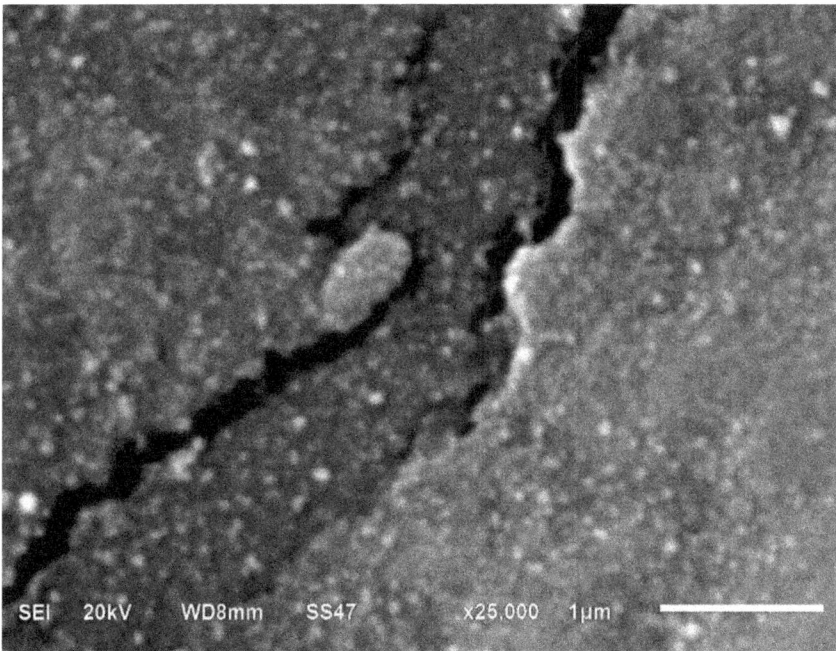

FIGURE 9.38 Image of Ti for cellulose nanofibril and nano-TiO₂ coating processes applied in aluminum with checker plate after second cleaning method for 100 cycles by SEM (magnification 25,000×) with SEI mode.

Source: Department of Science Service, Ministry of Higher Education, Science, Research and Innovation, Thailand [90]

white particles, assuming that they are nano-TiO$_2$ on the surface. These are similar to the characteristic of GFRP coated 'Solid' in Figures 9.17 and 9.18. It means that nano-TiO$_2$ remains enough on the surface of aluminum with a checker plate. For all these reasons, as explained before, the adhesive bonding efficiency for cellulose nanofibril and nano-TiO$_2$ coating processes applied in PVC antistatic is appropriate for the ambulance interior, especially in a part of the floor.

9.7 CONCLUSIONS

The critical characteristic of TiO$_2$ is the photocatalytic mechanism, which is the action of killing microorganisms and viruses: gram-negative bacteria, gram-positive bacteria, fungi, algae, protozoa, and viruses.

This chapter focused on the study in antimicrobial/antiviral nano-TiO$_2$ coatings for medical applications. Currently, nano-TiO$_2$ is widely used in several applications. From the size analysis by DSC, the average of nano-TiO$_2$ (PCO-001-IPC) was 37.30 ± 0.13 nm. Nano-TiO$_2$ was great the ability to kill microorganisms: *S. aureus* (ATCC 6538), *E. coli* (ATCC 8739), *E. coli* (ATCC 10536), *S. typhimurium* (ATCC 14028), *L. monocytogenes* (ATCC 15313), *K. pneumonia* (ATCC 4352), and *S. choleraesuis* (ATCC 10708). It was also good in the ability to kill viruses: H1N1 and Coxsackievirus. As coronavirus (COVID-19) pandemic, nano-TiO$_2$ significantly killed *Human coronavirus*, strain 229E, ATCC VR-740. The evaluation of acute oral toxicity on rats was a well-gained bodyweight. It appeared normal, and the assessment of skin sensitization on guinea pigs was not reactions in the negative control group.

In addition, the development of the coating process for nano-TiO$_2$ was studied for medical applications, especially in the ambulance interior materials. There were two crucial factors for the nano-TiO$_2$ coating process. Firstly, it was dispersion well for the nanoparticles on the surface of materials. Secondly, it was the efficiency of adhesive bonding on the surface of materials. The solution to these problems was used both the electrostatic sprayer technique and the cellulose nanofibril coating.

An example of the cellulose nanofibril and nano-TiO$_2$ coating processes was applied into the ambulance interior for five materials: GFRP coated 'Solid,' PVC, stainless steel, PVC antistatic, and aluminum with checker plate. An example of this application is an innovation of a pilot scale, leading to a manufacturing scale in Thailand. To evaluate dispersion and efficiency adhesion of nano-TiO$_2$ on their materials, SEM and EDS techniques were used for the surface analysis and the quantity of Ti, respectively. In addition, there were two cleaning methods for the evaluation of efficiency adhesive bonding property, that there were 0, 20, 40, 60, 80, and 100 cleaning cycles for each technique. The first cleaning method was as follows: washing with some deionized (DI) water, wiping with a cleaning cloth, and drying by blowing the air. The second cleaning method was as follows: washing with some deionized water, wiping by a cleaning cloth, wiping by Sporeclear medical device disinfectant wipes, and leaving for a minute before wiping again by a cleaning cloth. GFRP coated 'Solid' with the cellulose nanofibril, and nano-TiO$_2$ coating processes was a good dispersion of nano-TiO$_2$, and it was also a tremendous adhesive efficiency of nano-TiO$_2$ on its surface. Besides, other materials of this work were not significantly different results of dispersion and adhesion. Therefore, five materials were appropriate for the application of the ambulance interior. The scientific data of this work may be helpful for the protection of the coronavirus (COVID-19) pandemic, which is relevant to the ability to kill microorganisms and viruses by the nano-TiO$_2$ coating processes. This advanced processing material may be able to use in other medical devices, and it may be further studies in other applications.

Moreover, it is possible to do further research to develop a new technique coating for nanomaterials, which may be applied in deep technology. These studies will be helpful in various applications and industries, which may improve our quality of life in the near future. Last but not least, the author and our research teamwork are hopeful that our works in this study will be useful to protect the disinfection of COVID-19 for a medical person who is a dedication to the public, and it will also be helpful to inhibit COVID-19 pandemic for humankind.

ACKNOWLEDGMENTS

This work has been partially supported by the Department of Science Service (DSS), Ministry of Higher Education, Science, Research and Innovation, Thailand, and TKD Fiber Co., Ltd. (Carryboy), Thailand. I would like to say thank you for supporting scientific information by Infinite Purity Coating Co., Ltd. (Thailand) and Titanium World Technology Sdn Bhd (Malaysia). I would like to say thank you to my colleagues (Advanced Materials and Modern Ceramics group) who worked hard in this study.

REFERENCES

1. Samat, M.H., Ali, A.M.M., Taib, M.F.M., Hassan, O.H., and Yahya, M.Z.A. 2016. Hubbard U calculations on optical properties of 3d transition metal oxide TiO$_2$. *Results in Phys* 6:891–896. doi:10.1016/j.rinp.2016.11.006.
2. Foster, H.A., Ditta, I.B., Varghese, S., and Steele, A. 2011. Mini review – photocatalytic disinfection using titanium dioxide: Spectrum and mechanism of antimicrobial activity. *Appl Microbiol Biotechnol* 90:1847–1868.
3. Wójcik, E.B., Szwajgier, D., Oleszczuk, P., and Mieczan, A.W. 2020. Effects of titanium dioxide nanoparticles exposure on human health—a review. *Biol Trace Elem Res* 193:118–129
4. Ben, M. 2007. *Wikimedia Commons File: Rutile-Unit-Cell-3D-Balls.png.* https://commons.wikimedia.org/wiki/File:Rutile-unit-cell-3D-balls.png (By Ben Mills-Own work, Public Domain, https://commons.wikimedia.org/w/index.php?curid=2036065) (accessed October 16, 2020).
5. Benjah, B. 2007. *Wikimedia Commons File: Anatase-Unit-Cell-3D-Balls.png.* https://commons.wikimedia.org/wiki/File:Anatase-unit-cell-3D-balls.png (accessed October 16, 2020).
6. Krizu. 2012. *Wikimedia Commons File: Brookite Axis.png.* https://commons.wikimedia.org/wiki/File:Brookite_axis.png.
7. Harper, J.C., Christensen, P.A., and Egerton, T.A. 2000. Effect of catalyst type on the kinetics of photoelectrical disinfection of water inoculated with *E. coli. J Appl Electrochem* 31:623–628.

8. Tatsuma, T., Takeda, S., Saitoh, S., Ohko, Y., and Fujishima, A. 2003. Bactericidal effect of an energy storage TiO_2-WO_3 photocatalyst in dark. *Electrochem Commun* 5(9):793–796. doi:10.1016/j.elcom.2003.07.003.

9. Butterfield, I.M., Christensen, P.A., Curtis, T.P., and Gunlazuardi. 1997. Water disinfection using an immobilised titanium dioxide film in a photochemical reactor with electric field enhancement. *Wat Res* 31(3):675–677.

10. Kikuchi, Y., Sunada, K., Iyoda, T., Hashimoto, K., and Fujishima, A. 1997. Photocatalytic bactericidal effect of TiO_2 thin films: Dynamic view of the active oxygen species responsible for the effect. *J Photochem Photobiol A* 106(1–3):51–56.

11. Sunada, K., Watanabe, T., and Hashimoto, K. 2003. Studies on photokilling of bacteria on TiO_2 thin film. *J Photochem Photobiol A* 156(1–3):227–223. Doi:10.1016/s1010-6030(02)00434-3

12. Sökmen, M., Candan, F., and Sümer, Z. 2001. Disinfection of *E. Coli* by the Ag-TiO_2 system: Lipid peroxidation. *J Photochem Photobiol A* 143(2–3):241–244.

13. Ryu, H., Gerrity, Crittenden, J.C., and Abbaszadegam, M. 2008. Photocatalytic inactivation of Cryptosporidium parvum with TiO_2 and low-pressure ultraviolet irradiation. *Wat Res* 42(6–7):1523–1530. doi:10.1016/j.watres.2007.10.037.

14. Yu, J.C., Tang, H.Y., Yu, J.G., Chan, H.C., Zhang, L.Z., Xie, Y.D., Wang, H., and Wong, S.P. 2002. Bactericidal and photocatalytic activities of TiO_2 thin film prepared by sol-gel and reverse micelle method. *J Photochem Photobiol A* 153(1–3):211–219.

15. Dunlop, P.S.M., Byme, J.A., Manga, N., and Enggins, B.R. 2002. The photocatalytic removal of bacterial pollutants from drinking water. *J Photochem Photobiol A* 148(1–3):355–363.

16. Liu, H.L., and Yang, T.C.K. 2003. Photocatalytic inactivation of *Escherichia coli* and *Lactobaccillus helveticus* by ZnO and TiO_2 activated with ultraviolet light. *Proc Biochem* 39(4):475–481. doi:10.1016/s0032-9592(03)00084-0.

17. Sato, T., Koizumi, Y., and Taya, M. 2003. Photocatalytic deactivation of airborne microbial cells on TiO_2-loaded plate. *Biochem Eng J* 14(2):149–152.

18. Choi, Y.L., Kim, S.H., Song, Y.S., and Lee, D.Y. 2004. Photodecomposition and bactericidal effects of TiO_2 thin films prepared by a magnetron sputtering. *J Matter Sci* 39(18):5695–5699.

19. Pal, A., Pehkonen, S.O., Yu, L.E., and Ray, M.B. 2008. Photocatalytic inactivation of airborne bacteria in a continuous-flow reaction. *Ind Eng Chen Res* 47(20):7580–7585. doi:10.1021/ie701739g.

20. Dunlop, P.S.M., Sheeran, C.P., Byrne, J.A., McMahon, M.A.S., Boyle, M.A., and McGuigan, K.G. 2010. Inactivation of clinically relevant pathogens by photocatalytic coatings. *J Photochem Photobiol A* 216:30–310.

21. Watts, R.J., Kong, S., Orr, M.P., Miller, G.C., and Henry, B.E. 1995. Photocatalytic inactivation of coliform bacteria and viruses in secondary wastewater effluent. *Wat Res* 29(1):95–100.

22. Kim, B., Kim, D., Cho, D., and Cho, S. 2003. Bactericidal effect of TiO_2 photocatalyst on selected food-borne pathogenic bacteria. *Chemosphere* 52(1):277–281. doi:10.1016/s0045-6535(03)00051-1.

23. Muszkat, L., Feigelson, L., Bir, L., Muszkat, K.A., Teitel, M., Dornay, I., Kirchner, B., and Kritzman, G. 2005. Solar photo – inactivation of photopathogens by trace level hydrogen peroxide and titanium dioxide photocatalysis. *Phytoparasitica* 33(3):267–274.

24. Kim, S.C., and Lee, D.K. 2005. Inactivation of algo blooms in eutrophic water of drinking water supplies with the photocatalysis of TiO_2 thin film on hollow glass beads. *Wat Sci Technol* 52(9):145–152.

25. Sawada, D., Ohmasa, M., Fukuda, M., Masuno, K., Koide, H., Tsunoda, S., and Nakamura, K. 2005. Disinfection of some pathogens of mushroom cultivation by photocatalytic treatment. *Mycosci* 46(1):54–60.

26. Kashyout, A.B., Soliman, M., and El-Haleem, D.A. 2006. Disinfection of bacterial suspensions by photocatalytic oxidation using TiO$_2$ nanoparticles under ultraviolet illumination. *AEJ – Alexandria Eng J* 45(3):367–371.

27. Yao, K.S., Wang, D.Y., Chang, C.Y., Weng, K.W., Yang, L.Y., Lee, S.J., Cheng, T.C., and Hwang, C.C. 2007a. Photocatalytic disinfection of phytopathogenic bacteria by dye-sensitized TiO$_2$ thin film activated by visible light. *Surf Coat Technol* 202(4–7):1329–1332. doi:10.1016/j.surfcoat.2007.07.102.

28. Cheng, Y.W., Chan, R.C.Y., and Wong, P.K. 2007. Disinfection of *Legionella pneumophila* by photocatalytic oxidation. *Wat Res* 41(4):842–852. doi:10.1016/j.watres.2006.11.033

29. Tsuang, Y.H., Sun, J.S., Huang, Y.C., Lu, C.H., Chang, W.H.S., and Wang, C.C. 2008. Studies of photokilling of bacteria using titanium dioxide nanoparticles. *Artific Organs* 32(2):167–174. doi:10.1111/j.1525-1594.2007.00530.x.

30. Cohen-Yaniv, V., Narkis, N., and Armon, R. 2008. Photocatalytic inactivation of Flavobacterium and *E. coli* in water by a continuous stirred tank reactor (CSTR) fed with suspended/immobilised TiO$_2$ medium. *Wat Sci Technol* 58(1):247–252. doi:10.2166/wst.2008.664

31. Luo, L., Miao, L., Tanemura, S., and Tanemura, M. 2008. Photocatalytic sterilization of TiO$_2$ films coated on Al fiber. *Mater Sci Eng B* 148(1–3):183–186.

32. Cheng, C.L., Sun, D.S., Chu, W.C., Tseng, Y.H., Ho, H.C., Wang, J.B., Chung, P.H., Chen, J.H., Tsai, P.J., Lin, N.T., Yu, M.S., and Chang, H.H. 2009. The effects of the bacterial interaction with visible-light responsive titania photocatalyst on the bactericidal performance. *J Biomed Sci* 16(7):10.

33. Erkan, A., Bakir, U., and Karakas, G. 2006. Photocatalytic microbial inactivation over Pd doped SnO$_2$ and TiO$_2$ thin films. *J Photochem Photobiol A* 184(3):313–321. doi:10.1016/j.photochem.2006.05.001.

34. Pal, A., Mint, X., Yu, L.E., Pehkonen, S.O., and Ray, M.B. 2005. Photocatalytic inactivation of bioaerosols by TiO$_2$ coated membrane. *Int J Chem React Eng* 3:14.

35. Pal, A., Pehkonen, S.O., Yu, L.E., and Ray, M.B. 2007. Photocatalytic inactivation of Gram-positive and Gram-negative bacteria using fluorescent light. *J Photochem Photobiol A* 186(2–3): 335–341. Doi:10.1016/j.jphotochem.2006.09.002

36. Hu, C., Guo, J., Qu, J., and Hu, X. 2007. Photocatalytic degradation of pathogenic bacteria with AgI/Tio$_2$ under visible light irradiation. *Langmuir* 23(9):4982–4987.

37. Sheel, D.W,. Brook, L.A., Ditta, I.B., Evans, P., Foster, H.A., Steele, A., and Yates, H.M. 2008. Biocidal silver and silver/titania composite films grown by chemical vapour deposition. *Int J Photoenergy*. Article ID 168185, 11 pp. Doi:10.1155/2008/168185

38. Skorb, E.V., Antonouskaya, L.I., Belyasova, N.A., Shchukin, D.G., Möhwald, H., and Sviridov, D.V. 2008. Antibacterial activity of thin film photocatalysts based on metal-modified TiO$_2$ and TiO$_2$:In$_2$O$_3$ nanocomposite. *Appl Catal B* 84(1–2):94–99.

39. Matsunaga, T., Tomoda, R., Nakajima, T., and Wake, H. 1985. Photoelectrochemical sterilization of microbial cells by semiconductor powders. *FEMS Microbiol Lett* 29(1–2):211–214.

40. Kakita, Y., Kashige, N., Miake, F., and Watanabe, K. 1997. Photocatalysis dependent inactivation of Lactobacillus phage PL-1 by a ceramics preparation. *Biosci Biotechnol Biochem* 61(11):1947–1948.

41. Kakita, Y., Obuchi, E., Nakano, K., Murata, K., Kuroiwa, A., Miake, F., and Watanabe, K. 2000. Photocatalytic inactivation of Lactobacillus PL-1 phages by a thin film of titania. *Biocontrol Sci* 5(2):73–79.

42. Kashige, N., Kakita, Y., Nakashima, Y., Miake, F., and Watanabe, K. 2001. Mechanism of the photocatalytic inactivation of *Lactobacillus casei* phage PL-1 by titania thin film. *Curr Microbiol* 42(3):184–189.

43. Choi, J.Y., Kim, K.H., Choy, K.C., Oh, K.T., and Kim, K.N. 2007a. Photocatalytic antibacterial effect of TiO$_2$ film formed on Ti and TiAg exposed to *Lactobacillus acidophilus*. *J Biomedl Mater Res B* 80(2):353–359.

44. Cho, M., Choi, Y., Park, H., Kim, K., Woo, G.J., and Park, J. 2007a. Titanium dioxide/UV photocatalytic disinfection in fresh carrots. *J Food Prot* 70(1):97–101.

45. Chen, W.J., Tsai, P.J., and Chen, Y.C. 2008. Functional Fe$_3$O$_4$/TiO$_2$ core/shell magnetic nanoparticles as photokilling agents for pathogenic bacteria. *Small* 4(4):485–491.

46. Shiraishi, F., Toyoda, K., Fukinbara, S., Obushi, E., and Nakano, K. 1999. Photolytic and photocatalytic treatment of an aqueous solution containing microbial cells and organic compounds in an annular flow reactor. *Chem Eng Sci* 54(10):1547–1552.

47. Kozlova, E.A., Safatov, A.S., Kiselev, S.A., Marchenko, V.Y., Sergeev, A.A., Skarnovich, M.O., Emelyanova, E.K., Smetannikova, M.A., Buryak, G.A., and Vorontsov, A.V. 2010. Inactivation and mineralization of aerosol deposited model pathogenic microorganisms over TiO$_2$ and Pt/TiO$_2$. *Environ Sci Technol* 44(13):5121–5126.

48. Suketa, N., Sawase, T., Kitaura, H., Naito, M., Baba, K., Nakayama, K., Wennerberg, A., and Atsuta, M. 2005. An antibacterial surface on dental implants, based on the photocatalytic bactericidal effect. *Clin Implant Dent Relat Res* 7(2):105–111.

49. Cheng, T.C., Chang, C.Y., Chang, C.l., Hwang, C.J., Hsu, H.C., Wang, D.Y., and Yao, K.S. 2008. Photocatalytic bactericidal effect of TiO$_2$ film on fish pathogens. *Surf Coat Technol* 203(5–7):925–925. doi:10.1016/j.surfcoat.2008.08.022

50. Nagame, S., Oku, T., Kambara, M., and Konishi, K. 1989. Antibacterial effect of the powdered semiconductor TiO$_2$ on the viability of oral microorganisms. *J Dent Res* 68(special issue):1697–1698.

51. Kühn, K.P., Chaberny, I.F., Massholder, K., Stickler, M., Benz, V.W., Sonntag, H.G., and Erdinger, L. 2003. Disinfection of surfaces by photocatalytic oxidation with titanium dioxide and UVA light. *Chemosphere* 53(1):71–77.

52. Maneerat, C., and Hayata, Y. 2006. Antifungal activity of TiO$_2$ photocatalysis against *Penicillium expansum* in vitro and in fruit tests. *Int J Food Microbiol* 107(2):99–103. doi:10.1016/j.ijfoodmicro.2005.08.018.

53. Koide, S., and Nonami, T. 2007. Disinfection efficacy of a plastic container covered with photocatalyst for postharvest. *Food Control* 18(1):1–4. doi:10.1016/j.foodcont.2005.08.001.

54. Veselá, M., Veselý, M., Chomoucká, J., and Lipenská, M. 2008. Photocatalytic disinfection of water using Ag/TiO$_2$. *Chem Listy 102* (special issue)(15):s507–s508.

55. Giannantonio, D.J., Kurth, J.C., Kurtis, K.E., Sobecky, P.A. 2009. Effects of concrete properties and nutrients on fungal colonization and fouling. *Int Biodegrad* 63(3):252–259. doi:10.1016/j.ibiod.2008.10.002.

56. Linkous, C.A., Carter, G.J., Locuson, D.V., Ouellete, A.J., Slattery, D.K., Smith, L.A. 2000. Photocatalytic inhibition of algae growth using TiO$_2$, WO$_3$ and cocatalyst modifications. *Environ Sci Technol* 34(22):4754–4758.

57. Peller, J.R., Whitman, R.L., Griffith, S., Harris, P., Peller, C., and Scalzitti, J. 2007. TiO$_2$ as a photocatalyst for control of the aquatic invasive alga, Cladophora, under natural and artificial light. *J Photochem Photobiol A* 186(2–3):212–217.

58. Lonnen, J., Kilvington, S., Kehoe, S.C., Al-Touati, F., McGuigan, K.G. 2005. Solar and photocatalytic disinfection of protozoan, fungal and bacterial microbes in drinking water. *Wat Res* 39(5):877–883. doi:10.1016/j.waters.2004.11.023.

59. Peng, L., Wenli, D., Qisui, W., and Xi, L. 2010. The envelope damage of Tetrahymena in the presence of TiO$_2$ combined with UV light. *Photochem Photobiol* 86(3):633–638.

60. Navalon, S., Alvaro, M., Garcia, H., Escrig, D., and Costa, V. 2009. Photocatalytic water disinfection of Cryptosporidium parvum and Giardia lamblia using a fibrous ceramic TiO$_2$ photocatalyst. *Wat Sci Technol* 59:639–645.

61. Sjogren, J.C., and Sierka, R.A. 1994. Inactivation of phage MS2 by iron aided titanium dioxide photocatalysis. *Appl Environ Microbiol* 60(1):344–347.

62. Lee, S., Nishida, K., Otaki, M., and Ohgaki, S. 1997. Photocatalytic inactivation of phage Qb By immobilized titanium dioxide mediated photocatalyst. *Wat Sci Technol* 35:101–106.
63. Belhácová, L., Krýsa, J., Geryk, J., and Jirkovský, J. 1999. Inactivation of microorganisms in a flow-through photoreactor with an immobilized TiO$_2$ layer. *J Chem Technol Biotechnol* 74(2):149–154.
64. Otaki, M., Hirata, T., and Ohgaki, S. 2000. Aqueous microorganisms inactivation by photocatalytic reaction. *Wat Sci Technol* 42(3–4):103–108.
65. Greist, H.T., Hingorani, S.K., Kelly, K., and Goswami, D.Y. 2002. *Using scanning electron microscopy to visualize photocatalytic mineralization of airborne microorganisms.* Proceedings of the 9th International Conference on Indoor Air Quality and Climate, 712–717, Monterey, CA, July.
66. Guimaráes, J.R., and Barretto, A.S. 2003. Photocatalytic inactivation of *Clostridium perfringens* and coliphages in water. *Braz J Chem Eng* 20(4):403–411.
67. Cho, M., Chung, H., Choi, W., and Yoon, J. 2004. Linear correlation between inactivation of *E. coli* and OH radical concentration in TiO$_2$ photocatalytic disinfection. *Wat Res* 38(4):1069–1077.
68. Cho, M., Chung, H., Choi, W., and Yoon, J. 2005. Different inactivation behaviors of ms-2 phage and *Escherichia coli* in TiO$_2$ photocatalytic disinfection. *Appl Environ Microbiol* 7(1):270–275.
69. Sato, T., and Taya, M. 2006a. Enhancement of phage inactivation using photocatalytic titanium dioxide particles with different crystalline structures. *Biochem Eng J* 28(3):303–308.
70. Sato, T., and Taya, M. 2006b. Kinetic consideration of the effect of organic impurities on photocatalytic phage inactivation with TiO$_2$. *Kagaku Kogaku Ronbunshu* 32(3):288–292.
71. Vohra, A., Goswami, D.Y., Deshpande, D.A., and Block, S.S. 2006. Enhanced photocatalytic disinfection of indoor air. *Appl Catal B* 64(1–2):57–65. doi:10.1016/j.apcatb.2005.10.025.
72. Gerrity, D., Ryu, H., Crittenden, J., and Abbaszadegan, M. 2008. Photocatalytic inactivation of viruses using titanium dioxide nanoparticles and low-pressure UV light. *J Environ Sci Health A* 43(11):1261–1270.
73. Ditta, I.B., Steele, A., Liptrot, C., Tobin, J., Tyler, H., Yates, H.M., Sheel, D.W., and Foster, H.A. 2008. Photocatalytic antimicrobial activity of thin surface films of TiO$_2$, CuO and TiO$_2$/CuO dual layers on *Escherichia coli* and bacteriophage T4. *Appl Microbiol Biotechnol* 79(1):127–133. doi:10.1007/s00253-008-1411-8.
74. Yu, K.P., Lee, G.W.M., Lin, Z.Y., and Huang, C.P. 2008. Removal of bioaerosols by the combination of a photocatalytic filter and negative air irons. *J Aersol Sci* 39(5):377–392. doi:10.1016/j.jaerosci.2007.12.005.
75. Guillard, C., Bui, T.H., Felix, C., Moules, V., Lina, B., and Lejeune, P. 2008. Microbiological disinfection of water and air by photocatalysis. *CR Chim* 11(1–2): 107–113. doi:10.1016/j.crci.2007.06.007.
76. Han, W., Zhang, P.H., Cao, W.C., Yang, D.L., Taira, S., Okamoto, Y., Arai, J.I., and Yan, X.Y. 2004. The inactivation effect of photocatalytic titanium apatite filter on SARS virus. *Prog Biochem Biophys* 31(11):982–985.
77. Kato, T., Tohma, H., Miki, O., Shibata, T., and Tamura, M. 2005. Degradation of norovirus in sewage treatment water by photocatalytic ultraviolet disinfection. *Nippon Steel Tech Rep* 92:41–44.
78. Lin, Z.X., Li, Z.H., Wang, X.X., Fu, X.Z., Yang, G.Q., Lin, H.X., and Meng, C. 2006. Inactivation efficiency of TiO$_2$ on H1N1 influenza virus. *Gaodeng Xuexiao Huaxue Xuebao Chem J Chin Univ* 27(4):721–725.
79. Zan, L., Fa, W., Peng, T., and Gong, Z.K. 2007. Photocatalysis effect of nanometer TiO$_2$ and TiO$_2$-coated ceramic plate on hepatitis B virus. *J Photochem Photobiol B* 86(2):165–169. doi:10.1016/j.jphotobiol.2006.09.002.

80. AOAC OFFICIAL METHOD OF ANALYSIS 2016. *AOAC Official Methods 961.02.*
81. National Nanotechnology Center (NANOTEC), NSTDA, Thailand. 2020. Test Report No. NCH-PO556/DL63-304.
82. SGS (Thailand) Limited. 2016. Test Report No. 3223961.
83. Intertex Testing Service Hong Kong Ltd. 2017. Test Report No. HKGH0211938702.
84. Faculty of Medical Technology, Mahidol University. 2020. Test Report No. 2563-01-037.
85. Microbac Laboratories Inc, USA. 2018. Project No. 975-101.
86. Viroxy lab, Malaysia. 2020. Test Report No. VX-62-20-2020.
87. ESS. 2015a. *ESS Apple Duster – Science of Electrostatic Spraying.* www.youtube.com/watch?v=jPliFIgEWYU (accessed September 10, 2020).
88. ESS. 2015b. *TC-320 Electrostatic Sprayer System with Induction Charging Nozzle Technology.* https://dokumen.tips/documents/microbecide-tc-320-electrostatic-spraying-systems-ess-microbecide.html.
89. Department of Science Service, Ministry of Higher Education, Science, Research and Innovation, Thailand. 2018. Test Report no. L61/04866.1.
90. Department of Science Service, Ministry of Higher Education, Science, Research and Innovation, Thailand. 2020. Test Report no. L62/06274.1

10 Conducting Polymer Soft Actuators and Their Applications

M. Fuchiwaki

CONTENTS

10.1   INTRODUCTION: SOFT ACTUATORS BASED ON CONDUCTING POLYMERS

Scientists and engineers work diligently to produce zoomorphic and biomimetic robots with similar movements to those created by natural muscles. Toward that end, conducting polymers and electrochemically active materials currently constitute the foundation of promising polymeric sensing motors designed for use in zoomorphic and biomimetic robots [1–10]. In particular, artificial muscles or soft actuators based on conducting polymers have attracted significant attention in recent years.

Conducting polymers are applied in semiconductor devices, such as photovoltaic cells, luminescent diodes, transistors, and metallic conductors. The most significant characteristic of conducting polymers is their drastic enhancement of electroconductivity upon oxidation and reduction. Furthermore, conducting polymers can display changeable physical attributes such as expanding or shrinking [11]. These dimensional changes are produced by electrochemical oxidization and contraction that is called electrochemomechanical deformation (ECMD), which is

DOI: 10.1201/9781003143093-10

the property that makes it possible to use conducting polymers as artificial muscles and soft actuators [12–13)].

In artificial muscles or soft actuators based on conducting polymers, the oxidation and reduction of the conducting polymers drive an exchange of ions and solvent with the electrolyte, thus causing reversible volume variations. Consequently, they are reliable Faradaic motors because the actuation rate is a linear function of the reaction-driving current and the bending actuation amplitude under the consumed charge's linear control [14–17]. In other words, electrochemomechanical artificial muscles are polymeric motors driven by reversible electrochemical reactions generating reversible volume variations. A few millivolts of positive or negative potential increments can reverse both actuation and driving responses in operation. Moreover, artificial muscles or soft actuators based on conducting polymers are fabricated into thin-film forms that are small and lightweight, which means they can be driven with high response and have high levels of flexibility and durability, all of which are beneficial properties for actuators.

Several researchers have already reported on the development of artificial muscles or soft actuators based on conducting polymers such as polyaniline (PAn) [18–19], poly(o-methoxyaniline) (PmAn) [20–21], poly(3-alkylthiophene)s [22], and polypyrroles (PPy) [23]. Of these, ECMD-based artificial muscles or soft actuators fabricated from freestanding PPy films and constructed from the high-quality film have garnered particularly high levels of attention [24–27] because they can easily be obtained via electrodeposition and because the electrochemical activity of PPy films is broad from pH 3 to 10 [23].

Dimensional variations are induced by the ECMD electrochemical cycle (oxidation and reduction), two actuation modes: anion drive and cation drive. The electrochemical oxidation process is accompanied by anions from the electrolyte solution, which causes the expansion of conducting polymers by the volume of total inserted anions. In contrast, the electrochemical reduction process is accompanied by the expulsion of anions to the electrolyte solution, thereby resulting in the contraction of conducting polymers by the volume of total extracted anions, as shown in Figure 10.1.

In the case of a straight film of conducting polymer (anion drive actuation) attached with insulating tape in sodium chloride (NaCl) electrolyte solution, as shown in Figure 10.2, the soft actuator shows counterclockwise angular displacement during oxidation. In other words, the entrance of anions and water causes oxidation that swells the conducting polymer film. In contrast, the soft actuator shows clockwise angular displacement during reduction, which means the expulsion of anions and water causes the conducting polymer film to shrink. In cases of cation drive actuation, the soft actuator undergoes similar clockwise and counterclockwise angular displacements in reduction and oxidation, respectively, due to entrance and expulsion of cations and water. These actions result in bending movements of the linear conducting polymer soft actuator.

To make a sizeable bending movement, an asymmetric bilayer conducting polymer soft actuator consisting of anion-driven (right side) and cation-driven (left side) films [28–29] has been proposed, as shown in Figure 10.3. Here, the bilayer conducting polymer soft actuator performs a clockwise bending movement during oxidation. The anion-driven film swells due to the update of anions and water, and the

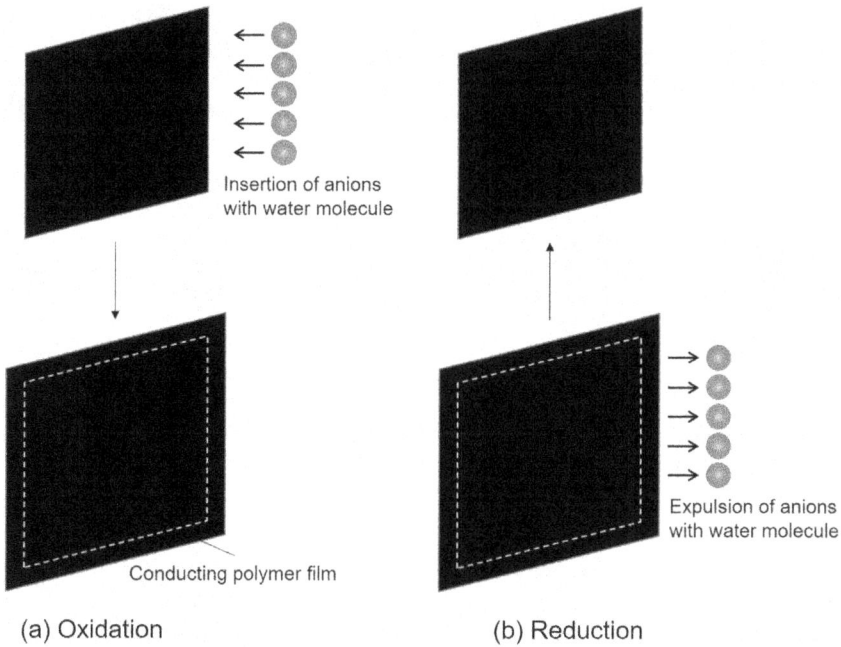

(a) Oxidation   (b) Reduction

FIGURE 10.1   Electrochemomechanical deformation of conducting polymer film.

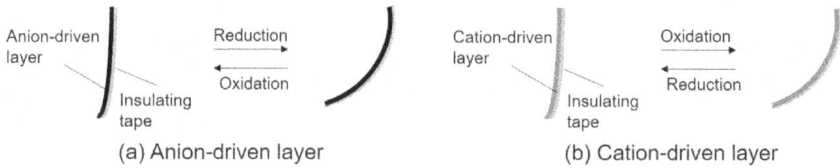

(a) Anion-driven layer   (b) Cation-driven layer

FIGURE 10.2   Electrochemomechanical deformation of a straight film of conducting polymer.

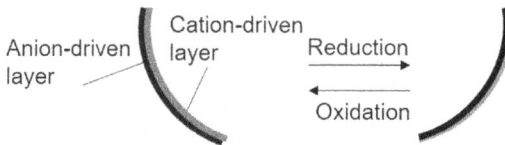

FIGURE 10.3   Electrochemomechanical deformation of an asymmetric bilayer conducting polymer soft actuator.

action-driven film shrinks due to the expulsion of cations and water. During the bilayer operation, the conducting polymer soft actuator performs a counterclockwise bending movement during a reduction. The anion-driven film shrinks due to the expulsion of anions and water, and the action-driven film expands due to the entrance of cations and water. In this case, the amplitude of the described movement is now a few times over that of the conducting polymer soft actuator attached with insulating tape in the same electrolyte solution.

An electrodeposition method and an evaluation method for the proposed conducting polymer soft actuator are introduced in the following sections. Additionally, a related mechanical application in which the conducting polymer soft actuators drive micropumps is described.

10.2   EXPERIMENTAL SETUP

The electrochemical experiments discussed in this chapter were carried out in a three-electrode electrochemical cell with a potentiostat-galvanostat, controlled via a personal computer (PC) [30–34]. A Julabo F25 cryostat (±0.1 °C) was used to provide temperature control. And a Metrohm Ag/AgCl (3 M KCl) is used as a reference electrode. Hence, every potential mentioned in this work is given about this electrode.

Pyrrole (PPy) was purified by distillation under vacuum using a diaphragm vacuum pump (MZ 2C, SCHOTT) and stored at −15 °C. Sodium chloride (NaCl, Panreac), sodium bromide (NaBr, Sigma-Aldrich), lithium bisimide (LiTFSI, Wako Pure Chemical Industries), paraphenolsulfonic (4-hydroxybenzenesulfonic) acid (HpPS) solution (Sigma-Aldrich), tetra-*n*-butylammonium bis (trifluoromethane sulfonyl), imide (TBATFSI, Tomiyama pure chemical industries), and dodecylbenzene sulfonic acid dissolved at 70 wt.% in isopropanol (DBSA, Sigma-Aldrich) were used as received. Ultrapure water was also used.

10.3   PREPARATION OF ANION-DRIVEN CONDUCTING POLYMER SOFT ACTUATOR

The anion-driven conducting polymer soft actuators (PPy.HpPS) were electrogenerated from 0.2 M PPy and 0.05 M paraphenolsulfonic acid (HpPS) aqueous solutions (50 ml). The stainless (SUS) plates were used as the working electrodes, and a constant current (0.5 mA/cm) was applied to the active electrodes for 1 h at 0 °C. After electrogenerated, the film on the SUS was washed with water and allowed to dry in the air for 1 h. After that, the film was peeled from the SUS, and the film borders were cut off. These free-standing films were then cut into smaller pieces, each of which, after weighing, was attached to a commercial double-stick insulating tape. A metallic clamp was used to ensure electric contact with the potentiostat-galvanostat [30–34].

10.4   PREPARATION OF CATION-DRIVEN CONDUCTING POLYMER SOFT ACTUATOR

Similarly, the cation-driven conducting soft polymer actuators (PPy.DBS) were electrogenerated from a 0.15 M pyrrole and 0.25 M dodecyl benzenesulfonic acid (DBSA) aqueous solution. A constant current (0.5 mA/cm) was applied to the working electrode (SUS) for 2 h at 0 °C. After electrogenerated, the film was washed and kept in deionized water for 24 h to rinse DBSA adhering to the film surface. After drying in the air for 24 h, the film borders were cut, and the films were peeled from the SUS. Those free-standing films were cut into smaller pieces, each attached to a commercial double-stick insulating tape. The metallic clamp was used to ensure electric contact with the potentiostat-galvanostat [30–34].

10.5   PREPARATION OF ASYMMETRIC BILAYER CONDUCTING POLYMER SOFT ACTUATOR

The working electrode (SUS) was first coated with a PPy.DBS film following the procedure described in the previous section and then washed and kept in pure water for 24 h to eliminate any organic acid molecules adhering to the film surface. Then, it was dried in the air for 24 h. In the next step, the dried PPy.DBS coated SUS was immersed in 50 ml of 0.05 M HpPS and 0.20 M pyrrole aqueous solution and PPy.HpPS was electrogenerated by following the procedure described already. After generating, the PPy.HpPS/PPy.DBS bilayer was washed with water and dried in the air over 24 h, after which the film borders were cut off and the PPy.HpPS/PPy.DBS bilayer film was peeled from the SUS [30–34].

10.6   CYCLIC VOLTAMMETRIC AND COULOVOLTAMMETRIC RESPONSE FOR ELECTROCHEMICAL CHARACTERISTICS

The three different conducting polymer soft actuators, PPy.HpPS/tape, PPy.DBS/tape, and PPy.HpPS/PPy.DBS was given 40 continuous voltammetric cycles between −0.4 V and 0.7 V at a scan speed of 10 mV/s in a 0.5 M sodium bromide (NaBr) aqueous solution. After successive voltammetric cycles, any previous structural memory [35–38] from the film was cleared.

Cyclic voltammetry (CV) is a type of potentiodynamic electrochemical measurement typically used to study electrochemical properties. The graph peaks refer to the oxidation and reduction states of the conducting polymer soft actuators. The author has already reported that, in the case of the PPy.HpPS/tape, the PPy.DBS/tape, and the PPy.HpPS/PPy.DBS [31], the oxidation and reduction peaks appeared clearly in all cases. Based on the CV responses, the electric charges Q were calculated using a time integration of electrical current I, as shown Eq. (10.1), called the coulovoltammetric response. The electric bills refer to the number of anions or cations being entered or expelled during the oxidation and reduction processes.

$$Q = \int I dt \qquad (10.1)$$

In the coulovoltammetric results obtained from the PPy.HpPS/tape, the PPy.DBS/tape, and the PPy.HpPS/PPy.DBS's general shapes of the coulovoltammetric results are similar for all three conducting polymer soft actuators [31]. The closed coulovoltammetric loop indicates that reversible oxidation and reduction are present. In all the cases, the minimum 1 and the maximum 3 values correspond to changes resulting from reductions to the oxidations and from oxidations to the reductions, respectively.

In the PPy.HpPS/tape, anions and water molecules are entered into the PPy.HpPS from 1 to 3 during oxidation and are expelled from the PPy.HpPS from 3 to 1 during reduction. In contrast, in the PPy.DBS/tape, the cations and water molecules are expelled from the PPy.DBS from 1 to 3 during oxidation and entered into the PPy. DBS from 3 to 1 during reduction. Additionally, in PPy.HpPS/PPy.DBS, anions, and water molecules are entered into the PPy.HpPS and cations and water molecules are expelled from the PPy.DBS from 1 to 3 during oxidation. While anions are discharged from the PPy.HpPS and cations are entered into the PPy.DBS from 3 to 1 during reduction [31].

In other words, an optimum level of asymmetric cooperation is achieved when one of the films exchanges anions while expanding and shrinking during its respective oxidation and reduction, respectively, and the second film exchanges cations are inducing shrinking and expanding during oxidation and reduction, respectively. These combined effects are due to the asymmetric simultaneous expanding and shrinking processes driven by the simultaneous oxidation of the two films and the concomitant reverse asymmetric shrinking and expanding driven by the reduction of those films [31–32]. Moreover, the shape gradient is slightly different in all three cases, so the electrochemical properties are different. The Q/E (Charge/Potential) gradient refers to the entrance/expulsion speeds of anions or cations or electrochemomechanical deformation speed.

10.7 APPLICATION OF CONDUCTING POLYMER SOFT ACTUATOR TO MICROPUMPS

In this section, the author explores the application of conducting polymer soft actuators to mechanical uses. The most significant advantage of conducting polymer soft actuators is that their thin-film forms are minimal and lightweight. In addition, they can be driven with high response and have high levels of flexibility and durability, all of which are favorable properties for an actuator. Accordingly, since conducting polymer soft actuators are particularly suitable for use as micropumps, the author will introduce two pump types in which such actuators are used to provide the necessary driving force.

10.8 MICROPUMP DRIVEN BY A PLANATE CONDUCTING POLYMER SOFT ACTUATOR

Planate conducting polymer soft actuators have been reported (28) and were electrodeposited from aqueous solutions in which paraphenolsulfonic sulfonic acid (HpPS) and dodecylbenzene sulfonic acid (DBS) provide the supporting electrolyte for the electro generation. In the fabrication process, electro generation is first performed on the central part of titanium (Ti) plate employed as a working electrode from 0.15 M PPy and 0.25 M HpPS aqueous solution. The PPy.HpPS actuator was electrogenerated on the central part of the Ti as an anion layer. Next, the electro generation was performed from 0.15 M PPy and 0.25 M DBS aqueous solution that electrogenerated the PPy.DBS on the Ti, ultimately producing the PPy.HpPS/PPy.DBS planate actuator, as shown in Figure 10.4. This planate actuator has a patterned bimorph structure with anion and cation layers [28].

In use, the planate bimorph conducting polymer soft actuator is operated in a 1.0 M NaCl solution. The CV response and displacement of the central part of the actuator from −1.1 V to 0.6 V and the scan speed of 20 mV/s were shown [28].

The oxidation and reduction peaks of the CV response are located at approximately 0.3 and −0.6 V, respectively. In the relationship between the CV response and the actuation of the conducting polymer soft actuator, the anion layer expands due to the entrance of the anion (Cl^-). At the same time, the cation layer shrinks due to the expulsion of cation (Na^+) in the oxidation. Moreover, the anion layer shrinks due to the expulsion (Cl^-), and the cation-layer expands due to the entrance (Na^+) in the reduction. Ultimately, the central part of the planate conducting polymer soft actuator bends toward the right during the oxidation and turns toward the left during the removal.

The planate bimorph conducting polymer soft actuator was then used to provide the driving force to the micropump. To accomplish this, an acrylic plate was placed in a tank to which a flow channel was connected. The actuator was then combined with the bottom of the tank, and a vinyl sheet was located between the actuator and the tank bottom. A 1.0 M NaCl aqueous solution was used to provide the electrolyte action. The tank and flow channel were filled with distilled water. This pump was not connected to a valve. Instead, the water level in the flow channel was oscillated by the planate conducting polymer soft actuator from ⁻1.1 V to 0.6 V and the scan speed of 20 mV/s.

The water level in the flow channel during the reduction and oxidation was also shown [28]. The apparent reciprocation of the water level is shown, and the flow rate was approximately 28 μl/min. The oscillating flow rate can be controlled by the electrochemical potential and the scan rate. Since it is well known that the required flow rates for micro total analysis systems (μ-TASs) and insulin pumps are from 1.0 to 50.0 μl/min [39–40], the micropump proposed in our study satisfies the required rates, and the author presumes that it can be used for those purposes.

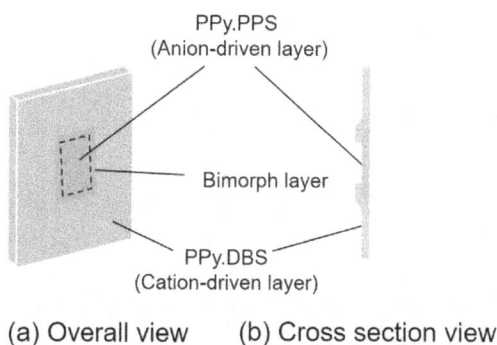

(a) Overall view   (b) Cross section view

FIGURE 10.4 Planate conducting polymer soft actuator.

10.9   MICROPUMP DRIVEN BY CLOSING–OPENING CONDUCTING POLYMER SOFT ACTUATORS

In the previous section, the successful development of a micropump driven by the planate conducting polymer soft actuator was discussed. However, that micropump could not transport the fluid continuously in one direction because the system does not have a valve. This section describes a proposed valve-less micropump system equipped with a conducting polymer soft actuator that can transport fluids in a single direction [29]. To accomplish this, the author first developed a bimorph-structured closing–opening conducting polymer soft actuator to provide the driving force for the micropump, which consisted of two actuators.

The closing–opening actuator was also created by electro generation. More specifically, electro generation was performed on a Ti from 0.15 M PPy and 0.25 M DBS aqueous solution. The resulting PPy.DBS actuator was electrogenerated on the Ti as the cation layer. Next, 0.15 M PPy and 0.25 M of tetra-*n*-butylammonium bis (trifluoromethane sulfonyl) imide (TBATFSI) aqueous solution were used electro generation the center of the PPy.DBS actuator, after which the PPy.TFSI actuator was electrogenerated on the PPy.DBS actuator as the anion-layer. Finally, the resulting bimorph-structured PPy.DBS/PPy.TFSI actuator was electrogenerated on the Ti.

Two PPy.DBS/PPy.TFSI actuators with slits were prepared and were placed face to face, as shown in Figure 10.5. Platinum sheets fixed the top and bottom parts of these films. The resulting actuator was driven in 0.5 M lithium bisimide (LiTFSI) solution from −1.2 V to 1.0 V and the frequency of 0.005 Hz.

The actuator opens widely and closes entirely due to oxidation and reduction, respectively, as shown in Figure 10.6. In the oxidation, the cation (Li^+) is expelled in the cation layer; thus, the cation layer shrinks. The anion ($TFSI^-$) is entered in the anion layer, hence the anion layer expands. In the reduction, the cation (Li^+) is entered, thus the cation layer expands, and the anion ($TFSI^-$) is expelled, thus the anion layer shrinks. As a result, the actuator closes. As a result, the actuator opens.

A closing–opening conducting polymer soft actuator provided the micropump. The micropump was capsule-type, and its length and diameter were 60 mm and 21 mm, respectively. The driving source is two closing–opening actuators placed inside the pump. A 5-mm-wide polydimethylsiloxane tube was incorporated and

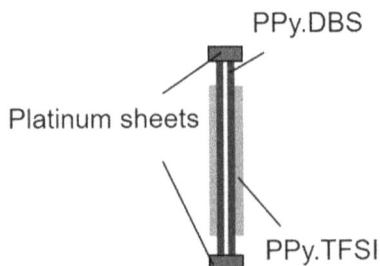

FIGURE 10.5   Cross-section of closing–opening conducting polymer soft actuator.

(a) Reduction

Cations are entered into cation layer

Anions are expelled from anion layer

(b) Oxidation

Cations are expelled from cation layer

Anions are entered to anion layer

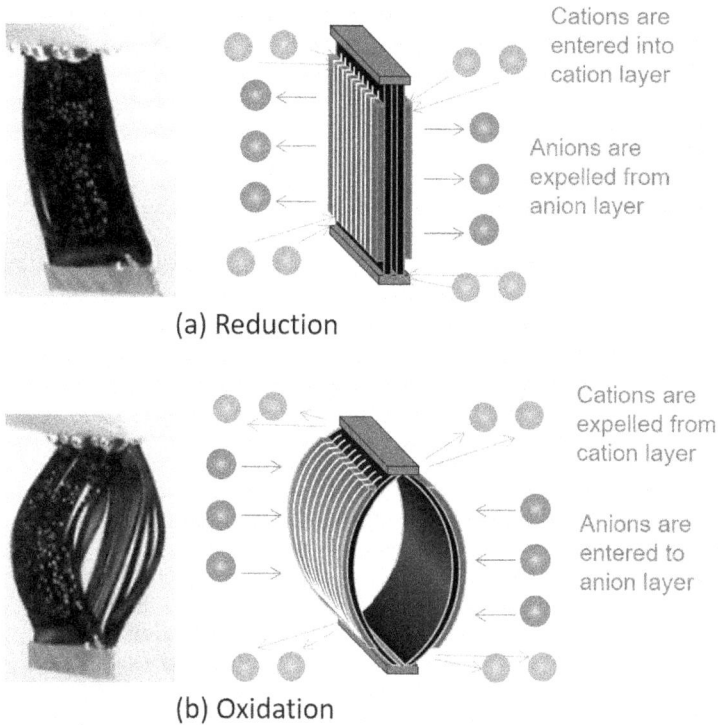

FIGURE 10.6 Closing–opening actuation of a bimorph conducting polymer soft actuator.

filled with the fluid to be transported, and a 0.5 M LiTFSI aqueous solution was sealed in the capsule. Although this micropump has no valve, it is connected to a tank at one end in a way that ensures the fluid in the tank is transported in just a single direction. The actuator near the tank is defined as A, and the actuator far from the tank (outlet side) is defined as B.

Since this pump is valveless, it needs the ability to transport fluid solely via the closing–opening actions of the actuators. A computational fluid dynamics (CFD) simulation using ANSYS-CFX was performed to realize an optimum one-direction fluid movement without a valve. In CFD, the governing equations of the fluid are the continuous and Navier–Stokes equations, as shown in Eqs. (10.2) and (10.3), respectively. A finite volume method was performed for the discretization. The computation grid was structured, and the total number was approximately 250,000. The boundary conditions at the walls and the tube ends were no-slip boundaries and open to the atmosphere, respectively. A laminar-flow model was used in this simulation because the Reynolds number is low.

$$\frac{\partial \rho}{\partial t} + \nabla \bullet (\rho U) = 0 \qquad (10.2)$$

$$\frac{\partial \rho U}{\partial t} + \nabla \bullet (\rho U \otimes U) = \nabla \bullet \left(-P\delta + \mu\left(\nabla U + (\nabla U)^T\right)\right) \qquad (10.3)$$

The micropump has two closing–opening conducting polymer soft actuators, with fluid transport in one direction achieved via the phase differences of the closing–opening movements. Figure 10.7 shows the opening lengths of the two actuators. The horizontal axis indicates the measuring times, and the vertical axis indicates the opening sizes. The solid and broken lines indicate Actuators A and B, respectively. As shown in this figure, the maximum opening length attained by Actuators A and B were $d_1 = 3.2$ mm and $d_2 = 1.4$ mm, respectively. Moreover, the phase difference between them was 180°.

Figure 10.8 shows the transport volume produced by the closing–opening actuators. The fluid is transported in a single direction without backflow. The transport volume, governed by the opening length of two actuators, is approximately 50 µl from $t = 0$ to 20 s. During $t = 0$ to 20 s, Actuator A is closed completely, and the fluid is propelled effectually downstream to the outlet by Actuator B. After that time, Actuator A opens gradually, and fluid is drawn into the tube from the tank. However,

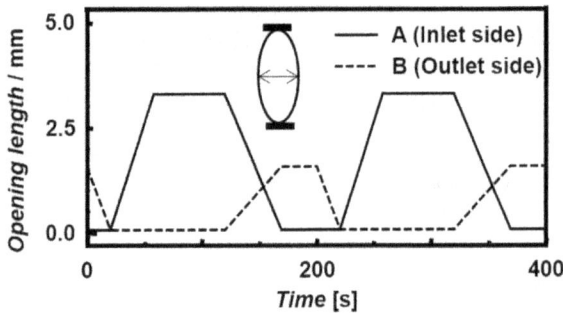

FIGURE 10.7   Opening lengths of two closing–opening conducting polymer soft actuators.

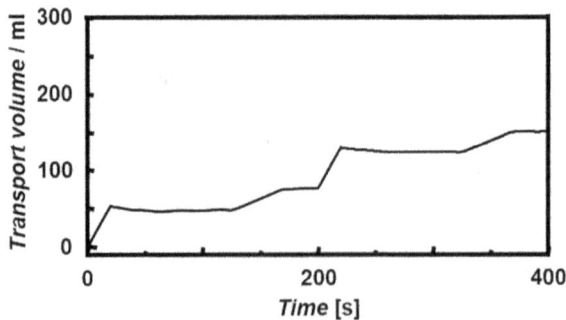

FIGURE 10.8   Transport volume of a micropump produced by a closing–opening movement of actuators.

Actuator B was closed yet, and the transport volume keeps constant. From $t = 110$ to 170 s, Actuator A is closing while Actuator B is opening, and the fluid is propelled again to the outlet. During $t = 110$ to 170 s up to the complete closure of Actuator A, the fluid volume is transported, approximately 75 μl. Then, with Actuator A closed, the liquid volume keeps constant without backflow until Actuator B begins to close again, thus completing the pumping cycle. In one closing–opening process of a pair of actuators, approximately 150 μl of fluid is transported. Repetitions of the pumping cycle ensure the fluid transport in a single direction with no backflow. Based on these results, the conducting polymer soft actuators were given the applied voltage to optimize closing–opening movements to produce micropump-driving force. The electrochemical potentials for Actuators A and B were −1.2 to 1.0 V and −0.6 to 0.5 V, respectively, and the frequency was 0.005 Hz. Furthermore, the two actuators had a phase difference of 180°.

The essential characteristic of the pump system is the relationship between the pressure head and the flow rate, which we have shown for our closing–opening actuator-based micropump [29]. PPy.DBS/PPy.TFSI means the closing–opening actuator acts as the micropump driver, PPy.DBS/PPy.HpPS means a system using HpPS instead of TFSI as the supporting electrolyte and double PPy.DBS/PPy.TFSI presents a case in which two closing–opening actuators (PPy.DBS/PPy.TFSI) are laminated. Our proposed micropump has a broad flow rate range of approximately 2.0–83.0 μl/ min, and the pressure head can be adjusted by either the supporting electrolyte or the number of layers. When HpPS is used as the supporting electrolyte, the radius of HpPS-is smaller than that of TFSI⁻, and the generative power of the actuator decreases. This reduces the pressure head.

On the other hand, the pressure head produced by two laminated actuators is approximately four or five times greater than a single layer. Since two laminated actuators were used, the generative power increased, and the pump delivered both a broader flow rate and a higher pressure head compared to the other micropump [29]. Furthermore, since our micropump uses volume variations to push the fluid, it can also transport high-viscosity liquids, including silicone oil, which has a viscosity level that is 300 or 400 times greater than that of water while maintaining almost the same high flow rates and pressure head. That is, our micropump can transport high viscosity fluid while keeping a broad flow rate range and a high-pressure head.

Energy consumption rates E_c (J/μl) and efficiencies η are important micropump characteristics and were calculated using Eqs. (10.4), (10.5), and (10.6). E, I, Q, t, and V mean the energy (J/s), the current (A), flow rate (μl/s), the time (s), and the voltage (V), respectively.

$$E = \frac{\int VIdt}{t} \qquad (10.4)$$

$$E_c = E/Q \qquad (10.5)$$

$$\eta = \frac{PQ}{E} \qquad (10.6)$$

The energy consumption rate and efficiency of the micropump were determined at approximately 28 μl/min [29, 41–44]. These results are compared with conventional micropumps driven by other materials, such as permanent magnets and piezo actuators. The energy consumption rate of our micropump is much lower than the traditional micropumps and has higher efficiency than the conventional micropumps. In our micropump, the electrochemical potential of the actuator was −1.2 V to 1.0 V. In contrast, the applied voltage range of the permanent magnet and piezo actuators of conventional micropumps were −10.0 V to 10.0 V approximately −100.0 V to 100.0 V, respectively. This indicates that the applied energy in our micropump was drastically lower than that of conventional micropumps, which is one of the essential characteristics of our conducting polymer soft actuator.

10.10   CONCLUSIONS

Conducting polymer soft actuators have a novel method of functioning that causes them to act similarly to natural muscles. Since they are fabricated from thin films, they are both small and lightweight and can be driven by the much lower applied voltage. They also boast high response and have high levels of flexibility and durability, all of which are valuable properties for an actuator.

However, conducting polymer soft actuators have not yet been applied to mechanical applications. In order to advance those possibilities, the author has developed various mechanical applications, one of which is using a conducting polymer soft actuator to provide the driving force in micropumps. Experiments were conducted to investigate that our proposed planate conducting polymer soft actuator achieved a fluid reciprocating motion. The electrochemical potential and the scan rate applied to the actuator could control the oscillating volume.

Furthermore, in addition to providing wide flow rates and a high-pressure head, the energy consumption rate of the micropump was found to be dramatically lower than conventional micropumps. Based on these results, a novel closing–opening actuator was fabricated and used to provide the driving force of a valve-less micropump. In this application, the closing–opening movements of the actuator were optimized by CFD so that liquid transport could be accomplished unidirectionally and without backflow.

Micropumps are widely used in broader fields, including chemical, biomedical, and mechanical engineering systems. They are vital components of the microelectromechanical system (MEMS) devices used in chemical analyses, such as μ-TAS, and medical instruments for insulin and hormone delivery. In such applications, micropumps transport liquids slowly at microflow rates. However, it has recently become necessary to widen flow rate, achieve higher levels of flow rate resolution, and provide continuous transport for specific flows. Unfortunately, it was difficult to satisfy these requirements because none of the available actuators were sufficiently small, lightweight, or capable of slow and accurate movements similar to those of natural muscles. From antimicrobial and antiviral delivery viewpoints, transdermal drug delivery systems (TDDSs), such as the recently developed next-generation systems that include drug storage tanks and microneedles, have been attracting significant attention in recent years. In such systems, the micropump is essential for transporting fluids from the drug storage tank to the microneedles, which means that a high-pressure head and highly accurate flow rate control are required. The micropump proposed in this chapter fully meets these requirements, and it is strongly anticipated that it will be incorporated in such systems in the future.

REFERENCES

1. Otero, T. F., Martinez, J. G., Arias-Pardilla, J. 2012. Biomimetic electrochemistry from conducting polymers. A review: Artificial muscles, smart membranes, smart drug delivery and computer/neuron interfaces. *Electrochimica Acta* 84:112–128.
2. Otero, T. F. 2015. Conducting polymers. In *Bioinspired Intelligent Materials and Devices*, ed. M. Shahinpoor, H. J. Schneider, 1–248. Royal Society of Chemistry.
3. Otero, T. F., Angulo, E., Rodriguez, J., Santamaria, C. 1992. Electrochemomechanical properties from a bilayer: Polypyrrole/non-conducting and flexible material-artificial muscle. *Journal of Electroanalytical Chemistry* 341:369–375.
4. Pei, Q., Inganas, O. 1992. Conjugated polymers and the bending cantilever method: Electrical muscles and smart devices. *Advanced Materials* 4:277–278.
5. Baughman, R. H. 1996. Conducting polymer artificial muscles. *Synthetic Metals* 78:339–353.
6. Smela, E. 2003. Conjugated polymer actuators for biomedical applications. *Advanced Materials* 15:481–494.
7. Spinks, G. M., Alici, G., McGovern, S., Xi, B., Wallace, G. G. 2009. Conjugated polymer actuators: Fundamentals. In *Biomedical Applications of Electroactive Polymer Actuators*, ed. F. Carpi, E. Smela, 193–227. Wiley.
8. Otero, T. F., Martinez, J. G. 2015. Physical and chemical awareness from sensing polymeric artificial muscles: Experiments and modeling. *Progress in Polymer Science* 44:62–78.
9. Jager, E. W. H. 2012. Actuators, biomedicine, and cell-biology, electroactive polymer actuators devices. *Electroactive Polymer Actuators and Devices (EAPAD) 2012, Proceedings* 8340.
10. Hara, S., Zama, T., Takashima, W., Kaneto, K. 2004. Artificial muscles based on polypyrrole actuators with large strain and stress induced electrically. *Polymer Journal* 36:151–161.
11. Salanek, W. R. 1991. *Science and Applications of Conducting Polymers*. CRC Press.
12. Otero, T. F., Rodriguez, J., Angulo, E., Santamaria, C. 1993. Artificial muscles from bilayer structures. *Synthetic Metals* 57:3713–3717.
13. Chen, X., Inganas, O. 1995. Doping-induced volume changes in poly(3-octylthiophene) solids and gels. *Synthetic Metals* 74:159–164.
14. Otero, T. F., Sansinena, J. M. 1997. Bilayer dimensions and movement in artificial muscles. *Bioelectrochemistry and Bioenergetics* 42:117–122.
15. Otero, T. F., Cortes, M. T. 2004. Artificial muscle: Movement and position control. *Chemical Communications* 284–285.
16. Conzuelo, L. V., Arias-Pardilla, J., Cauich-Rodriguez, J. V., Smit, M. A., Otero, T. F. 2010. Sensing and tactile artificial muscles from reactive materials. *Sensors* 10(4):2638–2674.
17. Valero, L., Arias-Pardilla, J., Cauich-Rodriguez, J., Smit, M. A., Otero, T. F. 2011. Characterization of the movement of polypyrrole-dodecylbenzenesulfonate-perchlorate/tape artificial muscles: Faradaic control of reactive artificial molecular motors and muscles. *Electrochimica Acta* 56:3721–3726.
18. Kaneto, K., Kaneko, M., Min, Y., MacDiarmid, A. G. 1995. Artificial muscle: Electromechanical actuators using polyaniline films. *Synthetic Metals* 71: 2211–2212.

19. Takashima, W., Fukui, M., Kaneko, M., Kaneto, K. 1995. Electrochemomechanical deformation in polyaniline films. *Japanese Journal of Applied Physics* 34:3786–3789.
20. Kaneko, M., Kaneto, K. 2001. Deformation of poly(o-methoxyaniline) film induced by polymer conformation on electrochemical oxidation. *Polymer Journal* 33:104–107.
21. Kaneko, M., Kaneto, K. 1999. Electrochemomechanical deformation in poly(omethoxyaniline). *Synthetic Metals* 102:1350–1353.
22. Fuchiwaki, M., Takashima, W., Kaneto, K. 2001. Comparative study of electrochemomechanical deformation of poly(3-alkylthiophene)s, polyanilines and polypyrrole films. *Japanese Journal of Applied Physics* 40:7110–7116.
23. Kaneto, K., Sonoda, Y., Takashima, W. 2000. Direct measurement and mechanism of electro-chemomechanical expansion and contraction in polypyrrole films. *Japanese Journal of Applied Physics* 39:5918–5922.
24. Madden, J. D., Cush, R. A., Kanigan, T. S., Brenan, C. J., Hunter, I. W. 1999. Encapsulated polypyrrole actuators. *Synthetic Metals* 105:61–64.
25. Hutchison, S., Lewis, T. W., Moulton, S. E., Spinks, G. M., Wallace, G. G. 2000. Development of polypyrrole-based electromechanical actuators. *Synthetic Metals* 113:121–127.
26. Fuchiwaki, M., Takashima, W., Kaneto, K. 2001. Comparative study of electrochemomechanical deformations of poly(3-alkylthiophene)s, polyanilines and polypyrrole films. *Japanese Journal of Applied Physics* 40:7110–7116.
27. Bay, L., West, K., Skaarup, S. 2002. Pentanol as co-surfactant in polypyrrole actuators. *Polymer* 43:3527–3532.
28. Fuchiwaki, M., Tanaka, K., Kaneto, K. 2009. Planate conducting polymer soft actuator based on polypyrrole and its application. *Sensors and Actuators A* 150:272–276.
29. Naka, Y., Fuchiwaki, M., Tanaka, K. 2010. A micropump driven by a polypyrrole-based conducting polymer soft actuator. *Polymer International* 59:352–356.
30. Fuchiwaki, M., Martinez, J. G., Otero, T. F. 2016. Asymmetric bilayer muscles: Cooperative actuation, dynamic hysteresis, and creeping in $NaPF_6$ aqueous solutions. *Chemistry Open* 5(4):369–374.
31. Fuchiwaki, M., Martinez, J. G., Otero, T. F. 2016. Asymmetric bilayer muscles: Cooperative and antagonist actuation. *Electrochimica Acta* 195:9–18.
32. Fuchiwaki, M., Martinez, J. G., Otero, T. F. 2015. Polypyrrole asymmetric bilayer artificial muscle: Driven reactions, cooperative actuation, and osmotic effects. *Advanced Functional Materials* 25(10):1535–1541.
33. Fuchiwaki, M., Otero, T. F. 2014. Polypyrrole-para-phenolsulfonic acid/tape artificial muscle as a tool to clarify biomimetic driven reactions and ionic exchanges. *Journal of Materials Chemistry B* 2(14):1954–1965.
34. Otero, T. F., Martinez, J. G., Fuchiwaki, M., Valero, L. 2014. Structural electrochemistry from free-standing polypyrrole films: Full hydrogen inhibition from aqueous solutions. *Advanced Functional Materials* 24(9):1265–1274.
35. Villeret, B., Nechtschein, M. 1989. Memory effects in conducting polymers. *Physical Review Letters* 63:1285–1287.
36. Sendai, T., Suematsu, H., Kaneto, K. 2009. Anisotropic strain and memory effect in electrochemomechanical strain of polypyrrole films under high tensile stresses. *Japanese Journal of Applied Physics* 48:051506.
37. Vorotyntsev, M. A., Skompska, M., Pousson, E., Goux, J., Moise, C. 2003. Memory effects in functionalized conducting polymer films: Titanocene derivatized polypyrrole in contact with THF solutions. *Journal of Electroanalytical Chemistry* 552:307–317.
38. Heinze, J., Rasche, A. 2006. The memory effect in solution. *Journal of Solid State Electrochemistry* 10:148–156.
39. Teymoori, M. M., Ebrahim, A. S. 2005. Design and simulation of a novel electrostatic peristaltic micromachined pump for drug delivery applications. *Sensors and Actuators A* 117:222–229.

40. Jeong, O. C., Konishi, S. 2007. Fabrication and drive test of pneumatic PDMS micro pump. *Sensors and Actuators A* 135:849–856.

41. Santra, S., Holloway, P., Batich, C. D. 2002. Fabrication and testing of a magnetically actuated micropump. *Sensors and Actuators B* 87:358–364.

42. Jang, L. S., Li, Y. J., Lin, S. J., Hsu, Y. C., Yao, W. S., Tsai, M. C., Hou, C. C. 2007. A stand-alone peristaltic micropump based on piezoelectric actuation. *Biomedical Microdevices* 9:185–194.

43. Geipel, A., Goldschmidtboing, F., Doll, A., Jantscheff, P., Esser, N., Massing, U., Woias, P. 2008. An implantable active microport based on a self-priming high-performance two-stage micropump. *Sensors and Actuators A* 145:414–422.

44. Fuchiwaki, M. 2014. Micro pump driven by a pair of conducting polymer soft actuators. In *Soft Actuators: Materials, Modeling, Applications, and Future Perspectives*, ed. K. Asaka, H. Okuzaki, 435–446. Springer.

11 The Recent Development of Antiviral Cold-Sprayed Copper Coatings against Coronavirus Disease Infection

Peerawatt Nunthavarawong

CONTENTS

11.1 INTRODUCTION

The recent outbreak of the novel coronavirus disease 2019 (COVID-19) is still problematic around the world. This respiratory disease is often transmitted to a new human host by airborne and physical contact transmissions from person to person, even by indirect fomite transmission as touching contaminated surfaces, such as medical devices and public equipment [1].

It is well known that copper (Cu) and a 60%-Cu alloy are officially registered as antimicrobial materials by the U.S. Environmental Protection Agency (EPA) used for the protective purpose of nosocomial infections and public areas [1–3]. They

DOI: 10.1201/9781003143093-11

have also disinfected microbial/viral pathogens via indirect fomite transmission; exceptionally, the virus responsible for the COVID-19 pandemic known as 'severe acute respiratory syndrome coronavirus-2 (SARS-CoV-2)' was rapidly incapacitated on copper surfaces. In the study of the airborne situation, previous work showed that the 99.9%-Cu inactivated SARS-CoV-2 and SARS-CoV-1 in aerosols testing after 4 and 8 hours, respectively [4].

In addition, the study of indirect fomite transmission, copper, and copper-nickel alloys has successfully incapacitated SARS-CoV-2 after 2 hours [5]. The release of Cu ions plays a significant role in destroying viral genomes and dispersing surface spikes [1, 6]. In contrast, COVID-19 survived on polymer and stainless-steel surfaces for a few days [4].

Also, traditional often-touched surfaces could be covered with Cu and Cu alloy coatings to inactivate viruses. In terms of fabricating these protective coatings, cold spray is a relatively new technique, which facilitates depositing large and several mm thick compared to other conventional deposition techniques.

Especially, it is deemed to be available for a high concentration release of Cu ions compared to these coatings produced over thermal spraying [2], as can be seen, more in detail in Sections 11.8 and 11.9, respectively; likewise, there have been shown beneficial coronavirus disease disinfection.

11.2   CONTACT-KILLING BY COPPER

As ancient knowledge, a very long time prior they recognized various pathogens, humans have known that copper is viable as a disinfectant. The report obtained by the Edwin Smith Papyrus, known as 'the oldest medical text,' described copper as a disinfectant agent from an Egyptian medical doctor circa 1700 BC. In Asia, by returning beyond an ancient Chinese as 1600 BC., the Chinese employed copper coins to treat bladder, stomach pain, and heart diseases. In addition, ancient people around the globe used bronze pots to disinfect diarrhea from their drinking water [7].

Until now, modern scientists and engineers have promoted copper and copper alloys as antimicrobial materials, by which EPA has registered other copper materials for more than 400 types [2, 8]. Antimicrobial copper is widely used to prevent hospital-associated infections. The use of copper and copper alloys on various touching surfaces decreases healthcare-acquired infections.

According to the Centers for Disease Control report, the cost of infectious cases was more than several 10,000 U.S. dollars per patient. However, infected cases decreased when often-touched surfaces in hospitals are made of copper, e.g., elevator buttons, push plates, light switches, bedside rails, tray tables, chair armrests, IV poles, faucets, and grab bars. For example, in the report of the Sentara Healthcare System in North Carolina and Virginia places, nosocomial infections were reduced by more than 80%. In addition, antibacterial copper is being used in healthcare centers, hospitals, and public transit systems found in several countries, such as Canada, Israel, Poland, Chile, and Peru [7].

Various copper alloys can utilize for antimicrobial/antiviral activities—key questions are as follows [1]:

- How long can it be inactivated?
- Will disease resistance happen?
- What kind of surface repair and maintenance methods are used for sustainable inactivation?

11.3 ANTIVIRAL MECHANISMS OF COPPER

Copper has specific atomic features and has quickly reacted as oxidation-reduction phenomena that provide superior killing power over gold and silver. As a result of Cu^{2+} ions, they can disable the components of viral cells, i.e., nonenveloped, enveloped, single-stranded RNA, double-stranded RNA, single-stranded DNA, and double-stranded DNA viruses [9].

For example, when viruses land on Cu surfaces, their cell walls are penetrated by Cu ions. Cu ions may damage viral proteins, and consequently, the generation of hydroxyl radicals destructs their RNA and N protein in cells, as illustrated in Figure 11.1.

The interaction of copper and human coronavirus 229E inactivated viral genomes and surface spikes [10]. Cupric (II) chloride dihydrate incapacitated the dengue virus replication [11]. The copper chelator ATN-224 promoted Cu^{2+} as destroying the oncolytic herpes simplex virus. The release of Cu^{2+} by the oxidative generation was harmful to the herpes simplex virus [6, 9].

Cu ions could inactivate the negative-sense RNA genome of the influenza A virus [6, 12]. Cu^{2+} ions and Cu oxide nanoparticles may incapacitate the viral mRNA, capsid proteins, and replication; they are possible to defeat the viable COVID-19 [6].

However, copper's antimicrobial/antiviral mechanisms are still being studied; they enclose concepts that [6]:

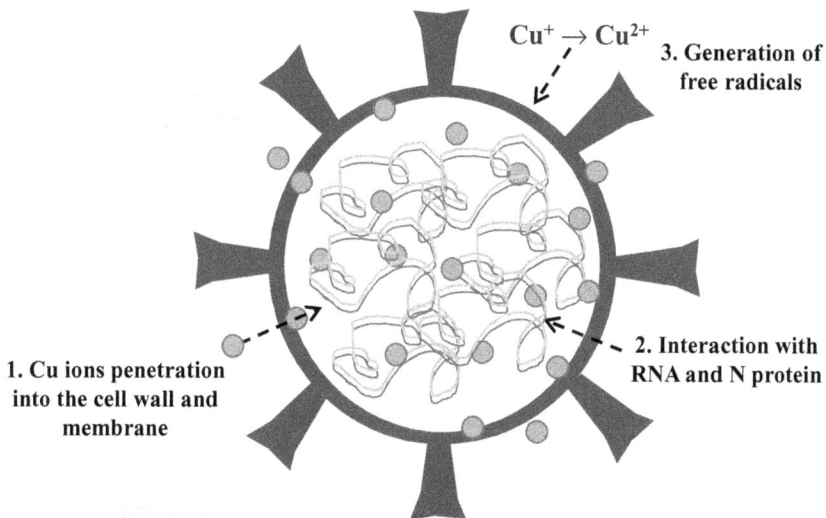

FIGURE 11.1 Contact-killing mechanisms of copper ions.

- Specific essential cell nutrients, i.e., potassium and glutamate, may be interrupted when high-dose Cu ions destroy the cell membrane wall.
- The leak of the weakening cell wall is experienced by osmotic imbalance.
- Excessive Cu concentrations do not need microbial cells, resulting in the significant loss of protein functions.
- In hydrogen peroxide and oxidative generation, Cu reacts as a 'Fenton-type reaction,' leading to the generation of toxic hydroxyl radicals wherein a chemical reaction is causing oxidative damage to the cell.
- Lipid peroxidation can cause cell death.

11.4 ANTIMICROBIAL/ANTIVIRAL ACTIVITIES USING BULK COPPER

Bulk copper processing consists of casting and mechanical processes. In the casting process, the melted copper is poured into the cavity to form solid copper. In contrast, wrought copper is made by several mechanical processes, i.e., rolling, extruding, and forging. These techniques made solid copper into plates, bars, and free-form contours as final shapes.

Cast copper alloys (95% Cu) have successfully killed *Escherichia coli* O157 for 6 hours of exposure at the operating temperature of 22 °C [13]. The traditional wrought copper (C11000) inactivated the influenza A virus for 6 hours at the incubation temperature of 22 °C. In comparison with stainless steel, the virus was made unable for 24 hours. Likewise, the influenza A virus was readily inactivated more than 10^3 times on the copper surface [12].

In the case of *Human coronavirus* 229E (Hu-CoV-229E), Hu-CoV-229E could survive on several polymer surfaces, i.e., polytetrafluoroethylene (PTFE), polyvinyl chloride (PVC), silicone rubber, even on glass, stainless, and ceramic tiles for several hours. In contrast, it was inactivated on wrought Cu alloy (C26000, cartridge brass) and wrought Cu–Ni alloys (C72500, C70600) for several minutes [10]. In the study of the novel coronavirus in aerosols transmission conditions, wrought copper surfaces (99.9% Cu) inactivated against SARS-CoV-2 and SARS-CoV-1 for 4 and 8 hours. In contrast, COVID-19 survived on polymer and stainless-steel surfaces for a few days [4].

11.5 ANTIMICROBIAL/ANTIVIRAL ACTIVITIES USING COPPER PARTICLES

Copper particle form is helpful for antimicrobial/antiviral activities, especially for nanoscale levels that are very powerful. For example, chitosan, composed of copper nanoparticles, could inactivate bacteria, such as *methicillin-resistant Staphylococcus aureus* (MRSA), *Salmonella choleraesuis*, *Pseudomonas aeruginosa*, and *Bacillus subtilis*.

Copper nanoparticles (Cu-NPs) and cuprous oxide (Cu_2O) had the ability of plasmid DNA inactivation [3]. Cu particles are available for inactivating viable viruses, i.e., noroviruses and influenza viruses. The use of Cu-NPs (copper iodide

CuI, 160 nm-diameter) has successfully incapacitated viral proteins of the influenza A virus.

Likewise, the production of hydroxyl radicals derived from cuprous oxide promoted viral inactivation [3, 14]. As a result of particle sizes on antimicrobial/antiviral activities, it should be noted that more minor is better. A very fine particle has greater penetration into the cell [3].

11.6   ANTIMICROBIAL/ANTIVIRAL ACTIVITIES USING COPPER THIN FILMS

The antibacterial activity of bulk copper and copper oxide films was compared against *E. coli and S. aureus. E. coli* was inactivated within 30 minutes on copper thin films.

In contrast, the viable *S. aureus* disappeared after 1 hour on both copper oxide thin films and bulk copper. This study has also remarked that the formation of the oxidation state of Cu_2O films did not decrease in antimicrobial efficacy [15].

For the anti-COVID-19 study, a copper-coated polypropylene filter face mask was studied. The copper thin film was produced about 20 nm thick using a vacuum coating system. With the use of the oxygen ion beam pretreatment, the coating adhesion improved and resulted in Cu_2O generation. Copper could also assist the filtration efficiency of more than 90%. In this study, the addition of the COVID-19 vaccine container (Vero cells) onto the copper-coated mask did not show the RNA replicase and SARS-CoV-2 envelope protein, thereby resulting in more than 75% reduction [16].

In contrast, the anti-COVID-19 study via indirect fomite transmission conditions compared with the antiviral efficacy, filoviruses, and SARS-CoV-2 were studied. Viral droplets placed on Luminore CopperTouch™ copper and copper-nickel surfaces for 30 minutes of exposure, thereby resulting in the anti-SARS-CoV-2 efficacy of 99% after 2 hours [5]. There has been a new report that copper alloys quickly inactivated COVID-19.

11.7   ANTIMICROBIAL/ANTIVIRAL ACTIVITIES USING COPPER THERMAL SPRAY COATINGS

In the past several years, antimicrobial copper coatings positively produced using thermal spray techniques, i.e., plasma spray and wire arc spray. The primary operating conditions for plasma spray consisted of temperature (1500–3500 °C), powder velocity (100–400 m s^{-1}), porosity (1–10%), and oxides (1–3%). Methicillin-resistant *S. aureus* (MRSA) testing of plasma-sprayed copper coatings was incubated for 2 hours of exposure at 20 °C and had the MRSA percent surviving more than 10.

When compared to arc-sprayed coatings, arc spray conditions had the temperature (1500–3500 °C), velocity (50–100 m s^{-1}), porosity (5–20%), and oxides (10–20%), thereby resulting in the MRSA percent surviving of below 10 [2, 8].

However, the reason for the higher antimicrobial efficacy experienced in the arc-sprayed coating over the plasma-sprayed coating has not been determined. Moreover, the use of thermal spray techniques for antiviral activities has not been published.

11.8   COLD SPRAY TECHNOLOGY

A solid-state deposition process, known as 'cold spray,' has been employed over the past few decades for use in a wide range of versatile coating applications [2, 17]. In this method, the deposited powder effectively produces large, several mm thick, and dense coatings onto various substrates, comparable to some high-temperature deposition techniques. There has been recently used for the past decade in medical applications.

Unlike a traditional thermal spray, the cold spray no needs the heat to melt the feedstock powder to produce the coating. Feedstock powders are transported to high velocities (300–1200 m s^{-1}) from low to high gas pressure (0.5–5 MPa) to deposit thick, dense coatings, resulting in minimum porosity coatings shown in Figure 11.2.

Cold spray deposition techniques are divided into two categories (i) high-pressure cold spray system (HPCS, pressure: 2.5–5 MPa, gas chamber temperature: up to 1100 °C, powder velocity: up to 1200 m s^{-1}) (ii) low-pressure system (LPCS, pressure: 0.5–1 MPa, gas chamber temperature: 300–550 °C, powder velocity: 300–500 m s^{-1}) [17], as shown in Figure 11.3.

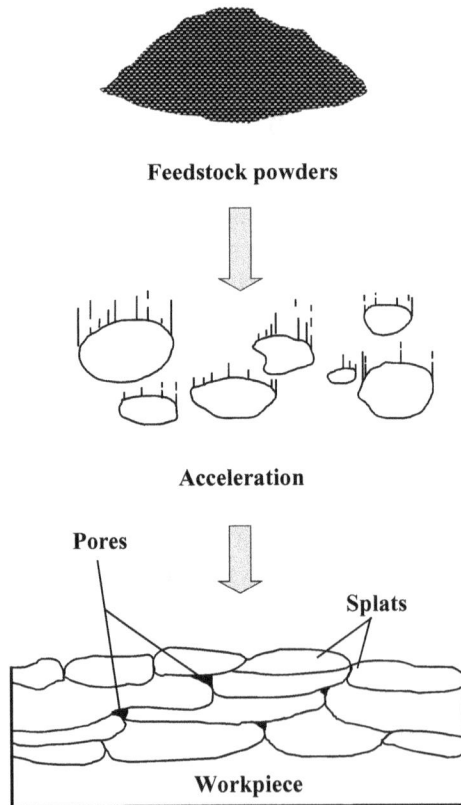

FIGURE 11.2   Principles of cold spray deposition.

High-pressure source

Powder feeder

Hot gas chamber

De Laval nozzle

Stand-off distance

Substrate

(a) High-pressure system

Low-pressure source

Hot gas chamber

Powder feeder

De Laval nozzle

Stand-off distance

Substrate

(b) Low-pressure system

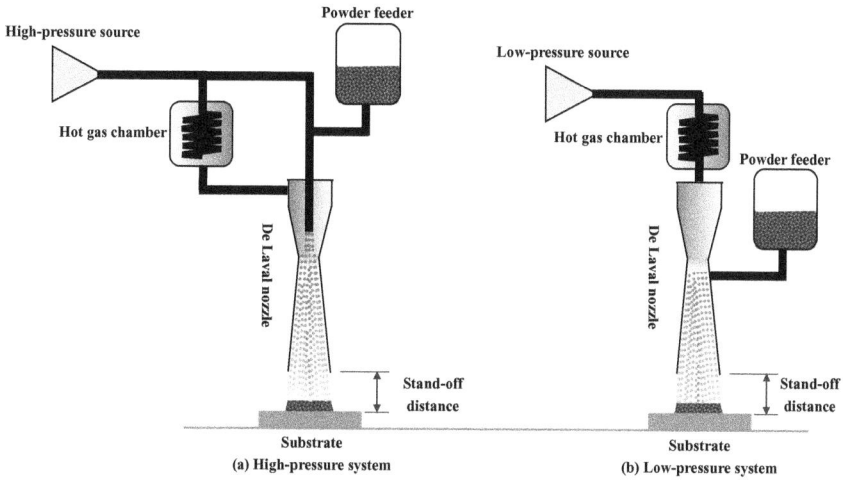

FIGURE 11.3 Categories of cold spray technology.

TABLE 11.1
The Categories of the Cold Spray System

Conditions	HPCS	LPCS
Process gas	N_2, He	Air
Pressure (bar)	7–60	6–10
Preheating temp (°C)	20–1100	20–650
Gas flow rate (m³ min⁻¹)	0.85–2.5 (N_2), max 4.2 (He)	0.3–0.4
Powder feed (kg h⁻¹)	4.5–13.5	0.3–3
Spraying distance (mm)	10–50	5–15
Electric power (kW)	17–70	3.3

The effect of spraying parameters, such as the carrier gas pressure, chamber gas temperature, powder feed rate, stand-off distance, gun transverse speed, spraying pattern, and overlap distance, on properties, e.g., mechanical, wear, corrosion resistance, and microbial properties need to be optimized for each application. As seen in Table 11.1, the categories of the two cold spray systems are listed.

The absence of high temperature during cold spray deposition methods does not cause detrimental properties, i.e., thermal oxidation, tensile residual stresses, phase transformations, and grain growth effects in the resultant coatings. In addition, compressive residual stress might also be made the coatings having longer fatigue life [17].

To date, the majority of the published research into the improvement of antimicrobial Cu and Cu-based coatings has employed using a high-pressure cold spray system: HPCS (N_2 and He as carrier gases), whereby achieving more extraordinary coating properties, in comparison with a low-pressure cold spray system: LPCS (air as carrier gas). In contrast, LPCS is deemed economical; it has achieved the cheaper and lower consumption of compressed air and the lower temperature in operation. Nevertheless, research on LPCS for these coatings is also limited.

11.9 ANTIMICROBIAL/ANTIVIRAL ACTIVITIES USING COPPER COLD SPRAY COATINGS

As the first report of antimicrobial activities by the U.S. Army Research Laboratory published in 2013, copper cold spray coatings have successfully inactivated against *methicillin-resistant S. aureus* (MRSA). The primary spraying conditions for a high-pressure cold spray system consisted of temperature (100–500 °C), powder velocity (600–1000 m s^{-1}), porosity (<1%), and oxides (<1%). The antimicrobial efficacy test had the MRSA percent surviving below 0.001 (incubation exposure of 2 hours at 20 °C).

Compared to copper thermal spray coatings, as previously mentioned in Section 11.7, the anti-MRSA efficacy of copper cold spray coatings was higher than 10^5 times [2]. In 2019, the copper cold spray coating (Cu ≥ 99%) produced using a high-pressure system was inactivating the *S. aureus* within 10 minutes of exposure. The optimum operating conditions had the gas pressure (3 MPa), chamber temperature (400 °C), nozzle surface speed (500 mm s^{-1}), and deposition layers (5 layers) [18].

In addition, antimicrobial copper-based cold spray coatings deposited onto polymer 3D printed parts were patented. Copper-based coatings were employed from the combination of silver, zinc, and aluminum-alumina and compared the coating properties on various substrates, such as acrylonitrile butadiene styrene (ABS), polylactide (PLA), and polycarbonate (PC). The optimum operating conditions used for a low-pressure system had the gas pressure (0.75–0.85 MPa), chamber temperature (190–210 °C), powder nozzle stand-off distance (5–15 mm), nozzle surface speed (10–15 mm s^{-1}), power feed rate (25–35%), and overlap distance (4–6 mm). Furthermore, the coatings, as mentioned earlier, were employed against *S. aureus* (ATCC 25923) dry contact testing, thereby resulting in colony reduction (15 minutes) of 99–100% [19]. Likewise, the combination of copper (>99.7% Cu) and silver powders (>99.99% Ag, 5 wt.%) produced antimicrobial coatings onto 3D printed acrylonitrile butadiene styrene (ABS) workpieces and had the bacterial inactivation within 5 minutes [20].

In contrast, antiviral activities employed by copper cold spray coatings using a high-pressure system have been reported since 2015. For example, copper cold-sprayed coatings produced from nanoparticle forms could inactivate 99% of the influenza A virus for 2 hours of exposure [21]. In addition, influenza A viruses were incapacitated with micropowder and nanopowder coatings as 97.8% and 99.5% of colony reduction, respectively [22].

For anti-COVID-19 testing, highly pure copper powders (99.9%, 5–60 μm in diameter) produced the coatings on stainless steel substrates using high-pressure cold spray deposition, thereby resulting in the anti-SARS-CoV-2 efficacy of 96% after 2 hours of exposure. The spraying parameters had the gas pressure (3 MPa), chamber temperature (500 °C), powder nozzle, stand-off distance (16 mm), and deposition angle (45°) [23].

11.10   THE RELEASE OF COPPER IONS BY MECHANICAL AND CHEMICAL INTERACTIONS

The ionic diffusion is more likely to respond to the release of Cu ions. For example, copper feedstock powders are transported at a very high speed to deposit cold spray coatings. As a result of severe plastic deformation, high strain rates during a deposition could increase the Cu ions diffusion efficiency through inevitable dislocations of deformed Cu grains, resulting in antimicrobial/antiviral properties [2, 8].

The diffusivity and dislocation density relationship related to ion diffusion can be calculated using Eq. (11.1), where D_e is the effective ionic diffusivity, D_0 is the lattice diffusivity, D_d is the pipe diffusivity, r is the average dislocation radius, and ρ_d is the dislocation density [8, 24].

$$D_e = D_0 \left(1 + \pi r^2 \rho_d (D_d/D_0{-}1)\right) \qquad (11.1)$$

The so-called 'strain hardening' or work hardening is a primary cold spray coating property where the dislocation density increases as the strain value increases: the higher dislocation density increases, the more increased microbial elimination [2, 8].

In addition, the release of Cu ions plays a significant role in destroying viral genomes and dispersing surface spikes. Hence, copper may have generated different oxide species of Cu_2O and CuO, depending upon diffusive Cu ions at different rates; likewise, Cu^{1+} and Cu^{2+} may have formed at the other oxide species [25].

Therefore, as the type of copper feedstock powders is considerable for cold spray processing for antimicrobial/antiviral activities, Cu_2O may obtain from the Cu spray-dried feedstock powder rather than from the Cu gas-atomized feedstock powder [26]. The Cu ions release rate of Cu_2O was greater than CuO, resulting in higher atomic diffusion and improving antipathogens by the contact-killing method [27]. Also, the release of Cu^{1+} ions is formed by cuprous oxide (Cu_2O) with aqueous solutions, as shown in the following reaction [26, 28]:

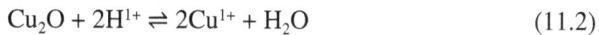

$$Cu_2O + 2H^{1+} \rightleftharpoons 2Cu^{1+} + H_2O \qquad (11.2)$$

Cuprous oxide responds to release Cu^{1+} ions, wherein this ion species could inactivate pathogens over Cu^{2+} [29].

However, the antimicrobial efficacy received by microscale copper cold spray coatings was more rather than the antiviral efficacy. The size mismatch between copper coating microstructures and viral sizes may decrease the antiviral effectiveness [8]. Likewise, it was attempted to describe the effect of grain sizes on the ion diffusion efficiency as expressed in Eq. (11.3) [26].

$$D_e = fD_i + D_l + (D_{gb}(t_{gb} (d_w - d)/d_w d)) + \rho_d a D_c \qquad (11.3)$$

where f is the atomic diffusion fraction through the additional interfacial pathways, D_i is the atomic diffusion coefficient through additional interfaces, D_l is the atomic diffusion coefficient through the lattice, D_{gb} is the atomic diffusion coefficient through the grain boundaries, t_{gb} is the thickness of the grain boundary, d_w is the line width, d is the average grain size, ρ_d is the dislocation density, a is the cross-sectional area of the dislocation cores associated with pipe diffusion, and D_c is pipe diffusion coefficient.

Also, since 2019, the nanostructured copper cold spray coatings have been studied to improve the ion diffusion efficiency against pathogen activities [26]; however, the virucidal test of the novel coronavirus has not been investigated.

11.11 CONCLUSIONS AND FUTURE PERSPECTIVE

Antimicrobial/antiviral copper materials play a significant role in the pandemic situation. Copper coatings produced using various deposition methods were suited to have been considerably applied on often-touched surfaces. In copper cold spray deposition, the Cu powder effectively produces large, several mm thick, and dense coatings onto various substrates, comparable to some high-temperature deposition techniques. Exceptionally, it is deemed available for a high concentration release of Cu ions compared to these coatings produced over thermal spraying. Remarkably, thick-film coatings have been economically made using low-pressure cold spray methods; nevertheless, research on the low-pressure cold spray (LPCS) system for these coatings is also limited.

Although great results are being obtained thus far for these LPCS coatings, there are still challenges to address. Hence, in future studies, they may be addressed the following questions:

1. What are the optimum spraying parameters of Cu and Cu-based coatings on varying the retention of reinforcing particles, hardness, wear, and antimicrobial/antiviral properties in LPCS coatings for each substrate?
2. What is the role of coating properties to the diffusive Cu ions response?
3. How can we obtain the accurate measurement of the inactivation period using a plaque assay for antiviral tests?
4. What are the sensitivity and repeatability of the existing wiping method and exposure to disinfectants on antimicrobial/antiviral activities and the appearance of contaminated coatings?
5. What is the virucidal efficacy evaluation using clinical studies compared to laboratory studies?

For the virological investigation, a study of destructive cellular COVID-19 structures by Cu ions toxicants does not appear to have been reported. Still, the destruction by the influence of Cu ions releasing has relied explicitly on the grain orientation, dislocation density, and hardness values of the cold-sprayed coating. Also, antiviral properties and understanding are crucial if antiviral copper-based LPCS coatings are used in household, hospital, healthcare, and general applications.

ACKNOWLEDGMENTS

The author would like to express gratitude and dedicate to the late Prof. Ionel Botef, University of the Witwatersrand, Johannesburg, South Africa, for all the collaborative research commenced. This work was funded by King Mongkut's

University of Technology North Bangkok, Bangkok, Thailand (Contract No. KMUTNB-63-KNOW-039).

REFERENCES

1. Michels, T. H., and A. C. Michels. 2020. Can copper help fight COVID-19? *Adv Mat & Proc* 1–4. www.asminternational.org/documents/10192/1630346/20_CopperCorona_ Digital_First.pdf/.
2. Champagne, K. V., and D. J. Helfrich. 2013. A demonstration of the antimicrobial effectiveness of various copper surfaces. *J Biol Eng* March 27;7(1): 1–6. DOI:10.1186/1754-1611-7-8.
3. Vincent, M., R. E. Duval, P. Hartemann, and M. Engels-Deutsch. 2018. Contact killing and antimicrobial properties of copper. *J Appl Microbiol* May;124(5): 1032–1046. DOI:10.1111/jam.13681.
4. van Doremalen, N., T. Bushmaker, D. H. Morris, M. G. Holbrook, A. Gamble, B. N. Williamson, A. Tamin, J. L. Harcourt, N. J. Thornburg, S. I. Gerber, J. O. Lloyd Smith, E. de Wit, and V. J. Munster. 2020. Aerosol and surface stability of SARSCoV-2 as compared with SARS-CoV-1. *N Engl J Med* 382: 1564–1567. DOI:10.1056/ NEJMc2004973.
5. Mantlo, E. K., S. Paessler, A. Seregin, and A. Mitchell. 2020. Luminore CopperTouch™ copper surface coating effectively inactivates SARS-CoV-2, Ebola, and Marburg viruses in vitro. *medRxiv*. Preprint. July 14. DOI:10.1101/2020.07.05.20146043.
6. Raha, S., R. Mallick, S. Basak, and A. K. Duttaroy. 2020. Is copper beneficial for COVID-19 patients? *Med Hypotheses* 142: 109814. DOI:10.1016/j.mehy.2020.109814.
7. Morrison, J. 2020. Copper's virus-killing powers were known even to the ancients. *Smithsonian Magazine* April 14: 1–3. www.smithsonianmag.com/science-nature/ copper-virus-kill-180974655/.
8. Champagne, K. V., K. Sundberg, and D. Helfrich. 2019. Kinetically deposited copper antimicrobial surfaces. *Coatings* 9: 257. DOI:10.3390/coatings9040257.
9. Sagripanti, J. L., L. B. Routson, and C. D. Lytle, 1993. Virus inactivation by copper or iron ions alone and in the presence of peroxide. *Appl Environ Microbiol* 59: 4374–4376.
10. Warnes, S. L., Z. R. Little, and C. W. Keevil. 2015. Human coronavirus 229E remains infectious on common touch surface materials. *mBio* 6: e01697. DOI:10.1128/ mBio.01697-15.
11. Sucipto, T. H., S. Churrotin, H. Setyawati, F. Martak, K. C. Mulyatno, I. H. Amarullah, T. Kotaki, M. Kameoka, S. Yotopranoto, and S. Soegijanto. 2018. A new copper (II)-imidazole derivative effectively inhibits replication of Denv-2 in vero cell. *Afr J Infect Dis* 12: 116–119. DOI:10.2101/2FAjid.12v1S.17.
12. Noyce, J. O., H. Michels, and C. W. Keevil. 2007. Inactivation of influenza A virus on copper versus stainless steel surfaces. *Appl Environ Microbiol* 73: 2748–2750. DOI:10.1128/AEM.01139-06.
13. Noyce, J. O., H. Michels, and C. W. Keevil. 2006. Use of copper cast alloys to control Escherichia coli O157 cross-contamination during food processing. *Appl Environ Microbiol* 72: 4239–4244. DOI:10.1128/AEM.02532-05.
14. Fujimori, Y., T. Sato, T. Hayata, T. Nagao, M. Nakayama, T. Nakayama, R. Sugamata, and K. Suzuki. 2012. Novel antiviral characteristics of nanosized copper(I) iodide particles showing inactivation activity against 2009 pandemic H1N1 influenza virus. *Appl Environ Microbiol* 78: 951–955. DOI:10.1128/AEM.06284-11.
15. Hassan, A. I., P. P. Ivan, Parkin, S. P. Nair, and C. J. Carmalt. 2014. Antimicrobial activity of copper and copper(I) oxide thin films deposited via aerosol-assisted CVD. *J Mater Chem B* 2: 2855–2860. DOI:10.1039/c4tb00196f.

16. Jung, S., J. Y. Yang, E. Y. Byeon, D. G. Kim, D. G. Lee, S. Ryoo, S. Lee, C. W. Shin, H. W. Jang, H. J. Kim, and S. Lee. 2021. Copper-coated polypropylene filter face mask with SARS-CoV-2 antiviral ability. *Polymers* 13: 1367. DOI:10.3390/polym13091367.

17. Nunthavarawong, P., N. Sacks, and I. Botef. 2016. Effect of powder feed rate on the mechanical properties of WC-5 wt%Ni coatings deposited using low pressure cold spray. *Int J Refract Metals Hard Mater* December; 61: 230–237. DOI:10.1016/j.ijrmhm.2016.10.00.

18. da Silva, F. S., N. Cinca, S. Dosta, I. G. Cano, J. M. Guilemany, C. S. A. Caires, A. R. Lima, C. M. Silva, S. L. Oliveira, A. R. L. Caires, and A. V. Benedetti. 2019. Corrosion resistance and antibacterial properties of copper coating deposited by cold gas spray. *Surf Coat Technol* 361: 292–301. DOI:10.1016/j.surfcoat.2019.01.029.

19. Botef, Ionel, Michael Lucas, and Sandy Van Vuuren. 2019. *Method of applying an antimicrobial surface coating to a substrate.* WIPO Patent 2019/064216, filed September 27, 2018, and issued April 4, 2019.

20. Lucas, M. D. I., I. Botef, R. G. Reid, and S. F. van Vuuren. 2020. Laboratory-based study of novel antimicrobial cold spray coatings to combat surface microbial contamination. *Infect Control Hosp Epidemiol* 41(12): 1–6. DOI:10.1017/ice.2020.335.

21. Sundberg, K., V. Champagne, B. McNally, D. Helfritch, and R. Sisson. 2015. Effectiveness of nanomaterial copper cold spray surfaces on inactivation of influenza A virus. *J Biotechnol Biomater* 22: 16753–16763. DOI:10.4172/2155-952X.1000205.

22. Sundberg, K., M. Gleason, B. Haddad, V. Champagne, C. Brown, R. Sisson, and D. Cote. 2019. The effect of nano-scale surface roughness on copper cold spray inactivation of influenza A virus. *Int J Nanotechnol Med Eng* 4(4): 1–8.

23. Hutasoit, N., B. Kennedy, S. Hamilton, A. Luttick, R. A. R. Rashid, and S. Palanisamy. 2020. Sars-CoV-2 (COVID-19) inactivation capability of copper-coated touch surface fabricated by cold-spray technology. *Manuf Lett* 25: 93–97. DOI:10.1016/j.mfglet.2020.08.007.

24. Mehrer, H. 2007. *Diffusion in Solids.* Berlin: Springer Nature.

25. Sousa, B. C., C. J. Massar, M. A. Gleason, and D. L. Cote. 2021. On the emergence of antibacterial and antiviral copper cold spray coatings. *J Biol Eng* 15(8): 1–8. DOI:10.1186/s13036-021-00256-7.

26. Sousa, B. C., C. J. Massar, M. A. Gleason, and D. L. Cote. 2020. Understanding the antipathogenic performance of nanostructured and conventional copper cold spray material consolidations and coated surfaces. *Crystals* 10(504): 1–43. DOI:10.3390/cryst10060504.

27. Hans, M., A. Erbe, S. Mathews, Y. Chen, M. Solioz, and F. Mücklich. 2013. Role of copper oxides in contact killing of bacteria. *Langmuir* 29(52): 16160–16166. DOI:10.1021/la404091z.

28. Palmer, D. A. 2011. Solubility measurements of crystalline Cu_2O in aqueous solution as a function of temperature and pH. *J Solution Chem* 40: 1067–1093. DOI:10.1007/s10953-011-9699-x.

29. Mathews, S., R. Kumar, and M. M. Solioz. 2015. Copper reduction and contact killing of bacteria by iron surfaces. *Appl Environ Microbiol* 81(18): 6399–6403. DOI:0.1128%2FAEM.01725-15.

Index

Note: Page numbers in *italics* indicate a figure and page numbers in **bold** indicate a table on the corresponding page.

For Product Safety Concerns and Information please contact our EU
representative GPSR@taylorandfrancis.com
Taylor & Francis Verlag GmbH, Kaufingerstraße 24, 80331 München, Germany

9 780367 697495